LOST IT!

And Loving It!

love yourself and live your life.

Julie & Martin

Julie and Martin Carrick

First Edition published 2020 by

2QT Limited (Publishing)
Settle, North Yorkshire BD24 9RH United Kingdom

Printed in the UK by Ashford Colour Press

Cover image: J & M Carrick

DISCLAIMER

This book is based on the authors' personal experiences and any suggestions or advice expressed or implied is intended for information only and is NOT given as professional medical/health related advice nor intended to treat, cure or diagnose any medical/health related condition. It in no way constitutes or replaces professional advice or recommendations. If you have a health problem, medical emergency, or a general health question, we always recommend you should consult your doctor.

A CIP catalogue record for this book is available from the British Library

ISBN - 978-1-913071-81-3

Contents

Introduction

Firstly, for those of you who haven't read our first book, 'Losing It', allow me to introduce ourselves.

We are Julie and Martin Carrick, sixty and sixty-two years old respectively. We are both now retired and live in the Yorkshire Dales, having moved there from Sheffield, almost ten years ago.

We are both ex police officers. Julie retired some time ago now, following a fairly serious road accident and subsequent prolonged illness with non-Hodgkin lymphoma, from which she has, finally, been given the 'all clear'.

I retired in 2006 having completed all my service in Sheffield and South Yorkshire.

We have two grown up boys, one living in Scotland and the other in Leeds, and almost as we began our new lifestyle in 2018, we were made proud grandparents for the first time.

I am a very keen cook and Julie is a very keen and talented baker. Apart from the occasional takeaway and meals out, we have always cooked from scratch and brought both our children up to do the same.

We have always been very sporty and keen about keeping fit, healthy and eating healthily. I played rugby for a long period of my life and Julie has always been a very keen swimmer, athlete and runner. We have always kept up our training, even when we had actually stopped taking part in our respective sports. Despite our fitness efforts, we have always had a problem keeping the weight under control and for a long time we were just known and referred to as 'Big people'. My nickname for a long period of my life was, in fact 'Tiny', which I certainly wasn't!

The heaviest I reached was almost twenty-one stones. Julie went up to seventeen and a half stones and it was around this time, following an emergency stay in hospital after suffering chest pains, that I was diagnosed with very high blood pressure, high cholesterol and because of this, had to start taking three lots of medication to keep it all under control. Julie had also begun having blood pressure and thyroid problems, along with high cholesterol. She was also prescribed medication to control these conditions.

This was almost twenty years ago and we did decide to try and lose some weight. We both lost weight, but not enough. And certainly not enough to get off the medications at that time and we continued to have to take all our tablets until just eighteen months ago.

I'm now off all my medication and Julie only takes her thyroid medication.

Shortly before moving to The Yorkshire Dales, I was diagnosed with stage 3(a) chronic kidney disease. I was told there was no cure and no medication I could take to control it, the prognosis being a gradual deterioration leading to eventual kidney failure.

As there aren't any symptoms to keep you aware of it, I'd completely forgotten about it until just a few months ago. I was given a blood test during a routine annual check up and found it had completely disappeared!!

In our opinion, this is entirely due to the fact we have now lost all our excess weight and, rather than going back to our previous ways of eating and piling back on all the weight we had lost, we continued to eat the same foods, but this time only very slightly increased the amount of food we ate and experimented with different recipes and new foods. We are now continuing to enjoy the massive benefits of that weight loss and we both feel we have regained the same health we had back in our youth. Again, this is proof enough for to us to absolutely believe that, 'It's not what you eat, but what you don't eat' that matters and we will continue eating 'OUR' healthy foods every day for the rest of our lives.

We began our programme in March 2018 and by the end of the year I was down to 13st 7lbs and Julie was 9st 13lbs. Julie lost a total of seven stones and I lost five stones. We're still those weights now, almost two years on and as we write this second book, still can't believe how wonderful we feel.

We both still feel absolutely fantastic. It was, and still is, a feeling we have tried and failed, on numerous occasions, to explain to other people. When we do try, it's a very emotional experience for both of us.

If we could convey that feeling, which is both a mental and physical feeling, world obesity would not be the problem it now is. It's certainly something we keep trying to pass on to other people, because the results are so amazing and life changing.

We're constantly met with comments like, 'you're only here once, enjoy life while you can'. 'Life's too short to worry about dieting. I'm fat and happy with the way I am'. Well, in our opinion, that's generally rubbish and there are many, if not thousands, of people who are very fat, very unhealthy and very unhappy.

We know how they, and you, feel. We also know how we feel now. We both know where we want to be now and for the rest of our lives. It's certainly not the fat option. We're more than happy to miss out on our previous 'feeding frenzies' and just eat the way we do now. We really don't feel that we're missing out on anything and find it very easy to just say no to all that nutritionally empty food we used to eat.

It's actually no effort at all not to eat the rubbish we used to eat and we have very few cravings at all nowadays for those types of food. Hand on heart, we really aren't tempted, any more, by those cakes, chocolates, bread and other products destined to make you fat.

We decided to write our first book, 'Losing It', because along the journey to our success, people had begun to notice our 'transformation' and asked us what we were eating and whether we could share some of the recipes we have developed from the foods we now eat with them.

It became difficult to just give people the recipes, without explaining why we were using specific foods and ingredients and why we no longer ate certain foods. We therefore began to transcribe a book from the diary we had kept and still keep, detailing our food intake along our way.

The truth of the matter is, as far as we're concerned anyway, the media, TV stars and world politicians can bang on all they want about 'Climate Changes' and becoming zero carbon countries, but if we don't do something about ourselves and our growing obesity problem, world wide, well, it won't matter about our planet because we'll all be dead through our overeating and the many associated illnesses and diseases brought about by being fat and eating the rubbish out there in the marketplace which is laden with sugars, preservatives and other ingredients requiring a science degree to understand what they are. There are so many processed and so-called healthy, low fat and supposedly good for you foods these days in shops and on supermarket shelves. They contain all sorts of chemicals, gums and additives. Common sense surely must tell us that they can't be good for us in the long run.

Almost everyone we know is more than just a bit overweight, or has a relative who is the same and has the associated 'being overweight' ailments like high blood pressure, high cholesterol, heart conditions or even worse, diabetes.

Unfortunately, doctors who are our first call when these problems arise, have virtually no training on the subject of nutrition and they often refer us to so called 'Nutritionists' who, themselves, have only studied the subject at university, via a manual or over the internet. Their 'knowledge' is gleaned from what they have read and not from what they have personally experienced or from experiments they have carried out on themselves.

This is where, I hope, we differ from all these so-called 'experts'.

Everything in our first book is based on OUR experiences with different foods and their effects on our weight, physique, mind, health and, in fact, our lives. That is why we are continuing with this lifestyle for the rest of our lives, hence this second book.

We hope this does not come across as a rant about doctors and 'experts' not knowing what they're talking about, because it really isn't and I'm sure there are some that do but I'm afraid it has to be said.

We don't want to become embroiled in arguments with medical, political or any other so called 'Expert Bodies' and their opinions. I'm sure there is a place for their opinions and knowledge, especially where there is documented science factored into the equation, because some of the science out there is pretty amazing. Some of it is very controversial where weight, nutrition, health and our bodies are concerned, even to the extent that renowned doctors and experts have been threatened with disciplinary action because of their ideas, opinions and results don't fall in line with government guidelines and the GMC (General Medical Council).

Doctors and medicine have come on in leaps and bounds over the past few years and the NHS is undoubtedly brilliant. However, there are far too many experts who appear to have far too many differing views and opinions about diet, exercise, food and how our bodies react to foods, and not enough solid facts confirmed by proper science, personal experience and reliable research. It all just leads to confusion. The current health problems brought about by our own unhealthy lifestyles can, in many cases, be reversed by a few simple lifestyle changes rather than by pills and potions.

There is also growing evidence that much information regarding diet, food, food processing, exercise and health issues, is actually covered up or withheld so that multi-billion pound industries don't lose money or go out of business! No names here, but the evidence is out there on the internet for all to see. Some of it may be false but not all of it, I'm sure.

Everything written in this book, our opinions and observations, are entirely based on our own experiments and experiences with food, diet and exercise. Some of our experiments have been total failures - when we've had some quite unusual and nasty reactions to some of the food we've eaten, or we've had to throw away complete meals when they haven't turned out right. We've also experienced minor setbacks where we have added on a few pounds. The good results are, however, ones that will work for you and others who find themselves in similar circumstances to those in which we found ourselves.

I know I keep talking about lifestyle changes, but that is exactly what has to be done. People make lifestyle changes when they decide to stop or cut down on smoking or drinking because it has become a problem in their lives. Many stop smoking and/or drinking completely and would never go back to it because of the vast improvement to their health, lives and, by the way, their bank balances.

There's no difference to adopting the same attitude towards food, eating and exercise. Change your food and way of eating and, I promise you, it will change your life in so many ways. Forever! I can't emphasise this point enough. If you really want the results, you have to make the change for life!

So, presuming you've already read our first book, 'Losing It', in this book we are going to explore a number of new topics and expand on several topics we've already touched on in that book, in order to help you maintain your new weight and the new you.

If you haven't read 'Losing It', you can still start from the beginning using the information in this book. However, 'Losing It' is still a good place to start your journey.

I'll be repeating myself several times during the course of this book when I say the advice we will give you is entirely based on our experiences and experiments with food, recipes and exercise over the last two years. We might, from time to time, touch on some scientific data that we have picked up along the way and think is relevant to our experiences and will be helpful to everyone

else. However, because we're not experts in nutrition, it will always be about something we've actually tried and tested ourselves and, therefore, we feel qualified to give an opinion.

All the recipes in this book have been tried and tested either in our kitchen at home or in different kitchens whilst we've been on our travels.

We took all the photos illustrating our recipes using our mobile phones in the kitchen where we have prepared that particularly recipe.

None of them have been taken in studios or airbrushed to make them look professional and glossy. We've done this in an attempt to portray authenticity and honesty. It's our food, not something we've had prepared by someone else or has just been devised for our book in order to boost sales. It's not sales we're really interested in (well maybe a bit!). It's about trying to pass on our passion and enthusiasm as to how it's totally possible to make some relatively small changes in relation to food that will ultimately make massive changes to your lives!

We will be looking at vegetarian and vegan options and the results of our trials of eating no meat.

Artificial sweeteners will be looked at in some depth. Do they have a place in our and your life?

The following is a list of some of the subjects we will be talking about in this book. I'm sure other items will crop up along the way though:-

EXERCISE and how much it contributes to weight loss and how weight loss affects exercise. We will also talk about nutrition in relation to exercise. How much do you really need to eat to still be able to train/exercise at an intensive level?

HOW DIFFERENT TYPES OF FOODS can affect your gut's microbes (gut bacteria), which, in turn, can immensely influence your bowels and their connection to the rest of your body. Things like mood, illnesses, sleeping, energy levels and general health are greatly affected by what you eat and what happens to the food in your gut. Hopefully we'll be able to explain this without getting too scientific, and make it easy to understand.

We will again be talking about other PEOPLE'S ATTITUDES to the decision you made to change your life, get slim, stay slim and keep healthy. People's attitudes are something that's really shocked us, both in positive and negative ways.

There will be a chapter dedicated to foods that we consider our 'DANGER FOODS' and foods we have either completely stopped eating, or only eat in very small amounts. These include some foods that are actually considered 'healthy' by most 'experts'.

STRESS. A minefield of a subject, but one so many of us encounters either personally or with someone close to you. This can be at home or in the workplace.

Another controversial subject we will be discussing is FASTING and the positive effects it has on our bodies and digestive system. You will be surprised at how even short fasts can have a massive influence on your body.

We have been doing a great deal of research over the last eighteen months, during which time we've accrued masses of interesting information, but also a lot of rubbish. Hopefully in this book we'll be leaving out the rubbish!

We hope that by the time you've made the decision to get slim once and for all, and read our first book, this book will keep you on that road to health and longevity.

Quite recently, Julie and I had been discussing the events in our lives that had life-changing consequences.

For me it was leaving school and starting work, meeting Julie, getting married and us having children. Stopping smoking and drinking were both up there as well.

For Julie it was much the same, although she has never smoked. Having had cancer and conquering it was high up there for her.

However, we both agreed that, finally, being slim, healthy and having that feeling of new found total freedom, ranked up there amongst the best of those events.

I know many people will be saying that hindsight is a wonderful thing and that's very true, but we both wish we could pass on that benefit of hindsight to other people and show them just how good it feels when you've made the decision to change and then succeed.

So now we're getting to where we address what we've done to carry on and maintain our success. I must again stress that we aren't experts, medically trained or have any scientific proof of any of the conclusions we have reached along our way. These are just our opinions and the conclusions and results are totally based on what we have done and observed with ourselves.

If you have any serious medical complications, you should always seek professional medical advice before embarking on anything that may have an adverse effect on your health.

During the course of this book we regularly refer to a number of retailers whom we favour, however we must emphasise that none of these retailers have had any influence or control over what we have written in this book.

Okay, let's get going with maintaining your success and continued health.

Chapter 1:
Calories In, Calories Out?

One of the main reasons for writing our first book was because we had heard the phrase, 'calories in, calories out', far too many times over the years, that this was the only way possible to lose weight properly, and everything else was just diet industry propaganda and a way to earn a fast buck. We know that there are thousands of people out there who have tried this, lost some weight and are still fat now and wondering what to do next.

Well, undoubtedly, you will lose weight by cutting your calories so they are less than your calorific maintenance levels. There is absolutely no doubting this at all. It's basic science. If you burn more calories than you ingest you will lose weight.

This means that, really, if you wanted to, and providing you didn't go over your basic calorie maintenance level, you could eat chocolate all day and you would still lose weight, providing you didn't go over your maintenance level and remained in calorie deficit.

Perhaps I should just say a little about calorie maintenance level. This is the amount of calories that your own individual bodies need to just get through your day. So, say for example, yours is 2000 calories, if you burn up more than 2000 calories or eat less than 2000 calories in a day, you will lose weight. If you don't burn up those calories or you eat in excess of 2000 calories you will put weight on. In essence this means, if you eat 2100 calories

you will, in fact, put weight on over time. When you think 100 grams of milk chocolate contains around 500 calories or a 50 gram bowl of so called 'healthy' muesli contains between 150 - 200 calories, it doesn't take long to add those calories up and go over your maintenance levels. Calorie counting just isn't sustainable for most people and they become very bored with weighing food and counting calories. Eventually the calories very slowly begin to add up again as you begin to start guessing how much food weighs. Remember, just 10 calories over your maintenance level will, over time, put that weight back on.

It's all well and good some of these diet companies telling you that no food is 'off limits' on their particular programmes. Obviously, you can eat a lot of low calorie food, but can have very little high calorie food. The problem with this type of dieting is that if you reach the ceiling of your daily allotted calories, say by lunchtime, because you've had just a few too many calories at breakfast or for your mid morning snack, it will mean you should not eat anything else for the rest of the day!

We wanted to be able to eat good food, plenty of it, and come up with some nice recipes. But most of all, we wanted to do something for the rest of our lives that was sustainable! Not go back to being fat, as well as not having to count calories! We also wanted something that didn't leave us still feeling hungry all the time and craving certain foods.

We truly believe that what we're doing now addresses all those factors.

We honestly don't miss sugar and the sweet stuff at all. Neither do we miss all the heavy carb-laden foods and meals we used to eat. We just don't have those cravings anymore. Yes, we cheat a little bit, but it's always with foods we regularly eat on our new lifestyle. Incidentally, they are not really cheat foods, but just foods we limit ourselves to eating every now and again that remain within the parameters of foods we now eat. (More about these foods later.)

We don't calorie count at all, but make sure all our food is nutritionally dense. This means that all the food we eat will fill us up, keep us satisfied for longer and feed our bodies properly.

There was an article on the news very recently stating that 'the powers that be' were going to not only label foods with how many calories are in a particular food, but also indicate how much exercise you would have to do in order to burn off those calories. That's basically fine, but 500 calories of one type of food will react with and be utilised by your body in a completely different way from 500 calories of another type of food. This will also vary dramatically from person to person.

A piece of cake or something similar could contain 500 calories and would probably not fill you very much at all, but 500 calories also equals a large plate full of veggies or salad. Accompanied by a little protein this would keep you feeling fuller for much longer than the piece of cake, as well as being far better fuel for your body.

So, hopefully I haven't completely confused you all. The point I'm trying to make is this. Everyone has different calorific needs and everyone reacts differently to different foods. We have experimented with a wide range of foods with very varied results.

Strangely enough, many of the so-called 'healthy' foods have caused quite severe reactions in both of us.

When I say 'severe' reactions, we've both suffered symptoms such as headaches, nausea, bloated stomachs, water retention and that feeling you get when you're catching a cold. Very similar to mild flu symptoms.

At first we thought that many of these

reactions were just imagined or coincidental. However, we both consumed exactly the same foods on all these occasions and suffered the same reactions. Anyway, more about this in a later chapter.

There's a saying, 'You are what you eat'. We agree with this whole-heartedly, but also believe it should include, 'but it's what you don't eat that matters'. It's becoming more and more apparent that there are quite a large number of eminent experts in the field of nutrition, diet and lifestyle who now agree that obesity will not be cured simply by the 'calories in, calories out' mentality. We humans are a far more complex species than we think we are.

We hope our continued experiments and experiences with ourselves and the food we eat and hopefully, you eat, will inspire you and others to stay on track for a long, long time. For always!

We don't want to be patronising, rude or disrespectful, but every time we see someone who is obviously struggling with their weight (we still find it difficult to call people fat, even though that's exactly what we finally had to admit to ourselves) we want to offer them some words of help or advice. It's difficult to hold back sometimes and not launch into 'preaching' mode. It's only because we now know how much better they would feel, both mentally and physically. We know that we could help them feel the same way as we do now.

On a lighter note, pardon the pun, this book includes a number of good recipes that we have developed, tried and tested both on ourselves, and our long-suffering guinea pig friends. We hope you will also enjoy and find them easy to make. You will see that none of them indicate calorie content or any other nutritional information.

So really this is just another recipe book with the addition of some facts and opinions based on what we have discovered along the way. It will definitely help you avoid the pitfalls we've experienced in order to help you along your journey to success.

We are both very passionate about food and get a great amount of pleasure from food and feeding people. Without trying to blow our own trumpets, most people are amazed by both the food and the amount we eat, especially those who have made snide remarks about us being too skinny and being borderline anorexics!

WE EAT PROPER FOOD AND PLENTY OF IT.

Chapter 2:
Having the 'GUTS' to Carry On

The purpose of this chapter is to both address your 'Gut' (digestive system) and your 'Guts' (courage).

The first part, your 'gut', is relatively easy to address. Again, I'm hoping that by the time you are reading this book, you'll have already read our first book, 'Losing It, It's Not What You Eat, But What You Don't Eat That Matters'.

'Losing It' was a transcript of our daily diary, outlining what we ate on a daily basis and a number of recipes that we had created in order for us to lose weight and stay healthy. A number of friends had asked us for some of the recipes and as they began to ask questions about the food we were eating, why we were eating some foods and not others, it made sense to write it down. It became obvious that we needed to offer more of an explanation as to why we were eliminating some food from our diet and lives, hence the book was written.

All the food we were eating and still eat now, are very important types of food which help to repair your gut, your gut's good/friendly bacteria, which in turn, gets the rest of your body working properly. They are all rich in nutrients and they are foods that feed, repair and heal your body.

Before our weight loss, I suffered from terrible heartburn every time I ate certain foods, namely, pastries, breads, both wholemeal and white versions, plus pasta, rice and numerous other high carbohydrate loaded foods. Fried foods, using grain based oils, also had the same affect.

Julie had problems with exactly the same foods but her problem was chronic constipation. When I say chronic, I mean not being able to 'poo' for several days, sometimes weeks, to the point, on occasions, where she was on the verge of being hospitalised. Prescribed laxatives just didn't do the trick.

Almost within days of us both changing the food we were eating, my heartburn disappeared and Julie no longer suffered with her constipation.

It would be nice to say we've never encountered these problems again. Unfortunately that hasn't actually been the case, but it hasn't been because of our wrongdoing.

There have been times when we've been forced, because of circumstances beyond our control, to eat food we wouldn't usually eat, the alternative being to go without and starve. These circumstances have been, in the main, when travelling and eating out, both at friends' houses and at restaurants. This is despite informing friends and restaurants that we don't eat certain foods prior to the event and even pre-booking meals on planes.

Both our 'gut' problems returned within hours of eating the food available. Luckily, by this time we knew what was causing the problems and we were able to get back to eating properly shortly afterwards.

The purpose of highlighting these 'gut' problems is to enforce how essential it is to get your 'gut' working properly and how sensitive it is to the effective working and maintenance of the rest of your body.

The lining of your digestive system is made from neurones, which is the same material as your brain and experts are now beginning to call your 'gut' 'Your second Brain'. They are beginning to realise that your 'gut' plays a far more important role in the way your body works and functions. The phrase, 'having a gut feeling' starts to take on a different meaning when you begin to consider this.

It's also why the experts are beginning to realise how important the right food and our gut and gut's bacteria are. Many problems and illnesses affecting sleeping, mood, energy/ strength/activity levels, irritable bowel syndrome and so on can be completely reversed, or at least vastly improved, without the use of medication, simply by eating the correct food. Doctors are performing 'faecal transplants' on patients who are suffering from gastrointestinal conditions such as irritable bowel syndrome and many other conditions.

These transplants are basically 'poo' samples obtained from people with good healthy gut bacteria, which are implanted into the gut of people with certain conditions and whose gut bacteria is poor or lacking in health.

Other related illnesses that are closely linked to your gut's health are diabetes, arthritis, high blood pressure and high cholesterol, to name just a few.

I've recently read that there are some experts who consider your own gut bacteria to be as individual as your DNA or fingerprints. I'm not sure how true any of this is. What we do find strange though is this.

We, as a couple, nearly always eat the same food together, every day. Obviously we don't eat the same recipes each day, but Julie will have the same lunch and the same dinner as me every day. She reacts to that same food, cooked the same way, very differently to me. This is very evident the next morning when it comes to getting rid of your rubbish. Yes, I am talking about poo here!

If we've both eaten the same food the previous day and usually the previous week as well, why does the bathroom smell completely different after each one of us has got rid of our rubbish. It has to be down to what's in our gut and what's happening in our gut in order to make each of us function healthily.

I could get into more scientific rambling but I'm not an expert. What I do know is, get your gut and gut bacteria sorted and many of these associated illnesses could be things of the past. However, in order to achieve this, you need to eat the right food.

We continue to eat the way we did when we first started out two years ago. It's absolutely no hardship to us. It's far more of a bother to others who either don't, or are not prepared to just think and consider what they eat every day.

Whilst on the subject of 'Guts', this is probably a good time to introduce fasting or intermittent fasting.

Before you start yelling, 'First they want to stop us eating all our lovely sugar, cakes and goodies, now they want us to stop eating completely!' let me explain.

Intermittent fasting actually means that you fast between meals. It also means you don't snack in between meals. It can be a bit more involved than that, because some of the fasts can last between eighteen and twenty-four hours and some even longer, forty-eight to seventy-two hours!

There was a time, not so long ago, when it was acknowledged that a good way to control your weight was to have several small meals over the course of your day. Current research now suggests that this is not true - quite the reverse, in fact. Fasting over a period of twelve to eighteen hours does not slow down your metabolism, but in fact, maintains it and some of these experts are actually saying it can actually increase your metabolic rate!

We usually fast for eighteen hours and then eat during the remaining six hours. We have our evening meal between 6pm and 7pm, some dark chocolate and a cup of tea around 8.45pm - 9.00pm and then don't eat again until at least 1.00pm the next day. More often than not, it's usually about 2.00pm. Sometimes we don't begin eating again until between 6.00pm and 7.00pm, so it works out to either eighteen hours or almost twenty-four hours of eating nothing and only drinking water, black tea or black coffee.

We always do our training/swimming first thing in the morning, at about 7.30am in what is known as a 'fasted state', having eaten nothing since the previous evening.

I can hear you all saying, 'Where do you get your energy from? You can't train, do any fitness regime or manual type of work with no food in you. How will I get through a working day just having one or two meals a day?'

Well the truth of the matter is, you can. Oddly enough, you can train and work even harder and better than you used to do before. A friend of ours is a joiner and follows a similar regime to us and he sometimes does forty-eight and even seventy-two hour long fasts, but continues to work with no problems whatsoever.

We often do little painting and decorating jobs for locals. OK, it's not a full time job and more of a hobby, but we start our day at around 7.30am in the gym or swimming pool. We do our training for about and hour and a half, work until 5.00pm/5.30pm and then come home and cook a delicious meal. We don't feel lacking in energy at all, quite the contrary, in fact. Once you've changed your old habits, started eating properly and sorted out your old body, you really will take on a new lease of life.

In layman's terms, fasting allows your digestive system to sort out all the food you've previously eaten. It sends all the nutrition it derives from that food where it is needed and allows your body to absorb it all properly. Then it processes all the waste, begins to get rid of it from your body before you begin eating again. In essence, your digestive system initially has to work hard after food has been eaten, but then gets a rest before having to process all the food you will be eating for your next meal. It gives your body chance to have a good clean up, carry out any necessary repairs and absorb all the nutrients from the food you've just eaten. That's why you don't keep snacking between meals. You need to give your system a chance to rest and recover before it starts the whole process again.

After ten to twelve hours of not eating, your body enters a stage called 'Autophagy'. Basically autophagy means that your body begins to recycle itself, renew cells and tidy everything up. 'Auto' means self and 'Phagy' means eat. It means your body begins to literally eat itself. Don't worry, it is actually beneficial to your body and overall health as your body is just eating and recycling itself. It removes the body's rubbish, allowing it to get back to peak performance. Your body also produces human growth hormone during this stage, which has been shown to decrease inflammatory substances and also slows down your body's ageing process.

Again, let me emphasise, this is a very basic explanation of autophagy and it's a much more complex process than I'm qualified to write about in detail.

It can and does, help to restore and restart your whole body and actually, you really don't feel hungry whilst fasting after the first couple of days.

It's certainly helped us to keep on track and you do feel great when fasting. Completely the opposite to how I thought we would feel. I assumed we would feel weak, light headed and be absolutely starving all the time. In fact we're full of energy, our brains seem to work better, our heads are clearer and we're not constantly craving our next meal or wanting to snack all the time.

We were recently on holiday in Lanzarote for a month and decided to fast for twenty-four hours, having just one meal a day, over a prolonged period.

We ate at around 6.30pm every night, something very healthy, and then stopped eating at around 8.30pm that same evening. We then didn't eat anything else until the following evening, again at around 6.30pm. We finished eating at 8.30pm therefore we were fasting for around twenty to twenty-two hours per day. We only drank plain water or black tea and coffee throughout that time.

We did this for a full fifteen days. During this time we trained almost everyday in the apartment we were staying in, using our resistance bands. We walked at least five kilometres every day, but in the main, doubled that distance most days. Unfortunately we didn't have any scales to record any results regarding our weights.

We really didn't feel hungry at all and had no cravings for anything sweet or anything we don't usually eat.

However, towards our fifteenth day we both started to develop little pot bellies and felt slightly swollen/bloated. Our training didn't seem to have the same 'edge' it usually had and we both felt that something wasn't quite 'on point'. There was nothing major. No feeling weak, dizzy or anything else and nothing we could really put our finger on.

At this point we made the decision to revert back to our usual two meals a day. Instantly, within minutes, we felt much better and regained our normal 'buzz'.

Although we occasionally have days when we only eat one meal a day, usually we have two meals. This seems to suit us both best. Our first meal of the day, sometime after 1pm, is generally a fairly small meal and consists of some form of protein, nuts, tinned fish or leftover meat from the previous day plus an avocado and some olives.

Unbeknown to us, whilst we were in Lanzarote, Kitty, our social media advisor, was doing exactly the same as we were. Uncanny I hear you say. Even more uncanny is the fact she experienced exactly the same reactions as we did. She also noticed her mood and temper appeared to have deteriorated as well, which is something we didn't experience.

We have yet to do a forty-eight hour, or even longer, fast. Not completely sure it's necessary for us at this stage. Never say 'never' though.

I don't think we can really say anything further about gut bacteria and fasting because if we try and elaborate further, it becomes a bit too scientific for us and probably for most of you as well.

Anyway, give fasting a try and see the benefits for yourselves, unless you are pregnant, a small child or suffering from some specific illness that stipulates you have to eat three meals a day. The common advice about eating three meals a day for optimum health is, in our view, a total myth. You can easily get through the day on two, or even just one meal and you'll be amazed at just how good you will feel.

I know there'll be thousands of 'fasting experts' out there who will disagree with us and some already have. However, if your body doesn't feel right doing something, you need to change what you're doing. After all, it wasn't just the odd day we did it, but fifteen consecutive days!

This leads me nicely on to the second part of this chapter. Having the guts to carry on. Having experienced the consequences of eating food that doesn't agree with us is one of the things that gives us the strength to carry on with our regime and maintain good health.

You've got to remember, what we are doing now is something we fully intend to carry on with for the rest of our lives and that's exactly what you have to do. This is not a quick fix in order to lose some weight before an upcoming holiday, wedding or similar event. It's a lifelong commitment that needs to be undertaken in order to stay the way you are now. We're not saying that you have to go to the same extremes we have, for example, giving up alcohol, or even being as strict as we are. You can still drink small amounts of red wine and some spirits and, if you think you have the willpower to get straight back on track the very next day or even next meal after you've had a wobble or cheat, well so be it. We find it much easier to just stay on track.

We are not very good at going off track, or at least, I'm not. Julie is marginally better than I am at being able to do this, but like me, there are thousands of people that find this almost impossible to do. In my opinion, this is proof of how addictive all the food you and many, many thousands were and are still eating, actually is. You wouldn't say to a drug addict or alcoholic, 'Go on, just one snort or just one pint won't do you any harm'. Well, in my opinion, it's the same with food. Some food just seems to force your body to crave more and more of the same, crave inducing food. In the end you just cave in and before you realise it, you're back to square one - fat and very unhappy.

In the past when we've attempted to lose some weight, we've always made a point of having a treat (cheat) day. This meant that on Sundays we would have some cake or a dessert. At first we were fairly strict with these rules, but slowly and surely these occasional treats became more and more regular until they just became the everyday norm. Your body just wants more and more and before you know it, all that hard work has been in vain.

The food we now eat doesn't make your body crave the foods we used to eat, thus making it very easy to maintain what we now eat. Maybe some people might consider this a bit sad or narrow minded, but trust me, because of the trials and tests we have done over the last eighteen months, it's far better to just eliminate these types of food completely.

Having said that, we do actually crave certain foods, but now it's all the sort of foods that keep us feeling healthy, slim and feel full of life. We never thought in a million years we would catch ourselves saying, 'I could really eat a nice big salad just now'! It was usually a piece of cake or some biscuits in the past.

Chapter 3:
Snacks and Snacking

This chapter actually links in with the previous chapter, in which we discussed your 'gut'. In this chapter we'll be talking about snacks and snacking. For many years it's been thought that 'healthy' snacking was not only great for maintaining and keeping your metabolic rate stable and working correctly, it was also a great way to control your weight because eating healthy snacks between meals would help you feel full and satisfied until it was time for your next meal.

The evidence currently being circulated around the diet industry now is actually contrary to this and it appears that complete abstinence, or fasting, between meals is the best way forward.

We've tried both, over fairly long periods of time, at least six to eight weeks each time and we have to agree with the latter!

As previously stated, we fast every day between our evening meal and our lunchtime meal the next day. We don't eat at all. Between lunch and dinner we usually don't eat anything again, however, we occasionally have a snack, usually nuts or nut butter. If we've been trying out new recipes, especially if it's some cake or dessert, we may try some of that as well, but usually only a very small portion between us.

We quickly discovered that if we made a regular habit of snacking, the weight began to creep back on. Because of this, snacking is kept to a minimum and any snacks we do have are **ALWAYS** from our 'Yes' list of foods and **NEVER** anything sweet or sugary!

There is some science behind the reason for not snacking and briefly, it's the same science involved with fasting.

If you don't eat between meals, your body and guts have a chance to catch up. As I've previously stated, you will digest whatever you've eaten for lunch and your guts get a rest and get prepared for your evening meal, therefore not forcing your digestive system to keep working overtime.

As far as we are concerned, this makes sense and it works very well for us. Any hunger we initially encountered when we first stopped snacking between meals is very quickly overcome. Within a day or so any hunger completely disappeared.

If you're still starving after a meal and providing you've waited for twenty minutes or so in order to allow your meal to settle, drink some more water. If this doesn't work, have a snack then. Just a few nuts or a spoonful of nut butter will help to make you feel full.

Don't wait for too long after a main meal before addressing this situation, because if you do, those few nuts or nut butter then becomes an additional snack or meal. Treat it as a dessert and then just don't snack any more.

Incidentally if you are hungry between meals, it's possible you are mistaking hunger for thirst. Always have a large glass of water before thinking of eating anything and you will be surprised how often doing this will make those hunger pangs disappear.

Whilst on the subject of water, make sure you drink plenty of it all day. I know it's sometimes difficult to drink plenty of water especially when you have limited access to a loo. It's a problem if you're working, driving, visiting people and places where toilets are not always available. Also when you first start drinking a lot of water, you'll find yourself waking up a couple of times during the night to use the toilet. Your body will adjust after a short time and you should find constant visits to the loo become less frequent. Your body will find its own levels, but make sure you drink plenty of water.

As a last resort if you find yourself caving in and having to munch on something, make sure it's something healthy like nuts, nut butter, a small amount of cold meat or make a small green salad and drizzle it with plenty of olive oil.

Something else we've tried, although it's not for the faint-hearted, is consuming oil. Either extra virgin olive oil or extra virgin coconut oil. That's it. On its own and from a spoon. I know many of you will turn your nose up at eating oil straight off a spoon, but it does make you feel full and both oils are actually very good for your guts. I actually like the taste of both oils and can easily consume both of them on their own, however, Julie isn't very keen on the flavour of coconut and prefers olive oil.

Just be mindful of snacks and snacking and if your weight is creeping up, cut back on them until you're back to normal. Keep any snacks healthy and in line with our 'Yes' foods list. Don't ever be tempted to resort to old habits and eat biscuits, cakes and crisps etc.

Chapter 4:
People's Attitudes

We are still astounded at people's attitudes with regard to health, food and their bodies. It's also been amazing how people reacted to us when we decided to change what we eat, lose weight and get healthy. We thought people would be happy that we had achieved our goals, but in quite a few cases, it was quite the opposite! It was as though we had somehow betrayed them by actually becoming slim and were now no longer paid up members of the fat club!

It was very much the same when we stopped drinking. It was as though we had left those particular 'communities' or 'clubs' and we weren't welcome back again!

After writing our first book, we did many promotional events around the country in different book stores, supermarkets, sports centres and establishments where we thought we would be able to promote our book. But most importantly, we wanted to spread the word about how we succeeded in losing our weight, actually changed our lives and hopefully, how we could inspire and help others to change theirs.

One of the things we didn't want to do, right from the start, was to come across as preaching or being evangelical, as many people seem to do when they achieve something hard or difficult in their respective lives. We sincerely wanted to hold out a hand to people and just tell them to read our book and see if it could maybe help and inspire them to achieve the same as we had, either by following the same methods we had, or something that suited their needs and lives. Our book was never intended to be a 'diet bible', nor that anyone who bought the book should follow what we had done to the letter! We wrote it with the intention of giving people help, inspiration and hope.

We met some very unhappy people during these promotions. Some worryingly unhappy! However, when we began to talk to them about what we had done and how we hoped we could inspire them to do the same, the same old excuses began to pour out. Mainly, it was excuses where they blamed other people in their lives. It was because of what these people may think or say about the fact they had actually made a decision, to take the bull by its horns and do something about their unhappy lives.

It was either the husband/wife who wouldn't be happy about them going on a diet or having to buy different food for the rest of the family. Or that their partners weren't happy about them stopping drinking for a while or not eating cereal any more and so on. It didn't seem to matter that that person was desperately unhappy about their weight and life, so long as they were keeping everyone else happy. We frequently meet people who are accompanied by their respective partners who ask us about our book and promotion who are obviously in need of some help regarding their current lifestyle. The conversation doesn't last very long before their other half suddenly butts in and begins to talk on behalf of their very unhappy partner. The conversation then goes something along the lines of '**WE** don't need to diet and **WE** don't need a book to tell us what to eat' and so on!

Honestly, there were a fair few people who were actually almost suicidal about their lives and their weight! It was pretty scary and very, very sad.

The fact is, you need to speak with family, partners and friends alike and just say, firstly to yourself and then to these people, 'I'm going to do this for **ME** so that I can then become a better person for **YOU**!'

I've mentioned this earlier, but if we don't all wake up soon and become a little more knowledgeable about food and the food we eat, we're rather rapidly heading towards our own demise. Sorry to sound so gloomy, but it has to be said. Do something for yourself and others will follow you. That includes your partner, family and friends. Trust me.

When others begin to see your huge changes, they will want to follow your example. Whether they achieve the same success as you will depend on those particular individuals. However, they will have your support and you'll be able to offer some sound advice as you've already been through the same process.

I know you can't just write off your friends and family just because they don't agree with what you are going to do for the rest of your life. In our experience, just get on with it quietly anyway and others will slowly latch onto what you're doing when that light bulb moment suddenly switches on.

Unfortunately it won't switch on for some, that's their decision and not something you need to feel guilty about. But most will want to get on board with you, even if they don't do it with the same gusto as you.

Don't worry about eating out. Ring restaurants up and tell them what you eat and don't eat. Ask them if they can cater for you. In most cases they will. If they refuse, just go somewhere else. Vegetarians and vegans have had this problem for years. However, now that some 'experts' and 'celebrities' are saying that it's good to eat plant based food and it's all over the news and television as the latest 'new trend', eating out veggie style is much easier for them now than it's ever been.

Find what works for you, stick to your guns, don't be swayed by others who may try and force you into doing something you don't want to do, which will just leave you feeling rubbish about yourself afterwards.

We've actually found that some old friends have turned their backs on us since we lost our weight. We have no idea what's gone wrong, or why they have done this, but can only attribute this to some form of jealousy in that we have achieved our success and they haven't. We haven't been able to come up with anything else despite attempting to address the situation, so unfortunately we've just moved on. Funnily enough a lot of them are still fat people!

The up side of this, however, is that we have now met many more like-minded people who have taken their place. Our weight loss and lifestyle change seems to have opened up many more opportunities and horizons, which includes lots of new friends.

We never, ever dreamed we would actually lose our weight, never mind, write a book about what we've done and here we are writing a second book.

Give yourself a chance and see where you can get to and what you can achieve!!

Chapter 5:
Stress

This is going to be a difficult subject to try to address. Everyone has ideas about what stress is and how to address it. They are all very different to the next persons' ideas.

Some people appear to have relatively stress free lives, whilst others just go from one stressful situation to the next. Many appear to actually thrive on stress, whilst for others it's a major cause for concern and can be very debilitating. It can be the cause of many associated mental and physical disabilities, one of them being over-eating which, in turn causes weight gain and obesity, which then causes that ever-increasing circle of getting stressed, eating to counteract that stress and then getting stressed about putting on weight.

We would be the first to admit that we're not the best at dealing with stress and over the years it's caused us a fair few problems, one way or another.

Having said that, though, we seem to have come out of the other side reasonably well. Stress can cause your body to enter into a 'Catch 22' situation. When you become stressed your body releases a chemical called cortisol. This puts your body into the 'fight or flight' condition, increasing adrenaline and shutting down other bodily functions in order to facilitate this. Two of these functions are the proper digestion of food, and sleep.

Then, because you are very stressed and you can't sleep, your body releases more cortisol and because you have too much of that floating around in your system you still can't sleep. An ever-increasing circle of stress develops.

Unless you can get your stress under reasonable control, it becomes a never-ending problem and too much cortisol definitely slows down your weight loss and damages your overall health.

In this day and age it's almost impossible to avoid stress, so it's a case of trying to deal with it the best way you can. We're still dealing with it, but think we're slowly getting there. Some of the best ways to deal with stress are by dealing with it naturally. Exercise, hobbies, holidays, time off from work, talking with a friend or your family, sometimes even a stranger, meditation and, in our opinion as a last resort, seeking medical help and medication. Don't get me wrong, doctors nowadays are very clued up about stress and the associated mental conditions. They offer some fabulous advice and help so don't let our opinion put you off speaking to a doctor about any problems you may have.

From our experience with seeking medical advice, it very often just resulted in certain medications being prescribed which only seemed to mask the problem and so any solution to the stress is only short lived. Many of the medications prescribed for stress can be very addictive, therefore causing you more anguish and stress when it's time to try and stop taking them.

I've personally experienced being prescribed medication for a sleeping/stress problem, which occurred shortly after I retired. I'm not sure if it was just the anticlimax of retirement or stress associated with our kids being in their late teens and trying to decide what to do with their respective lives. I just wasn't sleeping well at all. I visited the doctor, probably looking for a 'fast fix' and was prescribed some anti-depressants, the name of which I can't recall, sent away and told to come back in a month. Looking back now, I can now see how potentially dangerous those meds were as there were all sorts of warnings accompanying them. I had to wean myself onto them to reach the appropriate dosage and under no circumstances just stop taking them. Well, for that month, I just went about life in a total blur. Every morning I woke with a hangover despite not drinking, and my speech was slurred all day. I'm sure people thought I had been drinking. The most important thing though, was that they had no effect on my sleep whatsoever. I made my mind up to stop taking them. Full stop. No weaning myself off them or going back to the doctors and probably not the right thing to have done. I've never taken anything like it again and I hope I won't have to ever again!

Our answer has been, firstly, to address the cause of the stress and confront it. If it's a certain situation, a person or people, then try and reach an amicable solution with that particular situation or persons involved.

It often takes a lot of courage to do this. If you don't think you can do this on your own, have a friend or family member accompany you when you do it, not only for support, but to act as a mediator, if necessary. Having a colleague or friend with you can be especially important if you're attempting to address a work situation where workmates or bosses are involved. Many workplaces now have mediators, first contact personnel or mentors who receive very good training in dealing with this sort of thing.

Very often it's much easier and quicker to do this than you would think and afterwards you can be left thinking, 'well I wish I'd done that weeks ago!' Pluck up the courage and just try and sort it out. Even if you don't always reach a solution, the very act of doing something positive is sometimes enough to put your mind at rest and can actually sort the problem out completely.

Some situations just can't be sorted out, even by addressing them personally. Sometimes it's just a case of completely walking away from the issue/situation, locking it away somewhere in your head and never returning to it. This can be very difficult, especially where there's money, property or a love interest involved. Fortunately, most of these things can be replaced if need be, eventually.

The hardest emotion to deal with in many of these situations is that stubborn old thing called pride. Pride makes complex and problematic situations very difficult to either solve or just walk away from.

Unfortunately it's just something you have to do. Often, once it's done, it's amazing how easy it was to do. You just have to swallow that pride sometimes and get on with life. There's a lot of talk about keeping positive about life and the trials and tribulations life brings us. We like to think that being truly realistic about your goals and ambitions is probably much more effective and achievable than trying to be positive all the time.

Be realistic as to what you think you can do and achieve. Be <u>realistically positive</u>! At least when you're realistic about life, disappointments are fewer, less impactful and easier to solve.

As a last resort when trying to deal with stress, especially if it's become unbearable and natural remedies aren't working, seek out medical help, preferably in the form of some sort of counselling rather than medication.

The reactions in your body caused by stress have a tendency to build up little by little over time, until you suddenly feel like you're bursting. This is when people have breakdowns.

The results of stress on your body don't just disappear overnight, but build up and up inside you, so that what started out as a small problem ends up being a very serious problem for many people. A bit like how your weight goes up, little by little.

Funnily enough, since we've been eating the way we do, our brains seem to working in a much more logical way and dealing with stress has been much more manageable, again stressing the link between your gut and your brain!

Sorry, but there's no absolute answer to stress. Everyone has to deal with their stress as best as they can. But be aware, if you consider yourself to be one of those people who deals with stress well, but are experiencing some strange, unusual or unhealthy changes in yourself, there's a good chance it's stress that's causing them. Also, if you're finding your weight isn't coming off as you had hoped it would, or it's began to stall, or even started to go back on, it could very well be down to stress!

Chapter 6:
Exercise

We've both been closely linked or associated with sport, gyms, swimming, football and rugby, for most of our lives. Even before we met each other we were very 'sporty' people.

I started weight training in my teens to help with my rugby, field athletics and even then, my weight. I did, in fact, enter some body building competitions in my early twenties, but unfortunately lost out to the ever-increasing use of steroids within the body building scene. However, I just continued with the training because I really loved training with weights. In my opinion, there is no other exercise that has the same mental and physical benefits that weight/resistance training has. I know what mountain climbing, cycling, running and many other sports feel like. I've been there and done them, but, training with weights is very different and unless you've experienced it, you'll never know what it feels like. Many people have told me that they've tried weight training, but hate it, possibly because it's very hard work! It's pretty intense because it isolates the particular muscles you are targeting during a training session and exercises them much harder than many of the traditional types of exercise such as treadmills, exercise bikes and so on. It takes more than just one or two visits to the gym in order to understand what you're doing, how it works and why particular exercises work different muscle groups. My advice is, give it a go and give your body a chance to adapt to what you're doing and appreciate the results.

Julie has been a swimmer from about twelve years old and has been involved in athletics right up to having our kids.

She has represented Sheffield, Yorkshire, the Police and continues to swim now on a regular basis, and in some very cold pools that I wouldn't get into wearing a wet suit! I think you could say she is pretty dedicated to her swimming.

Exercise has kept us both mentally and physically fit, but unfortunately, not particularly slim. In fact, until just recently, we were quite fit, quite healthy, but FAT people.

I think we fell foul of the myth that if we did plenty of exercise, we could eat and drink what we wanted and the exercise would just burn off those unwanted, excess calories. I think that it's probably a well-known fact nowadays, that as a weight control method, exercise is probably not that effective or efficient.

However, before you start thinking, 'that's great, no more exercise', it's vital to stress that it is in fact, still important to keep mobile and remember that exercise keeps you toned, supple, improves your immune system and, more importantly, keeps your heart and mind healthy.

I recently read a report about older people, (that's people over fifty), and how, as you get older, you naturally begin to breath more shallowly, therefore your body doesn't always receive a good supply of oxygen. Apparently this is a natural ageing process and happens to everyone, due to the little branch-like vessels in your lungs shrinking because of immobility and ageing.

It can, however, be drastically slowed down, and even reversed somewhat, so they function normally again. By doing regular, daily exercise that causes you to get out of breath only slightly, the vessels are forced to increase to their normal size again, thus supplying your body with adequate amounts of oxygen.

Not so many years ago it was thought that the art of getting slim and staying slim was to concentrate on doing around 60-70% exercise and 40-30% diet. In our opinion and based on our own experiences, we believe it's totally the other way round, if not even more radical and something like 20% exercise and 80% diet. 'Experts' are now agreeing with this view that diet is now far more important than exercise.

Before starting any sort of exercise, especially if you've not done much previously, always consider consulting someone who has some good knowledge about training and exercise, especially in whatever exercise or training you decide you want to participate in. I don't necessarily mean turning up at your local gym and speaking to the personal trainer who works there, although that's always a good place to start, but speak to someone who's actually been participating in whatever sport you choose to do yourself.

In our opinion, experience is nearly always a better qualification than a certificate probably obtained by completing some sort of online course on the internet! No, we're not saying that all personal trainers aren't properly qualified. There are some brilliant trainers out there who are really passionate about what they do and who are extremely knowledgeable. However there are some very dodgy ones as well. Make your own decision and choose wisely. Listen to someone who looks and sounds like they know what they're doing.

Just be careful you don't choose the type of personal trainer who, for whatever warped reason, takes extreme delight in getting you in the gym and then making you do a workout that is far too strenuous, difficult and complicated for your own personal ability and leaves you feeling totally exhausted and even ill. There are some trainers out there who revel in that sort of thing for some reason. It will just put you off going back again. A workout shouldn't last much more than an hour in total. That includes some cardio, weights and even then, an hour should be after you've been training for at least four to six weeks. A good training session should leave you feeling exhilarated and refreshed, not being unable to walk out of the gym, or spending the last ten minutes in the toilet being sick. Take it at your own pace, but remember, you do have to put some effort into your workout and get out of breath somewhat!

This may sound silly, but it also applies to something as simple as walking. Speak to someone who you know does a lot of walking. It may be a neighbour who regularly walks their dog. Ask them about the shoes they wear. How far they walk. Where they walk and how often do they walk. More importantly, ask them if you can tag along with them from time to time. Don't be a nuisance though, as walkers can often be the type of people who use their walks to find solitude and deal with their own problems! Their daily walk is often their own stress reliever, so be careful you don't intrude in their special moments of 'time out'!

There are many articles on the internet about exercise and doing workouts in the privacy of your own home, using very little or no equipment. Have a look and see if that's something that would be suitable for you. When we're on holiday or away from home, we often do a short workout when we get up, after our morning tea of course, using just our own body weight or using resistance bands, or a bit of both. It just sets us up for the rest of the day, but more importantly, it keeps us in the exercise 'habit'.

I could bang on about exercise all day. It's something we both find very interesting, satisfying and therapeutic. There are many ways to exercise and there will be something to suit everyone.

It is, however, a very individual thing. Some people hate it with a passion, in all its forms. The thing is though, it has an important place in your life. We know people in their seventies who have done no exercise all their lives but, because of some medical condition, have been referred to the local gym or swimming pool, in order to receive some remedial or physiotherapy type of treatment. They have found themselves really loving their exercise programmes and wishing they had done it years ago. It just goes to show that it's never too late to start something new in your life.

Although I've already said it's not a particularly good method of getting and keeping the weight off, we both discovered that when we finally lost all our excess weight, underneath all the flab we had some pretty good muscle tone and the exercise we've done all our lives had obviously kept our skin and muscles in really good shape.

So the message here is this. Do something.

Every day. Even for just a few minutes. Get out of breath and get your heart beating. You will see and feel the rewards that come with exercise, almost from day one. Just keep at it!

A point now about exercise and nutrition. Nutrition in the exercise business is a massive industry. It's certainly a multi million, if not a billion pound industry. There are many so-called nutrition 'experts' making a fortune out of the products out there on the market, promising all sorts of wonderful results after taking their particular products and supplements, many of which have been supposedly endorsed by experts, doctors and celebrities.

The only supplements we take, or have taken during our weight loss period are magnesium, potassium, vitamins B12 and D.

We don't have anything else. No protein shakes or bars. Nothing, just good old food and really not that much of that any more in comparison to the amount we used to eat.

We're still undecided as to how useful these supplements are. We were recently away on holiday in The Canaries for a month and during that time we did not take any supplements at all. We were still eating well, not eating rubbish and we noticed no difference in ourselves at all. Maybe we'll stop taking them completely. At the moment the jury's still out.

During the course of my body building years I've eaten vast amounts of protein in many shapes and forms and I seriously think I've had more success over the last two years, eating a lot less food, especially protein, than I've had in all the previous years even though I'm now in my sixties. I hate to think how much money I've wasted on different products.

I've recently done some research about protein shakes which included smoothies, and found that the research hasn't been very favourable to either of them. Apparently they don't go through your digestive system in the same way proper food does because they enter your body already in liquid form.

Firstly, you don't need to chew them, eliminating the first part of the digestion process, namely mastication, and the shake or smoothie enters your system rather too quickly and then exits your system, equally as fast. Therefore your body does not extract the full amount of nutrition from the shakes or smoothies, thus rendering them pretty useless, contrary to popular opinion. There are some experts that actually deem protein shakes and smoothies to be expensive, unnecessary laxatives!!

We think you'll have to make your own minds up as to what you do. Personally, I'd advise you to save your money and eat proper food.

If, however, you are still keen to take either vitamin or protein supplements, be very careful what type you buy and where you buy them from. Some of the cheaper ones are far better than some of the more expensive ones endorsed by sports stars, celebrities and medical experts. There are some good health stores, chemists and even supermarkets that have their own cheaper brands that contain exactly the same ingredients as the more expensive brands.

If you want more information, advice or any other details regarding exercise or what exercises we actually do, feel free to contact us directly via our social media pages.

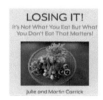
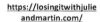

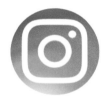
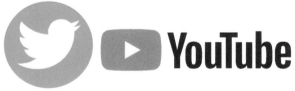

https://losingitwithjulie
andmartin.com/

Losing it with Julie and
Martin

losingitwithjulieandmartin

_Losing_It_JM

Chapter 7:
Alcohol

So, here we go!! Another very controversial subject, but one that needs to be discussed because of its effect on both weight control and overall health. I'll be brief and hopefully offer some sound advice in an unbiased way, as we've both been completely teetotal for the last twelve years, which means that most of the advice is given in hindsight. If only we were all good listeners of hindsight, I'm certain we would all be both wiser and wealthier people.

Assuming you've already read our first book, you'll know that the purpose of writing it was to help others lose weight and begin a new, healthy, slim forever, lifestyle. The purpose of this book is to help and inspire those same people and, hopefully, many others to lose weight, get healthy and then maintain their success and not resort to their old ways and habits.

Once again we must stress that what we write here are entirely our own opinions based solely on what we have experienced over the years.

We have had a very close, often dangerous and quite troublesome relationship and connection with alcohol in both a professional and personal capacity and for quite a long period of our lives.

We've both seen quite close friends and colleagues lose their lives directly through alcohol and alcoholism.

We've also been involved in very dangerous, life threatening situations and also extremely sad and moving situations. Again, these incidents have been directly linked with alcohol.

In May 2008 we both took the decision to stop drinking alcohol completely. We haven't drunk alcohol since that time. The decision to stop drinking was a far more difficult step to take than to actually stop drinking. I think that both of us had that same difficulty when we finally decided to lose weight. Once we had made the decision and got on with it, there was no stopping us. It was actually really easy.

We made our minds up, initially, to stop drinking Monday to Friday and then to just have a drink at the weekends. Well, we reached Friday evening and both of us realised that we just weren't bothered about having a drink. So we didn't and basically that was that!

People who knew us well were gobsmacked. We were quite heavy drinkers, especially me, and people couldn't believe what we had done. At first neither could I. It had been very easy to do, much easier than I had imagined. I personally believe that it was entirely due to adopting the right mindset from the beginning. If you want to do something or change something, no matter how big or small the change or challenge is, once your mind is made up, the rest is easy.

I'm not going to start being evangelical and start preaching, 'You shall not drink'. If you want to drink, drink. However, if you drink and you want to change your lives, lose some weight and get healthy, you will need to address both what and how much you drink.

There is absolutely no doubt about it. If you are starting out right at the beginning, you will need to stop completely, at least for a short period of time, probably two weeks or preferably longer.

Alcohol is empty calories. No matter whether it is wine, beer or spirits. It does not have any positive effect on your body. That's not only our opinion because most experts agree.

There's all sorts of stuff written about how red wine has many benefits. How it can act as an antioxidant and is actually good for your heart and circulation. It can help you relax at the end of a hard week at work and how it has many other so-called benefits.

We've managed much, much better without it and wish we'd done it years ago.

As I've mentioned, we haven't drunk alcohol for twelve years now and because of this we've lost track of how much booze costs because we very rarely frequent pubs or bars anymore. We couldn't tell you how much a pint is or how much people drink these days.

That was until we began researching different subjects for this book, alcohol being one of them.

We began talking to people who do drink and asked them where they drink, what they drink and how often they drink. It was quite obvious that many people found it extremely difficult and uncomfortable talking to us about their drinking and opening up about their drinking habits. It was apparent that many, or even most, people felt a little bit guilty about their drinking habits and probably didn't answer us truthfully. We weren't criticising or telling them their drinking was out of control, or that they should try and cut down on how much or how often they drank. We were not making any comments or judgements whatsoever. We were just asking the questions. We are still not making judgements. That decision is yours and yours alone.

However, what became very obvious was that people seemed to be drinking pretty excessively nowadays, probably more than ever. It was also apparent that drinking at home wasn't considered to be proper drinking, even though many people were drinking as much at home as they did in a pub at the weekend. Every night! It was also evident that just a couple of glasses of wine every night was actually a couple of bottles and more each night.

Alcohol is also something that affects all social groups and all parts of the country. It is not just associated with the rich, the poor, employed, unemployed, or people from the north or south. In our opinion it has quickly become a massive problem in this country for a great many people and is also adding to the huge obesity problem we now have.

So that's enough from us about alcohol except, if you want to make the changes, well, make them sooner rather than later.

Stopping drinking was definitely one of those life-changing decisions you make in life that completely changed our lives very much for the better. The day I stopped drinking I felt as though a massive weight had been lifted off my shoulders. Apart from no longer having that hangover and foggy feeling that lasted until mid-morning, there was never having to worry about who was drinking and who was driving. We both immediately started feeling more alive and far happier. Situations we previously considered stressful and problematic appeared far easier to deal with and far less stressful.

If you are a heavy, regular drinker, it's only a matter of time when, not if, you will start having some sort of alcohol related health problems!

If you are worried about the amount you are drinking and need any advice about alcohol, or you are toying with the idea of cutting down or even giving it up completely, we're more than happy to offer further advice if you contact us directly/personally via our social media pages, or we will be happy to point you in the right direction where you can get the help and advice you may need.

Chapter 8:
Sweeteners, Sugar and Carbohydrates

Sweeteners are obviously an alternative to natural and other refined sugars. Most alternative sweeteners are not natural products and are manufactured by some form of chemical process. Because of the unnatural processes involved in producing sweeteners, you would think that natural, raw cane sugar would be far healthier. Some years ago a well known sugar company actually ran a series of adverts on television, in which they made claims about how sugar was good for us and provided us with all our energy in order to get us through our busy days!

Unfortunately, in ours and in many experts' opinions, sugar is no better for us than many of the drugs that are peddled on our streets these days.

Simply, eating sugar signals your brain and subsequently your body, into thinking that sugar is the best possible fuel your body and brain can have in order to function at its optimum best. When those sugar levels begin to run low (your body burns sugar very quickly), it then demands more sugar, hence the craving for sweet things. That's when you get those slumps after eating a lot of sweet or carb- laden food. The cravings begin and you just want to eat more sugar or carbs. Carbs and sugar also don't leave you feeling full and satisfied like protein does.

The thing to remember, though, is that high carb foods like pasta, bread, rice and potatoes, to name just a few, are all sugar, albeit in a different form. Your body converts the starchy carbs into sugar and your body uses that sugar for fuel instead of burning your fat or the good fats you eat. In fact whatever carbs/sugar your body doesn't use up immediately, insulin will convert to it fat and store it up in your bodies.

Contrary to what a lot of people, including some experts, believe, you don't need sugar or carbs to function or survive. You are quite capable of living on very few or even zero carbs and moderate amounts of protein and fat. Your brain does need carbs/glucose to function properly, but if it doesn't get enough from the carbs you eat, it will convert some protein into glucose for that purpose. Your brain actually loves ketones, which are produced when you burn fat.

Inuits from Alaska used to survive on blubber and meat from seals, whales and fish and they survived with no trouble whatsoever. They ate very few vegetables or carbs. Some years ago it was considered that they were some of the healthiest people on the planet, however since they began to introduce fast food there, they've become like the rest of us. Obese and unhealthy!

Anyway back to sweeteners. Many of them contain no calories, no carbs, but plenty of chemicals. There is now growing evidence, though, that despite the zero calories and carbs attraction, it's actually the sweetness in the product that's the problem. The sweetness tricks your brain into thinking you're eating sugar/carbs, forcing your body to produce insulin and thus the fat storage process begins again. Unfortunately the research regarding this is still very conflicted. One side states that it's perfectly all right to consume these sweeteners and they have absolutely no adverse effects. The other side totally refutes this and states that the sweetness adversely affects our insulin production and blood sugar levels.

From experiments we've done on ourselves with different sweeteners, the latter appears to be correct!

You may think that once in a while it's OK to have a piece of cake, chocolate or a big plate of pasta, rice or a roast potato or two. The problem with this is that your body will immediately return to a carb/sugar burning machine and start laying down layers of fat

again, but in order to get your body back to a fat burning machine again it will probably take three to four days. So although your body can swap from fat burning to carb burning in a matter of minutes, the reverse takes much longer!

So in our opinion, it's just far easier to steer clear of the sweet stuff and carbs completely. In this book and our previous book, there are a number of dessert and treat recipes that call for the use of sweeteners of your choice. We always use Triple Zero Organic Stevia, which we buy from 'Grape Tree' as it seems to have the least after taste and fewest adverse effects/reactions on our bodies. It comes in a very 'sugary' consistency and can be used for baking. It contains zero calories and zero carbs, but does contain Erythritol, which is processed from sugar alcohol and is also an artificial sweetener.

Experiment to see what you like and which one suits you best. In our experience, though, consume too much, and you may see the pounds slowly creep back on and leave you wondering what you've done wrong.

There is a saying circulating within the diet/health industry that's quite apt. The best way to deal with sugar, in all its forms, is to 'Retreat from the sweet' completely. It's strange, but just a few days of not eating sugar totally transforms your taste buds and everything else tends to taste sweeter. We often segment lemons and stir them into salads, especially to accompany fish dishes and find they taste quite sweet and we can eat them like an orange. It's the same with limes as well.

So just to recap, eat too many carbs/sugar and your blood sugar spikes, more insulin is released, which is not absorbed by your cells properly. You then become hungry again, so you eat more carbs/sugar, more insulin is released and causes any extra calories to be stored as fat. So the never-ending circle continues, that is, until you cut out the sugar and carbs and you begin to burn your stored fat, or the fat you eat.

Once you do this you will have loads more energy and less of those slumps you get in an afternoon after your traditional lunchtime sandwich.

There is also a fair amount of evidence now that people who reduce their carbs and sugar consumption, especially those suffering from joint pain or arthritis, discover significant changes for the better once they've done this, sometimes even to the extent of being able to vastly reduce their medications or even completely stop taking them.

It was previously thought that this was down to just weight loss, which is completely understandable, considering that less weight and stress was being put on joints, ligaments and tendons etc. However there is a clear link that seems to establish that inflammation in your joints and body can be vastly reduced or even halted by reducing the amount of carbs and sugar you consume.

Chapter 9:
'Mid Lifestyle Crisis!'

This chapter is about what happens when you have a hiccup. Either when you've lost your weight and a few pounds have crept back on, or when you're still in the process of losing your weight, but have plateaued somewhat. Or if you have had a massive wobble and completely gone off the rails. This will happen to everyone at some stage. This is why we have added this chapter so that people are aware that it will happen and be able to take the appropriate action straight away. It's very disheartening when you do have a blip, but as long as you know it will happen, it's much easier to deal with.

That's why it's appropriate that this chapter appears midway through the book!

We had been experimenting with loads of new and different recipes for this book, gone through Christmas and been away on holiday/writing for a month. Subsequently we'd put on a few pounds. Not a lot, but more than we wanted to. Again, if this happens and there's a very good chance it will, those few extra pounds need to be addressed straight away.

Don't leave it until those few pounds mount up into a stone, then two and so on and so on.

As a result, we went right back to basics and started a week where we weighed all our protein again and got right back on track. It was no big deal, but hard fought success still has to be worked at and monitored closely, in order to maintain that success. We will never go back to being fat! Ever! Being slim and healthy is so much more fun, in so many ways. It does take some work, though, and there is no going back to the old ways.

We went back to the three day cleanse featured in 'Losing It', but this time we extended it for a full week, gradually adding a little bit more food in each day after the first three days. We again recorded everything we ate, firstly for the three day cleanse and then the subsequent four days. We also recorded our weight on Monday and then again the following Monday.

During this week we posted our daily food intake on our social media pages and recorded any relevant comments, observations and opinions throughout the week.

Kitty, our social media advisor, has lost a considerable amount of weight over the past year, some of it using our methods including several of our recipes from 'Losing It'.

However, during the previous few weeks she had found her weight plateauing somewhat, so she joined us for that week as well.

We asked everyone on our Facebook group to join in with us if they were experiencing the same problem, or were just starting out on our programme.

Christmas was out of the way and we were fast approaching Easter, so it was a good time for those people to come on board with us and get ready for spring and summer.

We got weighed the following weekend, after our three day cleanse, which actually turned out to be a four and a bit day cleanse. We'd weighed all our protein and been dairy free for the duration. No yogurt, cheese or anything dairy. We even limited our snacks between meals to the occasional few nuts.

I lost one pound and Julie stayed the same weight. We had both been convinced that we had lost weight. We both felt slimmer and absolutely full of energy. We'd had some really hard training sessions that week and had slept really well every night. It was a bit of a mystery why we hadn't lost more, although three days is perhaps not long enough to see any big numbers, especially as we didn't have that much to lose anyway. We were only talking about couple of pounds each!

It's does prove the importance of monitoring your weight on a fairly regular basis, maybe once a week. Keep working hard with your exercise and make sure you return to good eating after any cheat or hiccup the following day, or better still, your very next meal.

Chapter 10:
Vegetarians and Vegans

Being vegetarian or vegan is fast becoming very popular, especially, it seems with the younger generation. Unfortunately, both vegetarianism and vegan appear to have become one of the latest 'fashionable' trends, worldwide, which we feel is not how either should be viewed.

These 'trends' are often endorsed by the current favourite TV cooks, celebrities, doctors and people in the diet, food and health industries, who just seem to take any opportunity to make a fast buck from many of these current trends.

In our opinion, when someone has made the decision to stop eating meat, whether it be for ethical reasons, because of the taste or for any other reason, then that decision should be respected by everyone else and taken seriously. Unfortunately that doesn't seem to be the case and being a vegetarian is still looked upon as being 'hippie' or 'wacky' unless, as is the way nowadays, it's become the latest trend! We get the same reaction when we tell people we don't drink alcohol or eat certain food. We have been blatantly ridiculed, despite never trying to preach or force our opinions on to other people. We have been eating the way we do now for two and a half years and feel it's completely normal, easy and healthy. It's our way of life and a healthy life at that.

We aren't vegetarian or vegan, however, we do eat a fair amount of both vegetarian and vegan types of food and recipes. We regularly have meals that are totally devoid of any meat and animal associated produce. We have vastly reduced our consumption of meat nowadays and obtain much of our protein from sources like nuts, cheese, hemp, yogurt, eggs and of course, from the large amount of vegetables we eat. Yes, vegetables do contain protein, some more than others, but we know that most people aren't aware of this. We certainly weren't two and half years ago. We do eat some dairy products, but in very small amounts and usually only homemade Greek style yogurt, a small amount of double cream, crème fraîche, butter and a little cheese.

We recently carried out our own experiment by going totally vegetarian and partly vegan for a period of a month.

We are aware, at this point, all you veggies and vegans will be shouting, 'A month, is that all?' or words to that effect.

Well we discovered that our month of vegetarian and vegan food was very enjoyable, tasty and we didn't really miss meat BUT sadly found that our bodies seemed to be lacking in 'something'. That 'something' wasn't easily pinpointed either. We weren't sure what it was. We certainly weren't lacking in energy, but we were slightly weaker in the gym and when swimming. It just felt as though we weren't getting all the nutrition we were used to getting when we ate fish or meat. Maybe it takes more than a month for our bodies to adjust. We still continue with our vegetarian and vegan days on a regular basis and meat days are fast becoming less and less. However we still feel the necessity to consume some meat or fish from time to time.

One of the problems we did encounter was the fact that neither of us tolerated legumes, beans and pulses very well. None of them seemed to suit our guts and they gave us terrible wind, both those from cans and those we cooked from scratch.

Red kidney beans and chickpeas were the worst culprits. They left us both extremely bloated and windy. Out of all of them, butter beans suited us best, with red lentils cooked from scratch coming a close second.

The second problem we encountered was that both veggie and vegan recipes tended to be carb and sugar loaded. They use a lot of flours made from grains and they tend to include a lot of pasta, rice and bread, whole grain usually. These are all foods we avoid because of their tendency to cause weight gain, but also because of the way they are farmed and their high lectin content. Lectin is a protein found in many grains and some fruits and vegetables. Lectins interfere with the good bacteria in your gut and thus interfere with the proper digestion of your food and functioning of your body.

We were fine with all types of nuts, except peanuts, which, of course aren't nuts, but legumes. We use ground almonds and coconut flour in a lot of our vegetarian and vegan recipes to replace regular flours and we are perfectly fine with both of these. We are also good with flaxseed and have recently discovered how to make a 'flaxseed egg' in order to replace normal egg in some recipes. We have yet to conduct our experiments with this kind of 'egg' because we don't really eat that much food that we would use it in – baking for example.

We avoid soya products, mainly because of the methods used in processing probably most or even all, soya products.

However we still eat meat and will continue to do so until we can either find a low carb, zero soya, textured meat substitute or be educated otherwise.

We've tried to speak to quite a few veggies and vegans, in order to get their advice and their opinions about the food they eat and compare it with the food we eat, with little or no success. Many appear to be very reluctant to talk about their diet and the food they eat, perhaps for fear of being scoffed at or even ridiculed?

There are many veggies and vegans out there, who are not healthy, who are fat and who do not appear to actually know exactly what they are doing, but seem to have jumped on the current 'bandwagon'. Evidently their idea of being vegetarian is basically to consume anything that doesn't contain meat and this means chips, pasta, bread, rice with everything and actually, very few vegetables! Many are also unsure about what, if any, protein they're consuming, so long as they're not eating meat!

Having said that, I'm sure there are many veggies and vegans who do know what they're talking about. These are the people we need to talk to. We want to encourage them to read our book and join our Facebook group in order to advise and encourage people like us, and anyone else who wants to become either vegetarian or vegan.

We have read a fair bit about vegans and can definitely see where they are coming from, particularly with regard to the animal welfare side of it. It's something we all need to consider in this day and age because of the way meat, fish and poultry is raised and farmed in order to cater for our increasing desire for meat and fish. Some of the methods involved during raising and feeding these animals,

certainly leave a lot of questions unanswered and even many questions to be asked in the first place.

We have examined a number of vegan recipes, which we could and do eat on a regular basis, especially those containing nuts and hempseed. There are, however, many recipes containing sugar, albeit in forms like maple syrup, coconut sugar, honey and raw unrefined cane sugar. I know that these are all natural products, but at the end of the day they are just sugars and they have the same effects on our bodies as plain old processed, store bought sugar.

I have also seen a disagreement within the vegan community, as to whether eating honey follows the true vegan guidelines. My point is, though, honey is just sugar as well, despite how natural it is and sugar doesn't really have a place in our lives anymore. We feel so much better for not eating it.

Very recently, we've again been eating more vegetarian and vegan meals and on the days we don't eat meat we have both found that we don't sleep as well as on the days we eat some meat or fish. It hasn't just been the odd occasion either. It's been every time. We are wondering if it's something to do with not eating the essential amino acids usually found in meat and fish that your body cannot produce itself. We're open to advice and opinions about this subject.

I'm not trying to convert vegetarians and vegans and turn them into meat eaters, but it's important to listen to your body and if it feels that everything isn't working or functioning properly within it, have a look at what you're eating and make some adjustments. Very small omissions or additions of certain types of food can make some amazing differences to how you feel and function. Just remember, if you do make any changes to what you are eating, give your body a day or two to adjust to the changes before making any decisions about whether it's working or not.

So at this point in time and unless we can discover, or come up with anything plant based that suits our lifestyle and exercise regimes, we'll continue to be 'flexitarian', which means we'll lean towards the plant based way of eating but still eat meat and fish from time to time and in small amounts.

Chapter 11:
Danger Foods and Situations

In this chapter we'll be discussing 'danger foods' and 'dangerous situations'.

I've already mentioned some dangerous situations, these being eating out and eating with friends.

I've also glossed over some of our 'danger foods' in previous chapters, but in this chapter I'm going to explain, or attempt to explain, some definite NOs for us in terms of both food and certain situations.

Firstly, food. Our main danger food is carbohydrates. When I speak of carbohydrates, this includes sugar, bread, potatoes, pasta, rice, most fruit and some other vegetables that are carb and sugar loaded.

I know I've mentioned this before, but your body does not need carbohydrates to function. There are NO essential carbohydrates that your body needs. It will happily burn fat, either your own body fat or the fat/oil that you consume, for energy. In fact, in many experts' opinions and ours, your body will function much better without carbs, just burning fat.

As soon as we introduce carbs back into our diets, the scales start to move upwards again and we feel tired and lethargic. Within a few days of leaving them out of our daily food intake, we're back to feeling full of energy and the scales start to move back down again. Some of you will be probably saying, 'Well just don't eat them anymore' and that's exactly what we do. I'm not saying we're not sometimes tempted, because we are, but the more we just say no to them, the easier it becomes to not eat carbs and the healthier we feel. We NEVER crave carbs now. That's biscuits, sweets, bread or anything else that's carb loaded.

Other danger foods for us are most dairy products. We don't drink milk now, ever. We do have a small amount of full fat Greek yogurt and occasionally some crème fraîche or double cream. We also use some plain old butter, salted or unsalted, both in some of our savoury recipes and our pudding and cake recipes. We do eat some cheese - after all, we do live near the Wensleydale cheese factory. The dairy products we do eat are always full fat and there is a suggestion that the fermented types of dairy products, such as yogurt, kefir and hard cheeses, have much lower levels of lactose (sugar) in them. I think that reflects in the lack of any bad reactions we get from eating them. Blue cheese is our preferred option for cooking as it tastes much better when cooked and also the blue veins in cheese are good for your gut. However, dairy produce does tend to send the scales upwards for both of us, so we limit our consumption of all these products, not eating any for days, sometimes weeks at a time.

If, at this point, you're wondering where we get our calcium from, well we get all ours from the cruciferous vegetables (leafy greens, broccoli, spinach, cauliflower, salad veg and kale) we eat and from nuts, especially almonds.

There are a number of vegetables and fruits that cause us to have bad reactions when we eat them.

These are cucumbers, raw tomatoes, green peppers, although we do seem to be able to tolerate ripe, red peppers better, but only in moderation. Courgettes and squashes are other vegetables we don't eat, along with potatoes.

When we have eaten them over the course of the past two years, they have left us feeling very bloated, feeling slightly sick and experiencing mild flu type symptoms. This is, apparently, down to the 'Lectin' content in them. Many are related to the Deadly Nightshade family, which of course, is poisonous.

Therefore, we simply don't eat them anymore.

We concentrate on cruciferous vegetables such as leafy greens, cabbage, broccoli, sprouts etc., plus mushrooms, onions, loads of ginger, garlic and salad vegetables such as lettuce, radishes and celery.

Other 'danger foods' for us are beans and legumes. These also contain the protein Lectin, which appears hell-bent on destroying your good gut bacteria. The Lectins can be reduced by pressure-cooking, which is how beans and legumes are cooked when in canned form, but they really don't agree with us. Butter beans and red lentils are about the best for us out of them all. However red kidney beans and chickpeas are the worst and they give us both those mild flu symptoms I've already talked about.

We also don't have any problems with tinned tomatoes and we use these in curries and casseroles etc. It's probably because these are also pressure cooked in the canning process. We actually haven't tried cooking our own fresh tomatoes, yet!

I've mentioned Stevia and sweeteners already, but another quick word about it anyway. Really, the jury is still out and hasn't reached a definite decision about either Stevia or sweeteners.

We only use Grape Tree Triple Zero Organic Stevia, which does contain some Erythritol, which is a chemical and sugar alcohol. In our opinion, it has the least after taste of the many sweeteners in the market place today. It does not contain any calories or carbs and is therefore, not supposed to cause any weight gain. However, in our opinion, if you eat too much, your body can be tricked into thinking you're eating sugar and you may gain weight. Use it sparingly!

Dangerous 'food' situations will greatly differ from person to person. What one person perceives as a dangerous situation will be completely different to another. Eating out, either at a restaurant, friend's house, a celebration or special occasion, are the main dangers for us. I've already covered these in a previous chapter, however, there will be other situations you'll find yourself in, from time to time.

These could be when out shopping and the Deli counter has tasty treats to 'Try before you buy', or the butcher's counter has sausages or pie of the week, beautifully cooked and waiting to be sampled! Free! The supermarket or store may be running a promotion of one type of food or another from a different country. Even local farmers or food producers may have beautiful displays of tempting goodies to try.

It's so easy to just walk past, dip in and have a taste. Then to go back for a second, third and even fourth taste, readily encouraged by the young assistant behind the counter shouting, 'Please help yourself!' Sound familiar to you? I've already mentioned The Wensleydale cheese factory!

It's also very hard not to cave in and be tempted when you've had a long, hard day and the takeaway round the corner is advertising two meals for the price of one and even a free bottle of some sugary drink to wash it all down with. This includes a well-known high street store offering a bottle of wine to accompany a 'ready meal' for two. It sounds like an ideal remedy once the kids are tucked away in bed and there's also a bottle of something cold in the fridge.

All sound familiar!! It can be definitely scary and very hard to resist.

Fortunately, it does get easier. The more you commit to a regime or lifestyle and you see and feel the results for yourselves, the easier it becomes. Honestly!

We're still tempted sometimes, but we only sample the food we would eat every day. No cakes, pastries, sausage, pies or anything on our NO list.

We don't want to ever feel like we used to feel before we started our programme. Ever again. So that's why now we just walk on by.

Chapter 12:
Our 'CHEAT' Foods

The title of this chapter is slightly misleading, because we don't, or very, very rarely, cheat any more now. People have accused us of being far too disciplined; to the extent of being paranoid about not cheating and about the food we eat. We're constantly being told to chill out a little bit and eat some cake or something else we no longer choose to eat nowadays. We'll be the first to admit that we are slightly paranoid about what we eat.

However if you can understand how we feel now and how determined we are to never put that weight back on and be fat again, the term paranoid can be downgraded to just determined and passionate!

We do 'cheat', but we cheat by eating something from 'our' permitted foods. You will see that this is reflected in the recipes we have devised for this book.

We eat cake, puddings and even chocolate. Admittedly we don't gorge ourselves on these 'cheats'. Puddings and cakes are, in the main, reserved for special occasions. We keep having to tell people, and ourselves occasionally, that we are now slim people and intend to stay that way!

All our cheats are generally made from nuts, nut flours and nut butters. They are really delicious, very nutritious and they contain no sugar and only very little organic Stevia.

So there you are. It's a short chapter and hopefully you'll look at and try our recipes and agree with us how yummy they are. As I have already said, they are also very nutritionally dense recipes and not just useless calories that only clap on the pounds.

Chapter 13:
Treat Foods

Treat foods for us nowadays are where we just eat a little more of the foods we already eat! If we're really hungry in the afternoons, we may have some cabbage, lettuce or maybe some crudités with homemade nut butter or our homemade chocolate and hazelnut spread, which we call 'Notella'.

We always have a large stock of 85% cocoa solids dark chocolate, usually reserved for our supper with a cup of tea. However there are some beautiful sunny days when our view over Ingleborough just calls for an extra piece of the dark stuff with our afternoon tea.

For Easter, Christmas, parties and other special occasions we will have some homemade, sugar free truffles, chocolate fudge, walnut fat bombs or some flaxseed crackers and some lovely Wensleydale cheese. Although these don't sound particularly like diet or healthy foods, they are all made from our 'Yes' list of foods.

Again, check out the recipes in our first book, 'Losing It' and those in this book. I'm sure there will be plenty to satisfy everyone's tastes. Just remember, though, they are all free from traditional sugar and traditional flour, so although they are meant for treats only, they are allowed. Just don't overdo them!

Chapter 14:
Herbs and Spices

We're finally getting round to talking about food. Well, herbs and spices to be correct. Herbs, spices and recipes using these ingredients is one of our favourite subjects. It appears that many people generally buy herbs and spices for a specific recipe which has caught their eye in a magazine or that they have seen on the internet. Then they have either never made the recipe, or once they have, never used the herbs or spices again. Instead they are just stuffed in the back of a cupboard, to be dragged back out again when another recipe comes along, or when the cupboard is emptied because you're having a new kitchen installed! However, by this time they're probably two or three years past their sell by dates and don't taste of anything except dust.

I became interested in herbs and spices probably forty years ago. I was living in a flat and was just starting out on my culinary journey. Did I make some concoctions back in those days? You bet I did and more than just the odd dish ended up in the bin.

I can remember picking up a free chart after purchasing some dried Schwartz herbs and spices. I had seen a recipe for chicken curry in a magazine which I had seen somewhere and considered myself very exotic and daring back then. In those days, they were the largest producers of dried herbs and spices. The chart gave a list of all their products and outlined which herbs and spices were ideal accompaniments to different meats, fish, vegetables, fruit and desserts. It became my main cooking companion, as I couldn't afford cookery books and the only recipes I possessed were ones I'd made up myself and some that I had sneakily ripped out of woman's magazines in Doctors' and Dentists' waiting rooms and from the canteen at work.

I proudly displayed this chart on the back of a kitchen cupboard door and in no time at all, I had a large collection of different herbs and spices, which I used in everything I cooked. I truly believe that is was this chart and the subsequent herbs and spices I bought, that contributed to my lifelong love of cooking. The curry was a great success, by the way!

I have grown herbs for many years and still grow them today, mainly the easy to grow herbs such as thyme, rosemary, sage, oregano, chives and, with slightly less success, basil. Fresh coriander is also fairly successful. I've done this in our garden and in all sorts of containers, pots and even on the windowsill of our kitchen. I've grown great herb plants from the remains of those pots you buy in supermarkets. These aren't actually supposed to grow once they have all been cut. I replanted them out in the garden instead of just throwing them away, always wanting to make my contribution to recycling!

Even now, in the often very wild and windy conditions we experience where we live, I grow some herbs in an animal feed trough and just top them up a bit every spring/summer. I have a small bay tree in our garden, which I keep well pruned because they can grow pretty large if left to their own devices and use the leaves in curries, casseroles and tomato sauces.

I use an enormous amount of dried herbs as well, and there are some that I believe are nicer than the fresh versions when used correctly and for the right recipes. Herbs like thyme, rosemary and oregano are great to use dried, in long slow cooked casseroles, rubbed onto big joints of meat or sprinkled into vegetables for roasting.

Fresh herbs are great in salads, especially when used as an ingredient, rather than just a seasoning. Basil, thyme, chives and parsley are absolutely delicious used in great big bunches and mixed into salads. Don't be shy when using them, fresh or dried, and experiment with them in everything you eat. Generally, fresh herbs are best added right at the end of cooking and then just cooked through for a matter of a few seconds, but definitely no more than a minute or two. Many garden centres now have areas dedicated to fresh herb plants and quite often there are plants you don't often see in supermarkets. Herbs like borage, dill and fennel are great tasty herbs as well and can be grown in your garden.

Spices are a slightly different kettle of fish. You need to be a little more careful and precise with spices because one particular spice can easily overpower the next one. You need to be able to taste each spice and individual flavour in every bite.

I nearly always buy my spices from a good Asian supermarket. In my experience, staff in these places are usually really helpful and knowledgeable about advising you which different spices are available and which spices accompany different foods. There are literally hundreds of them, all having their own use and many also having great medicinal properties.

Don't buy too much spice at any one time because they do go 'off' and take on a slightly rancid taste if not used up fairly quickly. They only last a couple of months at the most!

When choosing your spices, if there are quite a few packets of the same spice on the display shelves, check the colour of them all. If some are darker shades than some of the others, choose the darker coloured packets, as the lighter ones are usually the ones that have been at the front of the display.

Experiment by mixing spices together to make your own 'curry' powder or 'spice' mix. Also buy some spices in their whole form, such as seeds like cumin, coriander, fennel, cardamom and fenugreek. Other whole forms of spices are cinnamon bark, cloves, star anise, nutmeg and mace (the dried skin of a nutmeg). Whole vanilla pods are also a lovely spice but they are quite expensive and there are some very good vanilla bean pastes available now. Spices like fennel and cumin seeds are lovely in roast veggies and rubbed onto joints of meat. They are also really tasty sprinkled into salads. Fennel, both the seeds and powder, accompanies fish and pork beautifully. Cumin is ideal with lamb, as is cinnamon, whole or powdered. Cinnamon is great with fruit such as Bramley apples and Comice pears. Coriander seeds, powder and fresh leaves, are ideal in carrot soup and other recipes containing carrots. Try a pinch of coriander powder in carrot cake.

Cardamom, again in seed or powder, is delicious with chocolate and lemon recipes. It also adds lovely flavour to chicken and cauliflower rice dishes.

Whole nutmeg, grated into cauliflower mash, mixed with grated cheese and used as a topping on baked dishes, adds a lovely savoury flavour.

Fenugreek is a very aromatic spice which makes your house smell like an Asian restaurant and gives your food that traditional Asian restaurant taste. Be careful with it though, it's quite powerful and can mask the other flavours you're using. Just half to one teaspoon is all you need. Also be careful to wipe up any spills of this spice because it will make your kitchen, if not the whole house, smell of curry for a good while!

Turmeric is a beautiful, subtle and very under-used spice. Admittedly, I've never used fresh turmeric, which looks very much like a piece of fresh ginger. Therefore I'm unable to comment if fresh is better than the dried powder form. I suspect it probably is and now that it's becoming easier to get in the large supermarkets, I'll be giving it a try very soon. It's really good rubbed on the skin of chicken thighs before roasting and on salmon fillets prior to pan-frying. It's also great to rub on meat and fish, prior to barbecuing.

I've recently seen an Indian recipe where it's been used in yogurt and dessert dishes. They have been infusing it in warm milk for centuries and using it as a medicinal drink for many ailments such as stomach upsets, relief from arthritis, heart complaints and high cholesterol It's also been added to that ever-increasing group of 'Superfoods' and has been marketed as the latest miracle food.

There's certainly some evidence that it's an extremely beneficial ingredient to add to food, however, that said, I just love the earthy, slightly floral taste is has! Again, be careful about spills. It does stain worktops and sinks if you don't wash it away immediately. It can make your hands yellow as well if you don't wash them immediately!

We try and buy 'East End' spices whenever we can, as in our opinion, they are probably the best and freshest. They certainly seem to be far superior to supermarkets' own brands.

Finally, fresh ginger and garlic have to be included as two ingredients we use very regularly, almost daily.

Both ginger and garlic have scientific backing as being extremely beneficial to our daily diets, both in terms of giving our gut bacteria a good boost and being good for combating inflammation in our joints and bodies. Fresh, grated, ginger adds a real zing in cakes and desserts, and garlic can be added to just about any main course, either raw or cooked. We rarely have complaints these days that we smell of garlic. I'm not sure if our bodies have just become so accustomed to it because of our very regular use of it over the years, but there aren't many days go by when we don't eat some garlic and ginger.

Garlic is another ingredient that's fairly easy to grow in your garden. Generally, the garlic you buy in shops for culinary purposes won't grow very well, if at all. I believe it's because they're usually hybrid versions and not intended to be grown on. However, garden centres sell bulbs that are grown specifically for planting out and it's as simple as planting one clove in a pot, waiting for it to start shooting and then replanting it out in your garden.

Remember, herbs and spices are the predecessors of many of our present day medicines and medications. They have tremendous benefits to our gut's health and health in general.

So in conclusion, use fresh and dried herbs and spices in abundance when preparing and cooking your food. Many, if not most, of our main course and accompaniment recipes contain herbs and spices.

Experiment with them and find the ones you like the best. Even a jar of just plain old mixed herbs will add great flavour to your food and recipes.

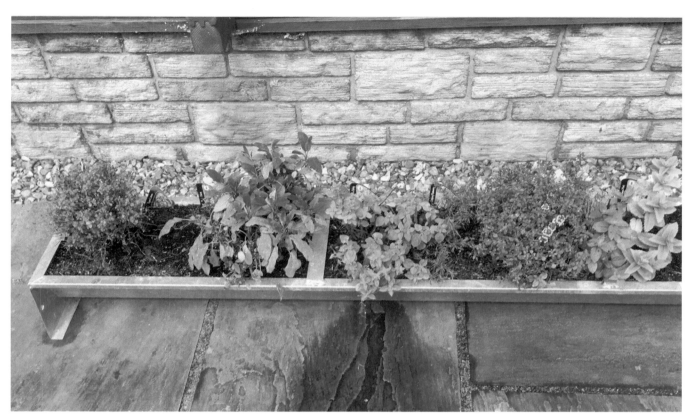

Our herb trough

Chapter 15:
Our Favourite Store Cupboard Ingredients

Our favourite store cupboard ingredients are closely linked with the previous chapter about herbs and spices.

As I write this chapter, I'm listening to the news, which is outlining the current status about Coronavirus and the desperate state we seem to be in. There's talk of fights taking place in supermarkets and shops, as customers clamour to fill their trolleys with pasta, rice, milk, flour and bread.

Well we went shopping ourselves, shamefully thinking that if we don't join them, we are going to be left with none of the food we eat.

Luckily for us and maybe rather selfishly, there was plenty of fresh veg and even frozen cauliflower, broccoli, sprouts and many other vegetables.

There also seemed to be plenty of fresh and frozen meat, fish and local fresh cheeses. However, the pizzas, pies, chips and ready meals shelves and freezers compartments, were completely empty, as were the pasta and rice shelves. Even the chocolate and sweet shelves were running out or in some cases, empty!

However, it was looking as though our store cupboards, fridge and freezers were not going to be running low any time soon.

We found ourselves queuing outside supermarkets in the cold and rain so that people could stock up on 'essential' booze and rubbish food. Instead of stocking up on real food, which was in some cases restricted to limited purchases, it appeared they were concentrating on buying rubbish. Very few people appeared to be buying the fresh produce. I began to think that this virus and the resulting food situation worldwide, might just be the answer to getting back to healthy eating and combating the global obesity problem. This isn't a book about politics or our political views, however there is definitely a link between politics, the massive food producing companies, and obesity.

Enough of our opinions, but unfortunately, I somehow doubt the situation will change any time soon. Here's hoping though. At least some people have seen it all as a wake up call and a good opportunity to change their lives.

These days our store cupboards contain far less than they used to.

Apart from the aforementioned herbs and spices, they tend to contain a lot of olive oil, both the refined type for cooking and extra virgin olive oil for using in dressings for salads and vegetables.

Dressings don't always have to be cold or laden with sugar, maple syrup or honey. I have read the labels on many jars of salad dressings and they read like a scientific formula.

Olive oil, mustard powder, dried herbs, vinegar or lemon juice, salt, pepper and maybe some crushed garlic are all you need for a delicious salad dressing. Tahini, which is sesame seed paste, mixed with garlic, olive oil, lemon juice and water, is great on many meat and fish dishes. Also try many of the different types of vinegars available nowadays. Just make sure there's no sugar in them.

Extra virgin olive oil can also be used to make warm dressings to smother over plain steamed veggies. Just warm the oil in a pan on a very low heat so the oil doesn't burn or overheat, add some crushed garlic, dried herbs, salt, pepper and it literally transforms plain old steamed vegetables into a delicious main course that you could just eat on their own.

We use coconut oil for cooking curries, especially Thai curries and occasionally in some cakes and biscuits.

We also use coconut oil as an after sun cream as it helps to stop us peeling and is very good for sunburn.

If you make a lot of stir-fried dishes, use avocado oil. Avocado oil can withstand high temperatures and doesn't have a strong after-taste, unlike some olive and coconut oils. It also makes delicious mayonnaise if you are proficient at making your own. I have had some great success with it, but unfortunately I have had more instances where it has split than successful attempts. Give it a go though. Just follow a traditional recipe, but use avocado oil.

We always have a stock of tinned tomatoes. As previously mentioned, we don't appear to be affected, 'gut' wise with tinned tomatoes. We use them in many different curries, Bolognese and casserole sauces. Just make sure that they don't contain any added sugar or any ingredients other than tomatoes.

Olives are always on a shelf in our cupboard. We have tried many different olives over the past two years from various parts of the world, both pitted and with their stones left in. Their prices vary greatly and, in our opinion, the more expensive ones were not necessarily the better tasting ones.

On a recent trip to Thassos, a Greek Island just off mainland Greece, we discovered their locally grown olives, which were very black and very crinkled when ripe. These are our absolute favourites. Unfortunately, it seems to be impossible to buy them here in the UK. We're hoping someone will read this and prove us wrong though. They are delicious.

We generally buy pitted green olives from Aldi.

They are cheap and tasty and we consume a lot.

We always have a bottle of 'middle of the road' quality Balsamic vinegar in stock. There is a lot of snobbery about what is the best Balsamic vinegar to use and buy. Again, the more expensive ones don't always seem to be the best. Always pick one that doesn't contain any added sugar and is just made from concentrated grape must. The very cheap vinegars are usually very thin and do not coat salad leaves and vegetables properly like the slightly more expensive versions do. When I say more expensive, don't go spending money on those that are vintage forty year old vinegars, just buy mid value ones, or the more expensive ones if they have been reduced or are on offer.

Use Balsamic vinegar in dressings and when sautéing or roasting veg. The vinegar will reduce and form a lovely sticky coating to the vegetables.

Tinned fish. Tuna, mackerel, salmon and sardines, either packed in olive oil or brine, are always in our food store.

They are great when you're a bit pushed for time and can be added into salads to make a quick tasty meal.

Don't choose the fish that's packed in sunflower oil or tomato sauce, just those in olive oil, water or brine.

Probably our biggest and favourite store cupboard ingredients are, nuts, nut flours, homemade nut butters, hempseed, Triple Zero Organic Stevia and flaxseed.

Try the dessert or treat recipes in this book. None of them contain traditional flours or sugar. Homemade nut butter tastes far superior to mass produced shop bought butters. You aren't able to tell how long some of these nut butters have been made. We just make a kilo at any one time. It certainly doesn't last long in our house!

If you are unfortunate enough to have a nut allergy, there are other flours that you can use, these being cassava, tapioca and tiger nut flour. Keep in mind, though, that these flours are rather high in carbs, so they are best avoided if you are just starting out on your weight loss programme.

We always have a good supply of tea, both fruit infusions and regular tea. We drink a lot of coffee, both instant and pods for use in our Nespresso machine. We do drink a lot of Nespresso and in our opinion it is the best of the lot.

Finally, just a quick word about fridges and freezers. Make sure your fridges and freezers are well stocked up.

Firstly your fridge. Have plenty of salad ingredients in the crisper. A block of Parmesan cheese, some ready made dressing in a bottle or a jar. A tub of Greek style yogurt, crème fraîche or double cream.

A couple of packets of fresh herbs. Some

salted and unsalted butter. Lastly, some fresh meat, chicken or fish for the next few days only. Do not buy and stock too much fresh produce in your fridge. You will only end up having to throw it in the bin when it is out of date or starting to go rotten.

In our freezer we always keep a stock of frozen cauliflower, broccoli, sprouts and spinach. There is always some frozen chicken, meat, fish, usually salmon, which we can either get out the night before for the next day, or we can just defrost in the microwave quickly on the day.

Frozen berries are worth stocking for a quick pudding, should you need some, along with a box or two of homemade sugar free ice cream.

We often make enough curry or casserole for four people and we freeze the rest in reusable plastic containers. They usually taste much better, second time round.

Soup also freezes well, so when you decide to make some, make sure you double the quantity you need and freeze the rest for a later date. Even small amounts of soup can be frozen and then added to casseroles to create richer, thicker sauces.

Use your freezer to its full potential. You will be surprised at what you can freeze. Just keep an eye on when you freeze something, (date marking is a good idea), and make sure you wrap food up properly or put it in sealable containers to avoid freezer burn or liquids leaking out and then sticking things together.

A final word on store cupboard ingredients, although this is about fruit bowls and not cupboards.

Always have a couple of lemons or limes, along with a couple of avocados in your fruit bowl.

We use both lemons and avocados on an almost daily basis. Lemons can be used as an ingredient in salads by peeling them, segmenting them and dicing them to add into salads as an accompaniment to fish. They add a nice touch of acidity to the meal, which is perfect with fish. Use the juice as a condiment to season your food. A good squeeze of lemon in any dish just before serving adds a real zing.

Don't forget the zest as well. It's great in cauliflower fried rice and in many desserts.

There aren't many days that we don't eat an avocado, either chopped up in salads, in our guacamole or just scooped out of its skin as a snack. We love them. It seems that supermarkets are all too ready to reduce them as soon as they feel only slightly soft.

We buy some that are still hard and always have a couple ready to eat straight away.

You are probably thinking that our food stocks are a little excessive for just two people. Well, maybe they are, but we like being prepared in order to avoid making those bad decisions we later regret, such as having to order a last minute takeaway or having to go out for tea because there's nothing in the fridge or cupboards!

Just have a stock of your own favourite food and foods that you are comfortable with cooking and eating. Make life easy and your meals tasty, not just for you and your family, but for visitors, whether they are the planned type or unexpected ones!

Chapter 16:
Essential and Favourite Kitchen Gadgets and Utensils

During the course of writing our first book, 'Losing It' and subsequently this book, a great many experiments have taken place in our kitchen, plus some of the kitchens we have found ourselves in whilst on our travels.

Consequently we've accrued a fair number of gadgets, utensils, pots and pans.

In this chapter I'm going to list some of those that we consider essential and those which are our favourites, along with a brief explanation as to why they are our essentials, favourites or indeed both, because some of them fall into both camps.

So here we go....

A good set of knives that are easily sharpened, plus a good steel or knife sharpener. These are definitely a 'must have' in your kitchen.

Don't be tempted to buy really cheap knives from some budget type stores because they are a waste of money (even if they do only cost £1.00!).

Also don't buy the very best, top end, professional chefs' knives. You don't need that type of quality and often they are only expensive because of endorsement by some well known chef. Unfortunately they're not always that good either.

Lakeland sell their own brand, which are excellent quality, stay sharp for a long time,

are easily sharpened, but most of all, are very reasonably priced. A set of three knives, which will cover just about any job in the kitchen, will cost around £50.00 and will last a lifetime.

A good electric hand mixer for mixing and whisking when baking, an electric hand stick blender for blending soups, making sauces, blending vegetables and so on, are both on our list of essentials.

Whilst on the subject of baking, which is Julie's area of 'expertise', a good selection of mixing bowls, both glass and plastic, that are microwave safe, are essentials. Both are inexpensive and will last for ages. It's a good idea to get plastic ones that have lids, which can double up to use for food storage as well.

Non-stick roasting trays and baking tins, in various shapes and sizes, are something we use on almost a daily basis, so are also essentials. Greaseproof cake tin liners are brilliant as they not only protect your tins, but save you having to grease the tins beforehand.

Invest in a decent set of digital scales, which have both imperial and metric units. Most supermarkets sell them in their homeware sections and they are fairly cheap items.

Have a variety of pans, sauté/frying pans/wok, and an all-purpose casserole/roasting dish that has a lid and can be used both on a hob and in the oven. One that can be used in the microwave as well is even better.

A good wooden spoon, spatula, measuring spoons and a measuring cup/jug, are all items we use everyday and for all sorts of purposes.

One last piece of equipment I feel I should mention is a yogurt maker. We've been using one for some time now and really love the yogurt it produces. The yogurt maker we bought is made and sold by 'Easiyo'. Basically it consists of a one litre pot which you fill with water and a premixed powder of whichever yogurt you prefer. You then mix it together and then place it in a larger container filled with boiling water. This is basically just a large thermos flask. We always have the full fat unsweetened Greek style yogurt. It takes between 8 - 12 hours, depending on the temperature in the room you leave the flask. The end result is a set, very creamy and tasty yogurt. There are many different flavours, both full and low fat versions and they all have the 'live' cultures that are so beneficial to 'gut' good health.

It's really easy to make and does save you money as well.

This is just a brief list of the items we consider essential for use in the kitchen. There will always be something else that you and others will consider to be their own essentials. It's your kitchen and your choice. Buy and use what you think will make life easy and practical but don't spend a fortune on stuff that will end up at the back of a cupboard somewhere in your kitchen, never to be used again.

A word now about our favourite, but not necessarily essential, gadgets and machines! We've experimented with a good quality blender and a 'Magimix ' food processor and we've found that the 'Magimix' is a lot better all round. It's more versatile and far more robust than most blenders.

There are other makes of food processors on the market, however, we have found that 'Magimix' ranks as one of the best. It's very easy to use, fairly easy to clean afterwards and has some attachments included with the very basic model.

Food processors are excellent for making nut butters, making puréed and mashed vegetables, blending soups to a super smooth consistency and chopping and slicing food. We use ours on a very regular basis. Without a blender or food processor, you won't be able to make your own nut butters. Lakeland sell their own brand of both these items at a very reasonable price.

We wanted to make some sugar free ice cream to include in our dessert recipes, however, had limited success without an ice cream maker. We ended up buying a 'Sage' ice cream making machine, which comes complete with a built-in compressor and eliminates the need to pre-freeze your ice cream mixing bowl prior to starting your recipe.

The results have been fabulous. We've tried and tested many different types of frozen desserts, including frozen yogurts and ice cream, some flavoured with fresh fruit, dark chocolate and even nut butter!

Again whilst trying and testing recipes, we discovered a multi-purpose pressure cooker that not only enables you to cook food incredibly quickly and safely (I can still recall some of the nightmare stories associated with older pressure cookers), but it has programmes that allows you to pre-brown food, prior to pressure cooking, long slow cooking and also a reheat function. It's a fabulous piece of equipment and something else we use on a very regular basis, however it cannot really be classed as an essential item of equipment.

The list of kitchen equipment could probably go on forever, everyone having differing opinions and ideas of what is and what isn't, essential or favourite equipment and gadgets. The aforementioned are just a few of our essential and favourite ones.

Some kitchen equipment and gadgets are very expensive and some are just, in our opinion, gimmicks. Don't be tempted by some of these gimmicky ones.

Just buy the things you need and will use on a daily basis, not something you may only use once a year! Don't be tempted by TV chefs or celebrities endorsing their 'own' or other company's gadgets. They get paid very handsomely by the manufacturers and very often they're not the best or even most useful item you will have purchased.

Lakeland, which we frequently use, and John Lewis have very good 'own brands' and are usually very competitively priced. Lakeland, especially, has an excellent 'returns and warranty' policy and will take back anything faulty or found to be unsuitable. The point is, shop around and make good useful purchases and don't waste money on items you won't use long term.

Chapter 17:
'YES' and 'NO' foods

In this book, we again have a 'Yes' and 'No' list of food that we do and don't eat. Both these lists are almost the same as the lists in our first book, 'Losing It'. But there are some additions, some subtractions and some maybes, although all three of these categories will depend on your own tastes and, or, any possible reactions you may, or may not encounter with certain food.

'YES' foods.

Again, apart from protein sources: meat, fish, nuts and dairy which should be weighed, and resistant starches, which are to be eaten in moderation, everything else is unlimited. So continue eating unlimited vegetables and reap their wonderful benefits!

Oils	Olive oil. Extra virgin for salad dressings, drizzling over cooked meats and veggies, and refined olive oil for cooking. Coconut oil - extra virgin. Avocado oil.
	All nut oils (except peanut oil) for use in salad dressings, e.g. walnut, hazelnut and sesame oil. These oils are also good for adding flavour to steamed vegetables, and we use sesame oil as a final dressing in stir-fried dishes.

We use a lot of oil, especially olive oil. Don't use it sparingly.

There's been a fair bit of research into olive oil and its benefits with ailments such as arthritis and conditions in the body that cause inflammation in joints and muscles. As I've said, we do consume a fair amount of olive oil and we tend to have very few aches and pains.

Sweeteners	Stevia. Erythritol. Xylitol. Remember what I've already said about sweeteners! There is a place for them, but be careful with them.
Nuts and seeds	Macadamia nuts, almonds, pecan nuts, walnuts, pistachios, pine nuts, coconut and unsweetened coconut milk and cream, chestnuts, hazelnuts, Brazil nuts, flaxseed, hemp seeds (preferably hulled. Apparently hemp seeds contain all the essential amino acids your body needs, one of the few plant based protein sources that does), sesame seeds.
NOTE:	Peanuts and cashew nuts are not allowed. Peanuts are a legume and don't grow on trees and can have severe reactions in people. Cashew nuts are also not truly nuts, even though they grow on a tree. They actually grow under a flower/bud on a tree and don't have the same sort of kernel as true nuts.
Olives	All olives except those stuffed with peppers or chillies.
Dark chocolate	Needs to be 75% cocoa solids or above. 25 grams per day. (Our favourite is Aldi 85%. It's really smooth and doesn't leave you wanting more. It's also pre-wrapped in individual 25 gram bars!) 95% cocoa solids chocolate tends to be quite bitter. However, grated or very finely chopped and sprinkled on top of Greek yogurt along with some berries, makes a lovely tasty, quick dessert. The bitterness in the dark chocolate seems to disappear when accompanied by other food.

	Cacao and cocoa are very similar, however, both start as cacao and then cocoa is derived from cacao by heating it at high temperatures, thus depleting the cacao of its nutrients. Cacao nibs have an intense bitter, dark chocolate flavour and are not to everyone's taste. They are however, low carb and have good nutritional properties. We add a few to desserts with cream or yoghurt for that added texture.
Vinegar	All vinegars including Balsamic, but read the labels to make sure there are no added sugars in any of them, especially the Balsamic and fruit vinegars.
Herbs and seasonings	All herbs and seasonings, including curry powders. Check pre-mixed curry powders as some contain rice and corn flour, as well as some other ingredients like ground lentil. We tend to buy 'East End' spices, which we find to be very good quality and taste very authentic.
Flours	Coconut flour and almond flour are the only flours we use. Cassava, tapioca and tiger nut flours are OK to use but we found they are not the easiest flours to bake with and we also think they have a strange taste. They are quite high in carbs so we've left them alone completely. Ground almonds and almond flour are our mainstays, with coconut flour being a close second. Ground almonds are a lot finer than almond flour, but either can be used to replace regular flour. (See our pie and dessert recipes using almond flour or ground almonds.)

Ice cream	There are some commercial brands of ice cream around that claim to be sugar free and dairy free, but in the main we found that they do contain sugar and/or sweeteners, gums and many other additives. There are some ice cream recipes in our first book that are very tasty and contain only Triple Zero Stevia, berries or other natural ingredients. Frozen yogurt is also very nice and can be flavoured with berries, some stevia and 85% cocoa dark chocolate chips.
Dairy products	We eat very little dairy produce these days. We usually limit our consumption of the dairy products listed below to special occasions and dinner parties. This is because, apart from the coconut based yogurts, most dairy produce does contain a fair amount of sugar in the form of lactose. Full fat double cream, crème fraîche and hard cheese all contain far less sugar than the other low fat versions. It's well worth keeping an eye on your dairy consumption though. 25 grams of cheese per day, preferably goats or sheep's cheese. Blue cheese is a better choice as the blue veining is good for your gut bacteria. Feta cheese. We use Aldi as it's good quality and made from sheep and goats milk. Butter. Yogurt. Goat or sheep's is best. Also there's a brand called CoYo which is made from coconut milk. It's quite expensive but very tasty. Full fat Greek yogurt. We make our own Easiyo Greek style set yogurt. Double cream. Full fat crème fraîche. Sour cream. Mascarpone cheese. Cream cheese.

Dairy continued	Parmesan cheese (a small amount grated goes a long way).
	Natural unsweetened kefir. Check the labels for added ingredients and sugars.
Wines and spirits	As previously stated, we're teetotal now. It's somewhat difficult therefore to advise people what to drink and what not to drink. Having said that, we would probably concentrate on small amounts of red wine or white spirits, mainly because of the lesser amount of sugar in these drinks. You need to bear in mind though, if your weight is beginning to creep up again, it could be down to your alcohol consumption slowly adding up, even by just one or two extra glasses a week. However, all alcohol, no matter how enjoyable you find it, is just empty, useless calories and in our opinion, better to leave alone until you've reached your desired weight goal!
Fruit	Avocado. Try and eat at least half of one everyday.
	All berries that are in season e.g. strawberries, raspberries, blueberries and blackberries.
	We grow our own rhubarb and have eaten that in season with a small amount of stevia and were surprised to find it not as sour as we remembered it was; a good sign that our sweet tooth has diminished greatly.
	Fresh lemons/limes, peeled and segmented, are also good for adding to all fish dishes and salads as a seasoning and extra flavour. Don't forget the zest of both of them as well. They're great additions to sautéed vegetables
	Ruby grapefruit is a new addition to this list. We add them, segmented and chopped, to salads. They add a real zing.
	We have started eating a small amount of 'in season' Bramley apples and Comice pears, in some of our dessert recipes.

Fruit continued	We're hopefully going to be experimenting with English eating apples, locally grown, but only when they're in season in the autumn. Fruit contains a lot of natural sugar called fructose and there's increasing evidence suggesting that fructose is actually one of the worst sugars you can consume! Most fruit also has a high carb content, so we avoid it or limit how much we eat as it tends to put our weight back on.
Vegetables	Cruciferous vegetables - These include broccoli, Brussels sprouts, cauliflower, all cabbage, kale, Bok Choy, Swiss chard. Chinese leaves. Spinach - We use it fresh in salads and the type that's frozen into small balls. With the small frozen portions it's really easy to use, because you can get out just the right amount you need for adding in curries or casseroles. Or defrost it in the microwave, squeeze out any excess water and use it to have with eggs in one form or another for breakfast or frittatas etc. Asparagus Garlic. Fresh ginger. Onions, red and white, including spring onions. Leeks Shallots All types of salad leaves, rocket, romaine, iceberg etc. Watercress. Radishes, including Asian radish. Fennel. Carrots. Mushrooms. Raw beetroot, grated on salads. We do use pickled beetroot but check it doesn't have any sugar in the pickling liquor.

Vegetables continued	Sauerkraut
	Chicory.
	Okra, or ladies fingers.
	Artichokes, both global and Jerusalem.
	All fresh herbs.
	Celery.
	Swedes (makes great chips).
	Tinned tomatoes.
	(Like us, you may now find you cannot tolerate fresh tomatoes. However, we are fine with tinned tomatoes and use them in curries and casseroles. A sign that you are intolerant to tomatoes or any other foods is that you feel very bloated, a little bit sick and either suffer constipation or diarrhoea. You may also experience slight flu symptoms, such as aches and hot or cold sweats. If you have any of these symptoms, omit the foods you think may be causing them. Check your diary and this food list.)
	Red peppers, cooked or raw.
	(Peppers are a new addition, which we tend to only eat whilst on holiday in Mediterranean countries. They don't seem to give us any adverse reactions when we eat them in the countries they are grown in, unlike the ones we buy and have eaten in the UK, despite being usually imported from abroad.)
	Dried red chillies, in moderation, and if you have no adverse reactions to them.
	Sauerkraut, read the label, make sure it is unpasteurised, and check for any added sugar content. (We make our own. It's really easy to make and you can experiment by adding your own secret flavourings. See our recipe under 'Sides Dishes and Accompaniments' in this book.)

Resistant Starches	In moderation only - maybe once or twice a week. We eat virtually no starchy vegetables these days, and only very occasionally eat those listed below
	Sweet potatoes.
	Parsnips.
	Celeriac (It makes great chips, fabulous soup but in our opinion is a borderline 'starchy' carbohydrate, falling between low and medium carbs.)

Protein

The following is a list of protein foods. Although it states 100 grams twice a day, it's perfectly OK to eat 200 grams in one meal, providing you haven't eaten any at your previous meals or any meals thereafter. So, for example, if you have a big salad at lunchtime and no protein at all, then you can eat your full daily allowance at your evening meal.

The only contradiction to this rule is, if you are doing a lot of exercise, four days or more a week, then protein amounts can be increased to 150 grams per meal. These weights refer to the weight of the cooked meat or fish, not raw and not the amount of protein found in that food. 100 grams of meat or chicken will provide approximately 25 - 30 grams of protein. The same amount of fish will provide approximately 20 - 25 grams of protein.

Nuts provide about half as much protein per the same 100 grams.

Poultry	100 grams twice a day. Chicken. Turkey. Duck. Goose. All game birds. Eggs (no more than 2 or 3 per day).
Meat	100 grams twice a day. Beef. (We don't seem to tolerate beef very well. We often feel bloated and have constipation the following day. Because of this, we only eat beef very occasionally.) Lamb. Pork. (Including a very small amount of bacon and we occasionally use some lardons in some of our tagliatelle dishes and occasionally some good quality rashers when we have our 'weekend breakfast/brunch'.) All game. No shop bought sausages or burgers unless you're absolutely sure what's in them. They shouldn't contain cereal or fillers of any kind. It's best to make your own from freshly minced meat, chicken or turkey. We don't skin our chicken, except in curries. We eat it. We also don't over-trim the fat from our meat. Fat is flavour. This isn't a low fat diet.

Fish	100 grams twice a day of any fresh fish or canned fish. Canned has to be in olive oil, brine or water. No tomato sauces or other types of oils. Canned tuna, salmon, sardines and mackerel are great because, generally, they come in just the right portion sizes for one person, give or take a gram, which certainly makes preparation easy! All shell fish, cooked or raw, but again, not in any sauces.
NOTE:	Over the past two years we have vastly reduced our consumption of animal based protein and eat many completely plant based meals. We have days where we don't eat any meat at all and we really enjoy these meals. In our opinion, we are reaping the benefits of doing so. We haven't noticed any deterioration in our training, whatsoever. In fact we both feel that it's vastly improved. However, as I've already stated, we do still eat meat and fish and will continue to do so, albeit in considerably less amounts than we used to.
Plant Based Protein	Some Quorn products. Check the labels because some contain sugar and a lot of preservatives and additives. Hemp seed tofu, if you can find it in shops. There are recipes on the internet for how to make it yourself. Hemp seed protein powder. Some veggie burgers. (Again check the labels for cereal and sugars).
	We've included a chapter about vegetarians and vegans and therefore can't really add a great deal more here. Experiment with beans and pulses etc., and find what suits you best.

'NO' FOODS

These are all the foods that you need to continue avoiding or eliminating from your diet. It's still more or less the same list as the one in our book 'Losing It', so some of those 'No' foods are still quite controversial. They are, however, foods that have a high content of lectins, are highly processed, have high carbs or have a high sugar content.

Refined starchy foods

We still haven't eaten any of these foods for well over two years. And probably never will. Ever!

Pasta, wholemeal, brown and white.

Rice of any kind, brown or white.

Potatoes and potato products like crisps.

All bread and bread products, including naan and other Asian type breads.

Pastries and all products using pastry made using traditional flours.

Any flours made from grains. This includes spelt and corn flour.

Quinoa, couscous, bulgur wheat and pearl barley.

Biscuits, crackers (except our flaxseed crackers). Ryvita etc.

Breakfast cereals. This includes porridge oats, muesli, granola, breakfast bars, biscuits and in other so - called 'healthy' foods.

All sugars, including most sweeteners. (Some Stevia is allowed, but you will have to judge for yourselves if it agrees with you).

All diet drinks, sodas and drinks claiming to have 'no added sugar' (juice concentrates).

Vegetables	Tomatoes, cucumbers, peas, sugar snap peas, mange tout, green beans, broad beans, chickpeas, soy and soy products like tofu and textured vegetable protein products. All beans and lentils. (Vegetarians will need to use lentils and beans for their sources of protein and will need to experiment with which works best for them. You may find that you are intolerant to some of them, especially if they leave you bloated, windy and feeling slightly 'off' after eating them). Aubergine, peppers of any colour (see 'Yes' foods regarding red peppers), courgettes, all squashes like butternut squash and fresh chillies (we do now use some dried red chillies).
Nuts and seeds	Pumpkin seeds, sunflower seeds, chia, peanuts and cashew nuts.
Fruit	All fruit except 'in season', berries. (Sparingly during your first six weeks. However, in our case, it wasn't until we achieved our goal weight. We continue to use fruit sparingly and when we do, it's always fruit that is in season, or fruit that was picked whilst in season and immediately frozen.) This includes melons, bananas, oranges, peaches, nectarines, grapefruit (we now eat some ruby grapefruit in salads), pears and apples. Again, if you're in your first six weeks of new eating, it's best to avoid all fruit. After that you can experiment by slowly adding in some fruit, but only a little at a time. Fruit is essentially sugar in a different guise! Some people find that when they start adding it back into their diets, the weight starts going back on. We have started eating some 'in season' Bramley apples and Comice pears, but only very occasionally.

Dairy products	All milk. (Unsweetened almond, hemp seed and coconut milk are allowed if you simply can't do without milk, however, we prefer to just not bother anymore.) All flavoured yogurts, including so-called low fat and those including grains and fruits. Keep to 25 grams of cheese, however, if you feel you can't stick to that small amount, you are probably best avoiding it completely, at least until you've lost your weight or feel more in control of your eating. Cottage cheese. Any sort of protein powders used, either for supplementation, or meal replacements. (The exemption here is hemp seed protein powder, which can be added to smoothies if you like smoothies and you are vegetarian or vegan.)
Oils	Rapeseed oil. Peanut oil (groundnut). Corn, sunflower or supermarket 'vegetable' oil (usually rapeseed). Margarine and all other so called 'healthy spreads', including the 'olive oil' and spreadable type spreads.
Meat	All processed meat products These are items such as sausage, chorizo, salami and all shop bought, pre-cooked meats, such as boiled ham, corned beef etc. All the sort of items you would probably buy for your normal packed lunches. Instead use your own cold cuts left over from roasts from the night before. One of our favourites for pack up is lightly toasted mixed nuts, left to cool, and then mixed in with salad. Either avoid bacon completely, or, restrict it as much as possible. We do use some lardons in our cabbage tagliatelle recipes, but only a small amount. Bacon contains a lot of nitrates and preservatives, which are not good for you and your 'gut'.

I recently went on a butchering course and part of this course involved us making our own bacon using a dry cured 'natural' method.

The ingredients were a piece of belly pork that was placed in an air tight container or plastic bag. A mixture of salt and saltpetre was added to the belly pork which we then took home and placed in the fridge for a week. The pork was turned and mixed in the curing mixture daily in order to cure the pork.

By the end of the week, the pork had taken on that pink colour that bacon tends to have and there was quite a lot of strange looking liquid in the bottom of the bag.

The meat is then washed and then hung to dry for a few days. That's your bacon!

The interesting fact here though is, 'saltpetre' has to be bought via a special permit because of its use in explosives etc. The ratio of salt and saltpetre has to be measured very carefully because saltpetre is actually dangerous to consume!

Most supermarket bacon, apparently, contains many more adverse ingredients than just the two I have outlined.

Anyway, it's your choice. Certainly food for thought though. A mushroom omelette for breakfast begins to sound very much more attractive I think!

As you will see, there still isn't a lot of fruit in there. Or starchy carbs. Or the cereals we have been told are 'healthy' for us. They are essentially all sugars, or at least they are after they have been through your digestive system. It's fuel that your body will want to use as energy/fuel, instead of fat, and the fat will be stored in your body if it isn't burnt up.

The general idea is that you get your body to start burning your fat and the fat/oil you eat for fuel, not carbohydrates and sugar.

Get your body burning its fat and you won't have the same cravings as it does when burning carbs. In fact you will start to crave food like salads and green vegetables etc.

There is also very little dairy. That's because of the lactose it contains, also a form of sugar. A large proportion of the world's population has difficulty digesting lactose because of having lactose intolerance. You may be surprised to find that you might be one of those and not realised it.

Don't worry about not getting your calcium. It's also found in almonds, kale, spinach and other cruciferous vegetables.

That's it. The foods we eat and the foods we don't eat. They are very much the same as in our last book, with only very slight variations.

Chapter 18:
Using up Odds, Ends and Leftovers

There is an enormous amount of media coverage at present, outlining the amount of food that we are all wasting. All over the world. Every day and by everyone!!

Please do not become one of those people and one of those dreadful statistics!

Buy, prepare and eat your food mindfully. Avoid buying some of those so called 'bargains' that many supermarkets advertise, but then you end up throwing away after a few days because you haven't had chance to use it and it's now gone rotten. You are just lining their pockets at the end of the day.

Just buy enough for you and your family for just two or three days. I realise that this can be difficult because of work and family commitments. However think of the money you'll save by just buying sufficient, and not having to throw the contents of your fridge in the bin at the end of the week when everything is past its sell by date and beginning to go rotten. Sound familiar?

Many people feel intimidated and are immediately put off eating healthily or by going on a new, healthy eating programme because of the idea that, in order to live that way, it will take up loads of time, involve vast amounts of shopping and pre-planning in order for you to succeed.

Well that's rubbish. You don't need to spend all day in the kitchen cooking and preparing meals for the next week or so and then spend the rest of your time at the supermarket buying all the ingredients.

Most summers we spend six weeks in Europe on a motorbike, travelling from place to place and the only pre-planning we do is to decide on the route we'll take the next day and what hotel we'll be stopping in.

In terms of food, we will more than likely have a bag of nuts in one of our panniers should we be unable to buy anything during the day whilst travelling to our next destination.

I know there's only the two of us to think about, but the point I'm trying to make is, don't let the idea of having to buy, cook and prepare food bog you down too much. Make it easy for yourself, in whatever way you can.

We often make enough food, especially meals like curries, casseroles, pies and roast vegetable dishes, for at least six people. We then either have the rest for lunch the next day or freeze it for another time, usually for when we're a bit pressed for time and a quick, easy tea is called for. It's just as easy to take your leftovers to work and even pack the kids' lunchboxes with some of your tasty leftovers.

Any leftover meat or chicken is great for adding to salads or shredding up into frittatas. We often make a 'Ploughman's type lunch' using cold meat or chicken with veggie crudités, liberally sprinkled with extra virgin olive oil, salt, pepper and some mixed dried herbs. If there are vegetables left over from the previous night, either roast or steamed, use these instead of crudités. You can substitute the meat or chicken with a small amount of local cheese, goat's cheese, grilled Halloumi, nuts or a spoonful of nut butter. These are just some of our favourites.

Providing you don't add salt, pepper, oil, or any other wet ingredients, you can make a big bowl of salad and whatever you don't eat straightaway can then be eaten for your next meal, or even the next day. Just place it in an airtight box and keep it in the fridge until required. When you're ready to eat it, just add an avocado, some salt, pepper, olive oil and then have it with whatever you've got planned for that meal. It saves loads of time and is just as delicious.

It takes no time at all to pack up a big salad for lunch the next day. You can even just take a pre-prepared mixed bag of salad to work and throw some nuts in the same bag and that way, you don't even have think about pack up boxes and any washing up. There's a tendency to buy large amounts of salad, not use much or even any of it and then throw the rest away.

Don't forget, the word 'salad' just means a collection of cooked or raw ingredients, although in my opinion, the ingredients should be cold when combined together in a salad. Use your imagination and experiment by putting your own favourite leftovers together to form really tasty dishes. Cold roast veg mixed in salads is really lovely. They add a nice caramel taste to what can be a bland tasting salad. If you've got some onions that appear to be going past their best, peel off any layers that look like they're not very nice, fry them in olive oil until slightly crisp and then allow to cool thoroughly. Stir them into a big salad and they give the salad a nice sweet, savoury taste.

We have actually served our 'leftovers' salad as a starter or side dish at quite a few dinner parties, or taken such a salad to barbecues or other peoples' dinner parties. Nobody realised they were eating leftovers (they know now though!) and they've thoroughly enjoyed it.

Leftover meat and chicken are great ingredients for making a quick curry. Make your own curry sauce and then throw in cold, leftover meat or chicken, providing you with your own midweek 'takeaway'. It works equally well using Chinese spices and flavourings.

I've recently read a lot about bone broths and how they're supposed to be really good for your gut's good bacteria. We've therefore compiled a few recipes that we call broths, but are actually just stews or casseroles that have no thickening agent in them. At first we thought they were going to be pretty tasteless. How wrong we were. They are in fact delicious, easy to prepare and cook, plus you can use up all sorts of leftovers - vegetables, meat (preferably with the bone left in for extra flavour and goodness) and chicken carcasses that have been picked over after Sunday lunches.

We've found that chicken and fish broths are the best because they cook really quickly, especially fish, and they're very filling as well.

Leftover chicken, meat and veggies are excellent ingredients that we use up in our pies, using low carb, zero sugar, gluten and traditional flour free pastry.

The main point is, don't waste your food. Don't be afraid to experiment with food using different herbs, spices, seasonings and flavourings.

Just make sure that any leftovers are left to go properly cold before freezing them or keeping them in the fridge. Cold meat will keep in the fridge for about four days in airtight boxes and vegetables a little longer.

Chapter 19:
RECIPES
That Help Us Maintain
Our New Lifestyle

Oven conversions

Gas	Fahrenheit	Celsius	Fan
1	275	140	120
2	300	150	130
3	325	170	150
4	350	180	160
5	375	190	170
6	400	200	180
7	425	220	200
8	450	230	210
9	475	240	220

BREAKFASTS

Granola

Serves 12

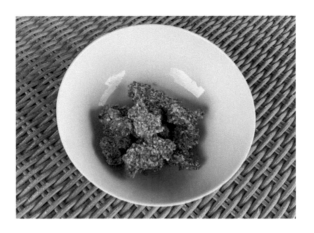

INGREDIENTS

120 grams unsweetened desiccated coconut or to taste
100 grams almond pieces, plus 100 grams of other crushed nuts of your choice,
eg walnuts, pecans etc
65 grams hemp seeds
65 grams sesame seeds
40 grams flaxseeds
20 grams stevia or sweetener of your choice (optional), or to taste
80 grams of home made nut butter
1 tablespoon cinnamon
80 ml water

METHOD

Preheat oven 150° / Fan 130° / 300° / Gas 2.
Pulse nuts and seeds in a food processor until you have larger and smaller pieces.
Place all ingredients into a bowl and mix until all combined.

Spread mixture evenly onto a prepared lined baking sheet and press down firmly with your hands or a spatula.

Bake for 25 - 30 minutes or until it is evenly browned, turn tray halfway through baking.

Tip: If the outside edges of the mixture brown quicker than the centre, you can always break the mixture up into large pieces and rotate them a bit so the centre becomes crunchy.

Leave to cool at room temperature on the baking tray, then break up the mixture into smaller pieces/clusters.

Note

Any nuts or seeds you like can be used from your storeroom cupboard, however they must not be salted/sugared.

Flaxseeds are very important as they absorb the water and help the mixture to form the pieces/clusters.

This recipe makes 12 portions, approximately 50 grams per portion.

Bacon, Eggs, Field (Portobello) Mushrooms

Serves 2

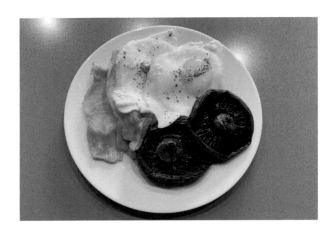

INGREDIENTS
4 x large field (Portobello) mushrooms
4 x large eggs
4 - 6 rashes of good bacon
4 tablespoons refined olive oil
Salt and pepper to taste

OPTIONAL
½ bag washed baby spinach
Knob of butter

METHOD
Preheat the grill to hot.
Place the mushrooms underside (gill side) facing upwards, onto the grill pan, drizzle the mushrooms with half the olive oil and season with salt and pepper.

<u>Either</u> fry the bacon in a frying pan, on a medium heat, until it is cooked as you like it or place the bacon on the other side of the grill pan, then grill both the mushrooms and bacon together turning to ensure they are cooked on both sides. The mushrooms may take a little longer.

Next, heat the remaining oil in another frying pan, on a medium heat, when the oil is hot, crack in the eggs and cook to your liking.

At the same time, if using the spinach as well, take a small pan with a lid, place on a medium heat, add the knob of butter and immediately add in the spinach. Lower the heat, cover the pan with its lid, wilt down the spinach, which will take approximately 45 - 60 seconds. Remove from the heat and remove the lid.

When everything is cooked, divide between two plates and serve.

Eat immediately and enjoy.

Special Weekend Breakfast Treat

Serves 1

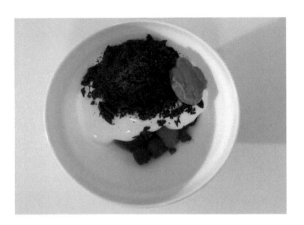

INGREDIENTS

2 rounded dessertspoons full fat Greek yogurt

1 rounded teaspoon homemade nut butter

6 fresh raspberries

15 grams 85% cocoa dark chocolate, grated or thinly sliced

20 grams mixed toasted nuts (optional)

Note

If you cannot get fresh raspberries, you can use frozen ones, <u>but</u> remember to get them out of the freezer a couple of hours before you need them, so they have defrosted properly.

METHOD

In a bowl, place in the Greek yogurt, then the raspberries, next the homemade nut butter, top it off with mixed toasted nuts (if using), plus the prepared chocolate.

Last Night's Leftovers Frittata

Serves 2

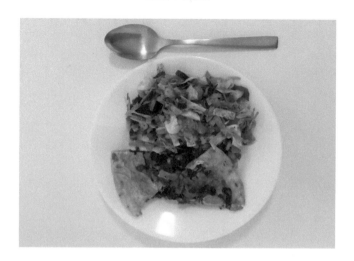

INGREDIENTS

4 - 6 large eggs

1 teaspoon of dried herbs of your choice (we think oregano is best)

1 tablespoon of refined olive oil <u>or</u> a knob of butter

2 tablespoons water or cream <u>or</u> milk (your choice)

Any leftover vegetables from last night's tea, e.g. roast <u>or</u> steamed vegetables, <u>and/or</u>

Any leftover meats from last night's tea, e.g. chicken, pork, lamb, beef cut into small (approximately 2cm) cubes

Salt and pepper to taste

METHOD

Preheat the grill to hot.

In a bowl whisk together the eggs, water <u>or</u> cream <u>or</u> milk, herbs of your choice, salt and pepper.

In a 28/30 cm frying pan add the knob of butter <u>or</u> olive oil over a medium heat. When butter <u>or</u> oil is hot add vegetables and/or meat and quickly just warm them through.

Make sure the vegetables don't burn, and do not stir them too much or they will turn into a mush.

Add the whisked egg mixture to the pan. Once it begins to set like an omelette, start to lift the edges of the egg mixture and tip the frying pan to allow the runny egg mixture in the middle of the frying pan to leak out to the sides.

<u>Don't stir the mixture or you will end up with scrambled eggs!</u>

When there is only just a little bit of runny egg left on the top of your pan, stick the pan under your preheated hot grill.

Continue to grill the frittata until the egg has completely set, turned golden brown and begins to soufflé up a bit.

Take the frying pan from under the grill, allow it to cool slightly before cutting into wedges, like pizza slices and serve.

This can be eaten for breakfast or left to go completely cold and taken to work for pack up.

It is delicious served cold.

Scrambled Eggs and Spinach
Serves 1

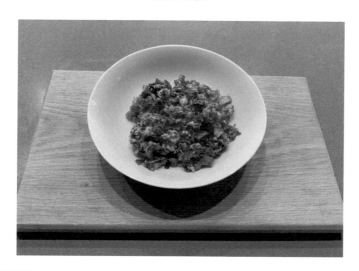

INGREDIENTS
   2 - 3 large eggs
   1 tablespoon water <u>or</u> cream <u>or</u> milk (your choice)
   Salt and pepper to taste
   A good handful of fresh washed baby spinach
   Knob of butter

METHOD
In a bowl, whisk together the eggs, salt, pepper, and water <u>or</u> milk <u>or</u> cream.
Heat the butter in a frying pan over a low heat.
When the butter melts and starts to foam, add the spinach and stir it around the pan until it wilts down.
Once the spinach has wilted add the whisked eggs to the frying pan and whisk in the pan continually, not allowing the eggs to set into an omelette.
<u>Don't</u> over cook the eggs.
They should still be slightly runny when you turn the heat off.

Serve on a plate with a little more baby spinach uncooked and drizzle with olive oil, salt and pepper.

VARIATION
This can be done with poached eggs if preferred.
Just poach the eggs in a poaching pan and wilt spinach in a separate frying pan with some butter.
Serve together sprinkled with salt and pepper.

REMEMBER
To serve 2 persons just double the quantities above.

Breakfast Raspberry Muffins
Makes 4 large muffins

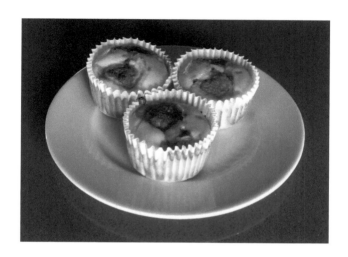

INGREDIENTS
100 grams almond flour
10 - 20 grams stevia, or sweetener of your choice to taste
65 ml milk of your choice
1 large egg
¼ teaspoon salt
10 - 12 fresh raspberries, depending on their size

OPTIONAL
Pinch of cinnamon or ½ tablespoon vanilla bean paste <u>or</u> vanilla extract to taste

METHOD
Preheat oven 180° / Fan 160° / 350° / Gas 4.
Line the muffin tin ready with muffin cases.
In a medium size bowl, mix all the dry ingredients until well combined.

Add the remaining ingredients <u>except</u> the raspberries and combine them well. Using a large spoon half fill the prepared muffin cases, then pop in a couple of raspberries depending on the size of the raspberries. Continue to fill the muffin cases with the remaining muffin mixture, try to fill them all to the same level.

I like to put a couple of raspberries on top of my muffins.

Place the muffins into the preheated oven on the middle shelf and bake for 18 - 20 minutes until cooked and the tops are turning slightly golden.

Remove from the oven, let them cool for a good 10 minutes so they firm up.

Serve with Greek yogurt, or a few more raspberries, or just on their own.

In our house they don't last long, but if you do have any leftovers they can be stored in an airtight container for later, or will freeze for up to a month.

Tips: If you are having young children visiting, this exact recipe will make 14 -16 mini muffins, <u>however</u> you only need to bake them for 12 -13 minutes, until cooked and slightly golden.

For teenagers, use the exactly the same recipe but use a bun tray, making 8 - 10 muffins, <u>however</u> only bake them for 15 - 17 minutes, until cooked and slightly golden.

In my experience young children and teenagers love these, especially when served with my homemade sugar free vanilla ice cream, and topped with a teaspoon of Martin's 'Notella' Chocolate and Hazelnut spread, (these recipes can be found in the Weekly Essentials recipe section of this book).

LUNCHES

Chicken Broth

Serves 2

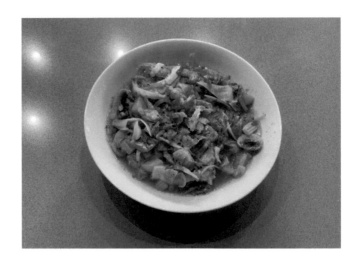

INGREDIENTS

4 chicken thighs, skinned, but leave the bone in
1 large carrot, diced small
1 medium onion, thinly sliced
1 stick celery, thinly sliced
6 - 8 mushrooms, thinly sliced
1 medium cauliflower, cut into florets including stalks
1 - 2 cloves of garlic, peeled, crushed, finely chopped
A couple of handfuls of kale, remove tough centre stems, chop finely
2 tablespoons refined olive oil
1 teaspoon dried thyme
1 teaspoon dried oregano
1 teaspoon dried rosemary
1½ litres of water
Salt and pepper to taste

METHOD

Prepare all the ingredients as above.

Heat the oil in a large pan on a medium heat, when oil is hot, add in the carrot, onion and celery, fry until they are soft but not browned.

Add in mushrooms, and garlic, continue to fry for a couple more minutes.

Next add in all the water, chicken, plus herbs of your choice and bring everything to the boil.

Once it is boiling cover the pan with a lid, turn to a low heat and simmer for 35 minutes. Add in the cauliflower and simmer, still covered, for a further 10 minutes.

Serve in big soup/pasta bowls.

Serve 2 pieces of chicken per person.

Note

If serving more than 2 people simply add more thighs to this recipe. All the rest of the ingredients stay the same.

REMEMBER

Drink all the broth - it is good for your gut and it fills you up too!

Celeriac Soup

Serves 6 - 8

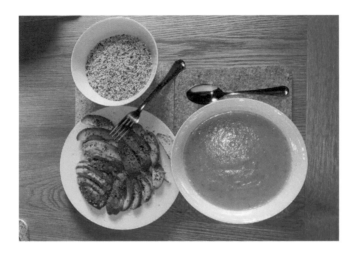

INGREDIENTS

1 full celeriac, peeled, chopped into 1½ cm cubes
2 medium celery sticks, finely chopped
1 medium onion, finely chopped
1 teaspoon mixed herbs <u>or</u> thyme
2 medium carrots, finely chopped
1 tablespoon refined olive oil
1 - 1½ litres of water
Salt and pepper to taste

METHOD

Prepare all the ingredients as above.
Heat the olive oil into a large pan, on a medium heat.
Add in onion, celeriac, carrots, herbs of your choice, fry until soft but not browned.

Add in the water, salt and pepper, bring up to the boil, then turn the heat down to low, put the lid on the pan, simmer until all ingredients are soft. Blend thoroughly with a stick blender, until soup is really smooth. A food processor or blender can also be used.

If soup is too thick, add extra hot water and stir it in thoroughly until the consistency is to your liking.

Serve and enjoy.

VARIATIONS

100 grams of pan-fried salmon can be placed in the middle of the soup, which turns it into a more substantial meal.

Huevos Rancheros

Serves 2

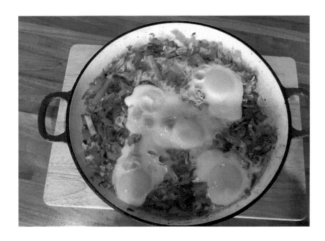

INGREDIENTS

4 large eggs (2 eggs per person)
Whole sweetheart cabbage, cut into 4, then thinly sliced
2 medium carrots, thinly sliced into ribbons
1 medium onion, thinly sliced
1 - 2 cloves garlic, peeled and roughly chopped
6 - 8 mushrooms, thinly sliced
2 dried chillies, crumbled
1 dessertspoon dried oregano
1 x 400 grams tin of chopped tomatoes
1 tablespoon refined olive oil
Salt and pepper to taste.

METHOD

Prepare all the ingredients as above.
Using a shallow casserole dish/sauté pan with a lid, heat oil over a medium heat.

Brown onions, carrots until soft, then add in cabbage, garlic and mushrooms, continue to brown gently for approximately 5 more minutes.
Add in tomatoes, oregano, salt and pepper, mixing well.
Turn heat down to low, when the mixture is bubbling in the pan, crack the eggs evenly around the pan on top of the mixture.
Keep heat on low, and cover with lid.
Cook on top of hob for approximately 10 minutes more, or until the eggs have just set. Keep checking every couple of minutes so that they are not overcooked or too runny.
Serve 2 eggs per person, dividing the mixture equally between the serving dishes.
Enjoy.

Broccoli and Pink Salmon Quiche

Serves 4 - 6

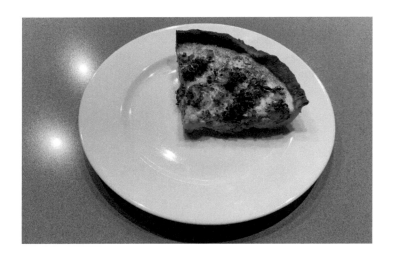

INGREDIENTS

For the Pastry
As per recipe under 'Weekly Essentials Section' of this book.

For the Filling
150 grams broccoli florets cut into small pieces (steam them before putting them into your quiche)

1 medium white onion sliced and softened

1 x 212 grams tin of pink salmon, well drained

125 ml milk (almond, coconut, sheep or goats milk can be used)

2 large eggs

2 teaspoons mixed herbs

Salt and pepper to taste

METHOD

For the Pastry

You will need a 23 cm/9 inch pie dish.

Make the pastry first and line the bottom and sides of the pie dish.

If you are not making the quiche straight away you can leave the prepared pie dish in the fridge until it is needed.

If using it straight away continue as below.

For the Filling

Preheat oven to 180° / Fan 160° / 350° / Gas 4.

Prepare the filling ingredients as above.

I steam the broccoli and soften the onion in the microwave. Whilst this is cooling, prepare the filling.

In a bowl place the eggs, milk, mixed herbs, salt and pepper, and whisk them together until they are well combined.

Next, place pieces of salmon into the prepared pasty case, add in the cooled broccoli and onion. Pour the egg mixture over the salmon and broccoli. (I cover the edges of my pastry with foil so they don't burn, but leave the centre of the quiche uncovered - if the centre starts to brown too quickly cover it with a separate piece of foil.)

Bake in preheated oven, on the middle shelf, until the centre of the quiche is golden brown and set, approximately 40 - 50 minutes.

Leave to cool slightly.

Serve with a salad or steamed vegetables and enjoy.

'Last Minute' Chicken Lunch

Serves 2

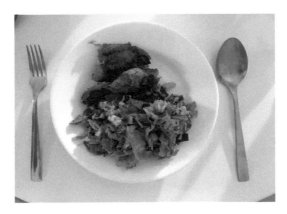

INGREDIENTS
I bought cooked roasted chicken
Salad

METHOD
Prepare a salad first.
Go to nearby spit-roasted chicken shop or supermarket and buy one.
Serve up a full leg, plus a wing per person, adding plenty of pre-made salad.

Note
Leftover chicken breasts can be used in a curry the next day for dinner.

Tip: Quite often supermarkets have deals where if you buy two cooked chickens you get them cheaper. It's always worth taking them up on the offer.
What we do is, take all the meat off the bones whilst it is still warm, then place the meat in an airtight box without its lid on to cool.
Once the meat is cold, cover with the lid and keep in the fridge to be used for quick meals when in a rush, or if unexpected visitors arrive, over the next few days.

Stir-Fry Turkey, Chicken or Quorn

Serves 2

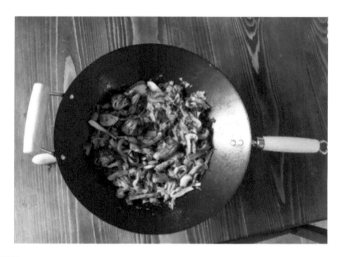

INGREDIENTS

200 grams thinly sliced turkey, chicken or Quorn
1 - 2 tablespoons refined olive oil or coconut oil
1 large onion, thinly sliced
1 large carrot, thinly sliced into batons
8 mushrooms, thinly sliced
¼ of white cabbage, thinly sliced
1 medium head of broccoli, chopped into small florets including stems
2 cm cube fresh ginger, peeled, finely chopped or grated
1 teaspoon sesame oil
Salt and pepper to taste

METHOD

Prepare all the vegetables before you start to cook.
Place turkey, chicken <u>or</u> Quorn pieces into a bowl, season with salt and pepper, mix thoroughly.

Heat oil in a wok or large deep sauté pan, on a medium heat.

When the oil is hot but not burning, add turkey, chicken <u>or</u> Quorn, stir-fry for approximately 3 - 5 minutes until slightly golden. Remove from pan with slotted spoon, retaining as much of the oil as possible in the pan. If needed add a little more oil to pan and reheat until hot.

Start adding the vegetables, onion, carrot and broccoli stems first, stir-fry until slightly brown.

Next add in the cabbage, broccoli florets, ginger and garlic, continue to stir-fry until these are going soft.

Next add in the mushrooms, continue to stir-fry until all the vegetables are beginning to soften, but not going to mush.

Return turkey, chicken <u>or</u> Quorn back to pan, stirring thoroughly.

When turkey, chicken <u>or</u> Quorn is heated through, remove pan from heat, add the sesame oil, stir thoroughly.

Check for seasoning.

Note

At this point a squirt of lemon or lime juice can be added to your pan. Serve and enjoy.

VARIATIONS

Cooked prawns, or any leftover cooked meat can be substituted for the raw turkey, chicken <u>or</u> Quorn in the above recipe, but <u>remember</u> these should be added at the end when all the vegetables are soft, to heat everything through.

Spicy Fried Rice (Cauliflower) with Paneer/ Feta Cheese

Serves 2

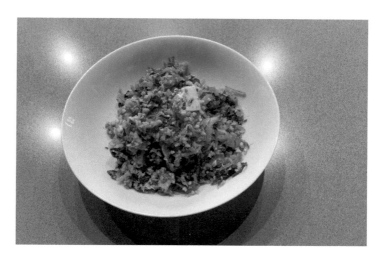

INGREDIENTS

100 grams Paneer cheese, cut into 1 cm cubes (this can be substituted with Feta cheese if you prefer)

300 grams cauliflower rice, (Aldi sells pre-prepared 300 grams tubs. Very handy)

1 medium onion, finely sliced

6 - 8 button mushrooms, finely sliced

1 medium carrot, grated

Good handful of fresh coriander, finely chopped

Thumb sized piece of fresh ginger, peeled and finely grated

2 large cloves garlic, peeled and crushed

1 dessertspoon whole cumin seeds

1 - 2 teaspoons good madras curry powder, depending how hot you like it

2 tablespoons of refined olive oil <u>or</u> 2 tablespoons coconut oil

½ teaspoon salt

½ teaspoon pepper

METHOD

Heat the oil of your choice in either a wok or a large deep frying pan, on a medium heat. When the oil is hot, add the cumin seeds, as soon as they start to sizzle, add the prepared onion, and fry until they start to brown.

Next add the prepared mushrooms, ginger, garlic, grated carrot, curry powder and continue frying for a couple more minutes.

Now add in the cauliflower rice and fry everything until any moisture from the vegetables has evaporated and all the ingredients are quite dry.

Quickly stir in the cubed cheese of your choice, stir around the pan until it is evenly distributed through the rice and then stir in the chopped coriander.

Add the salt and pepper. Check for seasoning and then serve it into warm bowls or plates.

Note

If you prefer your finished rice to be of a 'drier' consistency, before starting to cook this recipe, place the 'rice' on a baking tray, spread it out into one single layer and bake in a preheated oven 180° / Fan 160° / 350° / Gas 4 for approximately 10 minutes, giving it a stir every couple of minutes to ensure it does not burn.

Other vegetables can be used instead of the ones listed above, for example Spring onions, asparagus, red pepper, a crumbled up dried chilli, a handful of fresh roughly chopped spinach.

The cumin seeds could be swapped for fennel seeds or whatever else you fancy.

Broccoli Fritters

Serves 8

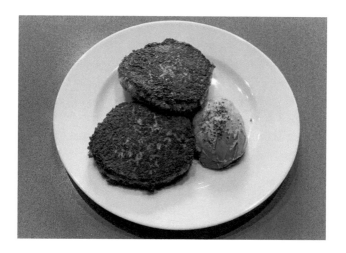

INGREDIENTS

2 medium heads of broccoli, chopped into florets, remove the stalks (approx 650 grams)

4 large eggs

75 grams almond flour

50 grams Parmesan cheese

1 - 1½ teaspoons chilli flakes to taste

½ onion, finely grated or chopped

1 clove garlic, peeled and finely crushed

1 teaspoon salt

½ teaspoon crushed black pepper

2 tablespoons refined olive oil or coconut oil

Note

Save the raw broccoli stalks which you can chop up and put into salads or make broccoli fries.

METHOD

Place the prepared broccoli florets into a food processor and pulse it until it becomes a rice like consistency, you may need to do it in two batches to get an even consistency. Place the broccoli rice into a large mixing bowl together with the rest of the ingredients <u>except</u> the oil. Mix well to combine them.
Leave it to rest for 10 minutes, then stir the mixture.
Heat a large non-stick frying pan on a medium heat, add half the amount of your chosen oil. Shape the prepared mixture into fritters, fry 2 fritters at a time in the frying pan for approximately 4 minutes on the first side.
<u>Do not</u> move the fritters whilst frying them on the first side, leave them to fry for the full time. Remember to check them near to the end of the frying time by lifting them slightly to make sure they are not burning. This prevents them falling apart and makes them really crisp.
Then turn them, continue to fry on the second side for a further 3 minutes or until they are golden brown.
You may have to alter the frying time slightly depending how big and thick you make the fritters.
Once golden brown and crisp, transfer them onto kitchen paper.
Repeat this process using the rest of the oil to fry the remaining fritters.

Note

This recipe makes 8 large fritters, 10 to 12 centimetres wide or 16 small ones. The mixture can be kept in the fridge for 2 days. I tend to make the fritters before I put them in the fridge on greaseproof paper on a baking tray.
Alternately they can be frozen on a baking tray, remember to put greaseproof paper on the baking tray as well as between the fritters so they don't stick together.
Once they have frozen place them into a plastic bag and label them. They can be kept in a freezer for up to a month.

DINNERS

Curried Chicken Thighs with Sweet Potatoes, Mushrooms and Broccoli

Serves 2

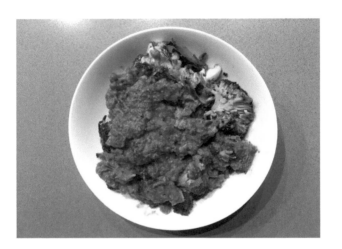

INGREDIENTS

4 chicken thighs (2 per person)

1 large onion, sliced

2 cloves garlic, peeled, chopped or grated

2 cm cube fresh ginger, peeled, finely chopped or grated

3 medium sweet potatoes chopped into 4 cm cubes

6 - 8 mushrooms, sliced

1 medium head of Broccoli cut into medium sized florets, including stalks

1 x 400 grams tin chopped tomatoes

2 tablespoons refined olive oil

2 teaspoons of bought madras curry powder <u>or</u> 3 teaspoons of homemade basic spice mix

Salt and pepper to taste

METHOD

Prepare all the vegetables.

If using a multi/instapot pressure cooker, heat up on browning programme for frying. Add oil, when hot, add onions, fry until they are brown at their edges, approximately 5 - 10 minutes.

Next add garlic, ginger and continue to fry for 1 more minute. Don't burn the garlic and ginger.

Add spices, salt, pepper, stir in well, then add all of chopped tomatoes, stir again.

Keep frying until most of the moisture goes from the tomato/onion mixture and it starts to form a paste.

Add chicken thighs, sweet potato cubes, and broccoli florets, stir well, then add enough water to bring the contents up to the minimum level indicated in pressure cooker or until everything is just covered by the liquid.

Cook on stew/meat setting for 25 minutes <u>OR</u>

25 minutes when full pressure is reached in a conventional pressure cooker. Release pressure and serve into bowls.

Note

This recipe can be cooked in a traditional shallow casserole dish with a lid. Use the exact same method but cook for 1 hour and add the broccoli and sweet potatoes half way through the cooking period on a low heat setting.

Serve and enjoy.

Easy Bolognese

Serves 4

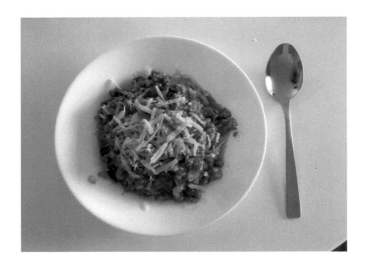

INGREDIENTS

  425 grams beef or pork mince or mixture of both
  1 medium onion, finely chopped
  1 large carrot, finely diced
  1 large stick of celery, finely diced
  6 - 8 mushrooms, finely sliced
  2 cloves garlic, peeled and crushed
  ½ - 1 red pepper, deseeded, finely chopped
  1 x 400 grams tin chopped tomatoes
  2 tablespoons refined olive oil
  2 tablespoons mixed herbs
  1 tablespoon tomato puree
  Salt and pepper to taste

METHOD

Prepare the ingredients.

In a sauté pan/frying pan with a lid, heat the oil on a medium heat, then fry onion, carrot, celery and pepper until soft but not browned (approximately 10 minutes).

Add the mushrooms, garlic, continue to fry until soft, add the tomato puree, mix thoroughly.

Next add the meat, stir well until all of the ingredients, including the meat are not clumped together.

Now add in the chopped tomatoes, mixed herbs, salt, pepper, mixing thoroughly.

Bring all the ingredients in the pan up to a simmer, turn the heat down to low, continue to cook slowly, cover with a lid and simmer for about an hour, or until the sauce looks rich, and the liquid has started to reduce.

If making this earlier in the day, <u>turn the heat off</u> and leave.

When reheating, remember to uncover it until the sauce reduces, so it's lovely, thick and no longer watery.

Serve with any type of vegetable, but a good idea is to have it with Cabbage Tagliatelle.

VARIATIONS

425 grams of any mince, e.g. chicken, turkey or Quorn.

Leek, Cauliflower and Broccoli Bake

Serves 2

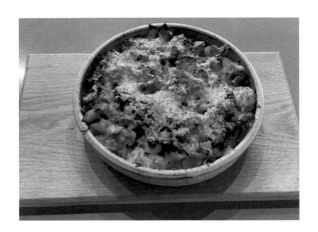

INGREDIENTS

1 medium head broccoli, cut into small florets including the stalks
1 medium head cauliflower, cut into small florets including the stalks
2 medium leeks, washed and thinly sliced
1 clove garlic, peeled and crushed
6 - 8 mushrooms, thinly sliced
50 grams pine nuts, toasted
75 grams strong cheese, grated (preferably a blue cheese or strong tasting cheese that melts well)
25 grams Parmesan cheese, grated
1 teaspoon mixed herbs
2 tablespoons refined olive oil
200 ml double cream
Salt and pepper to taste

METHOD

Preheat the oven 220° / Fan 200° / 425° / Gas 7.

Prepare all the ingredients as above.

Place the broccoli and cauliflower into a steamer, and steam them until they are just tender, approximately 8 minutes. Drain the broccoli and cauliflower into a colander and leave to cool. They can also be blanched in boiling water for 2 - 3 minutes and then left to drain and cool.

While waiting for these to cool, heat the oil in a frying pan over a medium heat. When the oil is hot, sauté the leeks until soft and just starting to brown. Next add in the mushrooms, mixed herbs, garlic and continue to fry until everything is soft and just starting to brown.

Turn off the heat, leave the pan to cool.

In a separate frying pan, over a medium heat, dry roast the pine nuts until golden brown, turn off the heat, leave the pan to cool.

Place all the cooled leeks, pine nuts, broccoli and cauliflower in a large bowl and mix thoroughly.

Place the mixture into a shallow ovenproof dish.

In a small bowl, mix your choice of strong grated cheese (not the Parmesan cheese), with the cream, add in salt and pepper to taste, then pour this over the vegetable mixture in the shallow dish.

Sprinkle the grated Parmesan cheese over the top of this mixture, then place in the preheated oven for approximately 30 minutes, until all the Parmesan cheese is golden brown.

Remove from the oven, leave to cool slightly.

Serve and enjoy.

We sometimes serve it with a big salad, but it is gorgeous just on its own!

Hunters Chicken

Serves 2

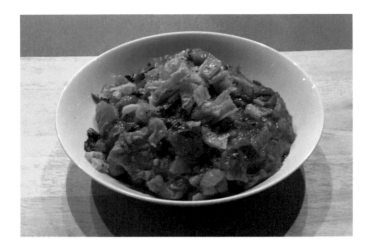

INGREDIENTS

4 x skinless chicken thighs, with bone in (2 per person)
I large onion, sliced thinly
I red pepper, sliced thinly
6 - 8 mushrooms, sliced thinly
2 large cloves of garlic, peeled, finely chopped
I x 400 grams tin of chopped tomatoes
I dessertspoon of mixed dried herbs
2 tablespoons olive oil
About 16 pitted green olives
Salt and pepper to taste
Small handful of fresh chopped flat leaf parsley
Approximately 300-450 ml water
I teaspoon of hot smoked paprika

METHOD

Prepare the ingredients as above.

Heat the oil in a large pan (which has lid), on a medium heat. When the oil is hot, add the onions and fry until light brown,

Then add in the red pepper and continue to fry until pepper is slightly soft.

Add the mushrooms, chopped garlic and once everything has softened and started to brown slightly, add all the remaining ingredients to the pan, except the fresh parsley. Add enough water to cover all the ingredients, including the chicken.

Put on the pan lid, turn heat down to low and simmer gently for about an hour. Once chicken is tender and just beginning to fall off the bone, take off the pan lid, increase the heat back up to medium.

Watch the liquid in your pan carefully, until it reduces slightly and just begins to thicken. Next add in the chopped parsley, check the seasoning and add more salt and pepper if necessary.

Serve with vegetables of your choice, we like to serve it with shredded cooked cabbage, or some roast vegetables.

Tandoori Chicken with Curried Roast Vegetables

Serves 2

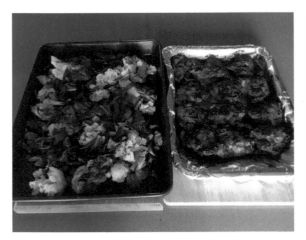 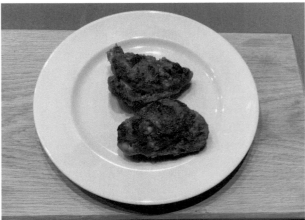

INGREDIENTS

4 skinless chicken thighs with the bone in (2 thighs per person)

2 - 3 tablespoons Greek yogurt

One batch of Tandoori Paste (recipe can be found in 'Weekly Essentials Section' of this book)

1 medium cauliflower, cut into small florets, including the stalks

1 medium head of broccoli, cut into small florets, including the stalks

¼ medium red cabbage, cut into 3 - 4 cm chunks

1 large onion, cut into chunks

2 medium carrots, cut into batons

6 - 8 medium mushrooms, halved and quartered

1 dessertspoon curry powder (East End is an excellent brand)

1 dessertspoon fennel seeds

2 tablespoons refined olive oil

METHOD

Prepare the chicken thighs, remove the skin, make slashes crossways on each thigh right down to the bone.

Mix tandoori paste with the yogurt in a large bowl until it is well combined, then place prepared chicken in the paste. Make sure you mix and push the paste into all the slashes. Cover this bowl with cling film, leave in the fridge for at least an hour, but we prefer to leave it overnight.

TO COOK

Remove the prepared chicken from the fridge at least 30 minutes before cooking, to allow it to reach room temperature.

Preheat the oven to 200° / Fan 180° / 400° / Gas 6. Place all the prepared vegetables into a large mixing bowl.

Meanwhile add the oil, curry powder, fennel seeds to the bowl of vegetables, mixing them well.

Spread all the vegetables out onto a non-stick baking tray, place on the middle shelf of the preheated oven, for approximately 45 - 60 minutes.

At the same time, place prepared chicken on a separate baking tray which we line with foil, place on top shelf of preheated oven, for approximately 50 - 60 minutes.

It is ready when both the chicken and vegetables have charred edges, just like tandoori chicken served in an Indian Restaurant.

Serve and enjoy.

Note

This can be eaten with the prepared roast vegetables as above or cauliflower rice, either way it is delicious!

Field (Portobello) Mushrooms and Red Onion Pie

Serves 6 - 8

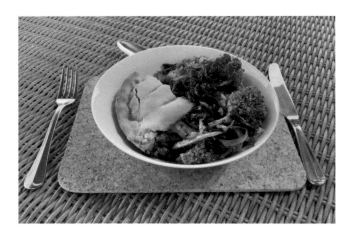

INGREDIENTS

For the Pastry
As per recipe under 'Weekly Essentials Section' of this book.

For the Filling
3 - 4 large field (Portobello) mushrooms, thinly sliced
1 large red onion, thinly sliced
1 - 2 teaspoons mixed herbs
1 tablespoon full fat crème fraîche
1 fat clove garlic, peeled and crushed
2 – 3 tablespoons refined olive oil
Salt and pepper to taste

METHOD

For the filling
Heat the oil in a large frying pan, on a medium heat, when oil is hot, add in
the onions and fry until they are soft, but not too brown, remember to put the

frying pan lid on whilst frying the onions.

Add the mushrooms, garlic, and herbs, continue frying (BUT leave off the frying pan lid) until all the vegetables are softened.

Stir in the crème fraîche, add salt and pepper, leave until cool before adding the mixture to the prepared uncooked pie case.

Place the prepared pie lid on top and press the edges together to seal the top of the pie to its sides, make a couple of slits in pie top, to let out the steam as it cooks.

Place the pie on to an oven tray. I cover the pie edges with foil to stop them burning.

(Note: sometimes the oil from the ground almonds runs out of the pastry, this is perfectly normal and the oven tray prevents it going all over your oven.)

Place the pie on the oven tray on the middle shelf of the preheated oven, bake for 40 – 50 minutes or until the pastry is golden brown.

Note

If the pie top starts to brown too quickly, cover it with a sheet of foil or greaseproof paper, to prevent burning the pastry. Remove the foil or greaseproof paper 2 – 5 minutes before completely cooked so the pastry top goes golden brown.

Remove from oven, allow to cool for 20 -30 minutes. I serve ours at room temperature usually with a large salad or sautéed vegetables.

Tips: This pie can be frozen prior to cooking or after it has been cooked, once it is completely cold, or if you make it the day before, it can be chilled it in the fridge, prior to cooking.

Remember to take the pie out of the fridge or freezer in plenty of time to allow it to reach room temperature before cooking it.

Pan Fried Pork Chops with Steamed Vegetables

Serves 2

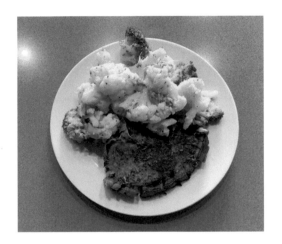

INGREDIENTS

1 pork chop per person approximately 100 grams per chop
1 large onion, finely sliced
2 cm cube fresh ginger, peeled, finely chopped or grated
Frozen cauliflower and broccoli florets, (a good handful per person, remember it is unlimited)
Frozen carrots and spinach, (these are also unlimited)
1 teaspoon mixed herbs
1 tablespoon refined olive oil
Salt and pepper to taste

METHOD

Prepare the ingredients as above.
Add the oil to a frying pan, on a medium heat, when oil is warm, add onion and fry until soft.
Next add the garlic and ginger to the softened onion, fry these until they are

also soft, then season with salt and pepper.

Meanwhile place all the frozen vegetables in a microwaveable bowl, cover with a plate, cook for 5 minutes in the microwave on full heat, or until soft.

Whilst this is cooking, prepare the pork chops by placing them on a plate, then add salt, pepper and mixed herbs to them.

Next, remove the softened onion, garlic and ginger from the frying pan on to a plate, return the frying pan to a medium heat, add a little more oil if necessary. When the oil is hot, add the pork chops, cook for 3 – 5 minutes on each side, depending on the thickness of the chops.

Spoon the cooked onions, garlic and ginger over cooked pork chops and serve with the steamed vegetables.

Once steamed vegetables are cooked, we add a knob of butter or some olive oil, mix thoroughly, then serve.

VARIATION

You could swap the pork chops for sirloin steaks, approximately 100 grams per steak per person, cook the steaks using the same method as above.

Chicken Kebabs

Serves 2

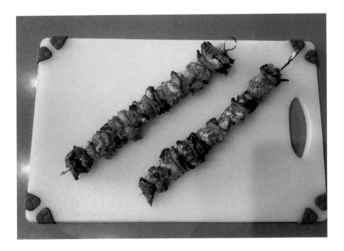

INGREDIENTS

2 chicken breasts, chopped into bite-sized chunks

I red pepper, chopped into bite-sized chunks

I medium onion, chopped into bite sized chunks

4 button mushrooms, left whole

Any other vegetables of your choice, chopped into bite-sized chunks can be used, if you do not like what we suggest

Pre-prepared Kebab Dressing/Marinade (this recipe can be found in 'Weekly Essentials Section' of this book)

Note

You will need 2 skewers, the prepared Kebab Dressing/Marinade, and a pastry brush.

If you are preparing the chicken breasts in the morning you can marinade the chicken in a bowl. Make sure all the chicken is well coated with the marinade.

Cover the bowl with cling film and store in the fridge until needed. Remember to remove the chicken from the fridge approximately 1 hour prior to cooking so it can reach room temperature.

METHOD
Preheat the grill on hot.
I put the prepared onions and peppers on a microwaveable plate and place them in a microwave on full power for approximately 2 minutes until they are just soft.
Skewer the chicken chunks, plus your choice of vegetables onto the skewers.
Using a pastry brush, brush the pre-prepared dressing/marinade onto the loaded skewers.
Grill for approximately 15 minutes under the preheated grill. Remember to brush the kebabs with the marinade whilst cooking.
Remember to keep turning the loaded kebabs to prevent them burning and allowing them to cook evenly.
Once cooked, serve immediately with a side salad, cauliflower rice or sauté vegetables

Feta Cheese and Red Onion Quiche
Serves 4 - 6

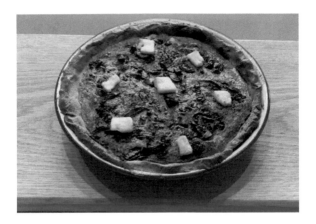

INGREDIENTS

For the Pastry
As per recipe under 'Weekly Essentials Section' of the book.

For the Filling
3 medium red onions, thinly sliced
75 grams feta cheese, sliced
2 large eggs
125 ml milk of your choice (almond, coconut, sheep's or goat milk) <u>or</u> for a richer filling use 125 ml double cream instead of milk
2 tablespoons refined olive oil
2 teaspoons mixed herbs
Salt and pepper to taste

METHOD

For the Filling

Preheat the oven to 180° / Fan 160° / 350° / Gas 4

Prepare the filling ingredients.

Sauté the red onion in a frying pan with the refined olive oil on a medium heat, until soft and slightly golden but <u>not</u> burnt, allow to cool down in the pan off the heat.

Whilst this is cooling prepare the filling.

In a bowl place the eggs, herbs, milk or cream if using it, salt and pepper, and whisk them together until they are well combined.

Place half of the cooled onions into the prepared pastry case bottom, then add in the slices of feta cheese, next place the remaining onions on top of the cheese layer.

Pour the egg mixture over the cheese and onion. (I cover the edges of my pastry with foil so they don't burn, but leave the centre of your quiche uncovered - if the centre starts to brown too quickly whilst cooking in the oven, cover it with a separate piece of foil.)

Bake in preheated oven, on the middle shelf, until the centre of the quiche is golden brown and set, approximately 40 - 50 minutes.

Leave too cool slightly. Serve with a salad or steamed vegetables.

Julie's Cheese and Onion Pie

Serves 6 - 8

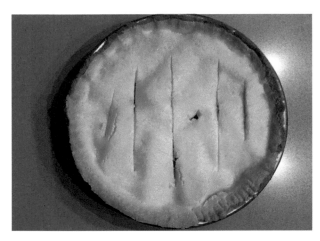 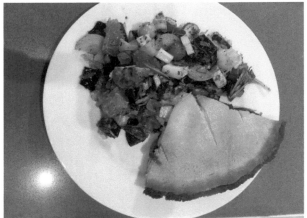

INGREDIENTS

For the Pastry
As per recipe under 'Weekly Essentials Section' of this book

For the Filling
25 ml refined olive oil
3 large onions, thinly sliced
200 grams grated or sliced cheese (I used either 200 grams of feta <u>or</u> 200 grams goats cheese)
Salt and pepper to taste

METHOD

Make the pastry first, remember to use approximately a third of the pastry mixture for the pie top, (leave to one side) then use the rest of the pastry mixture to line the bottom and sides of the pie dish.
If you are not making the pie straight away you can leave the prepared pie

dish/pie top in the fridge till it is needed.
If using it straight away continue as below.

Preheat the oven to 180° / Fan 160° / 350° / Gas

For the Filling
Heat the oil in a frying pan, on a low heat, fry the onions until they are soft.
Remember to put the frying pan lid on whilst frying the onions so that the
steam cooks them without burning them.
When the onions are soft, remove the lid, continue cooking the onions
until almost all the liquid in the pan has evaporated and they are slightly
caramelised.
Leave onions in the pan to cool.
Once they have cooled, cover the bottom of the prepared pie dish with a layer
of your choice of cheese, then a layer of cooled onions. Repeat both layers
until all the cheese and onions are used up.
Place pie lid on top and press the edges together to seal top of the pie to its
sides, make a couple of slits in pie top, to let the steam out as it cooks.
I always cover the edges of my pie with foil to stop them from burning. Place
the pie on an oven tray.
(Note: sometimes the oil from the ground almonds runs out of the pastry,
this is perfectly normal and the oven tray prevents it going all over your
oven.)
Place the pie on the oven tray on the middle shelf of the preheated oven, bake
for 40 - 50 minutes or until the pastry is golden brown.

Note
If the pie top starts to brown too quickly, cover it with a sheet of foil
or greaseproof paper, to prevent burning the pastry. Remove the foil or
greaseproof paper 2 - 5 minutes before completely cooked so the pastry top

goes golden brown.
Remove from oven, leave to cool for approximately 20 - 30 minutes before serving.
Serve the pie at room temperature, with a salad <u>or</u> sautéed vegetables.

This pie can be frozen prior to cooking <u>or</u> after it has been cooked once it is completely cool <u>or</u>, if making it the day before, it can be chilled in the fridge prior to cooking.

<u>Remember</u> to take out the pie from the fridge <u>or</u> freezer in plenty of time so the pie can reach room temperature before cooking.

SIDE DISHES AND ACCOMPANIMENTS

Celeriac Chips

Serves 2 - 3

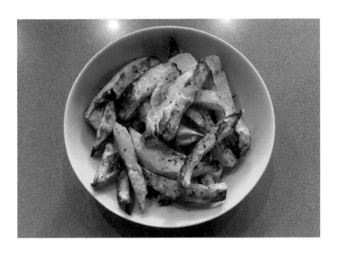

INGREDIENTS

I large celeriac, peeled and cut into I - 2 cm thick chips, not too thin

I - 2 tablespoons refined olive oil

Salt and pepper to taste

METHOD

Preheat the oven to 200° / Fan I80° / 400° / Gas 6

On a non-stick baking tray, spread out the celeriac chips.

Sprinkle with oil, salt and pepper. Mix well, place in preheated oven on the middle shelf. Cook for approximately 45 minutes, or until brown all over like traditional oven baked chips.

Remember to turn the chips over halfway through the cooking time. Serve straight from the oven and enjoy.

Note

We serve our celeriac chips with pan-fried salmon, or any fish of your choice (so long as it is not battered or covered in bread crumbs).

This is our version of homemade fish and chips, delicious with a big salad, or steamed vegetables, either fresh or frozen.

Chinese Style Sautéed Cabbage with Sesame Seeds.
Serves 2

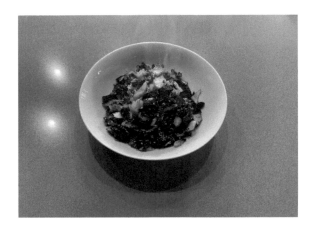

INGREDIENTS

Approximately ¾ of a cabbage, red or white, or a mixture of both, finely chopped into 2 cm pieces

1 large onion, finely chopped

1 - 2 dried red chillies, crumbled up

1 thumb size piece of fresh ginger, finely shredded into 3 cm long pieces

2 cloves of garlic, peeled, crushed

1 dessertspoon sesame seeds

1 dessertspoon sesame oil

2 tablespoons refined olive oil

1 teaspoon five spice powder

Salt and pepper to taste

METHOD

Heat the olive oil in a wok or deep frying pan, on a medium heat.

When the oil is hot, add the onions and fry until they are slightly brown.

Next add the chilli, continue to fry for a couple of minutes, then add the cabbage, ginger, garlic and the five spice powder.

Continue to fry all the ingredients until the cabbage is cooked and just tender.

Now add the sesame seeds, then the sesame oil, mixing well to combine all the ingredients.

Serve into prepared warm bowls.

Add the prepared avocado, herbs and olive oil. Mix ingredients thoroughly.

Sautéed Broccoli and Cauliflower
Serves 2

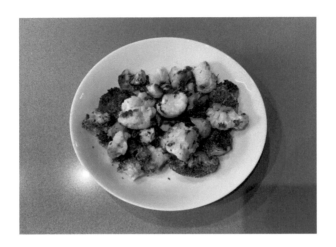

INGREDIENTS
    1 medium head of broccoli, cut into florets, including stalks
    1 medium head of cauliflower, cut into florets, including stalks
    1 medium onion, thinly sliced
    1 clove garlic, peeled, finely crushed or grated
    2 cm cube fresh ginger, peeled, finely chopped or grated
    6 - 8 mushrooms, finely sliced
    1 - 2 tablespoons of either avocado oil, refined olive oil <u>or</u> coconut oil
    1 teaspoon fennel seeds
    1 teaspoon dried thyme, oregano <u>or</u> mixed herbs
    2 tablespoons water <u>or</u> white wine
    Salt and pepper to taste

METHOD
Prepare the ingredients as above.
Place oil of your choice in a frying pan/sauté pan which has a lid, onto a medium

heat, when the oil is hot, fry onion, fennel seeds, broccoli and cauliflower stalks until soft.

Add the cauliflower and broccoli florets and continue frying.

Next add the mushrooms, garlic and ginger, frying until the vegetables begin to brown slightly and soften.

Add water or white wine.

TURN HEAT DOWN LOW

Cover with a lid.

Cook until all liquid has evaporated and all the vegetables are soft. Season with salt and pepper.

Serve and enjoy.

Steamed Vegetables with Onion, Garlic, Ginger and Sesame Oil Dressing
Serves 2

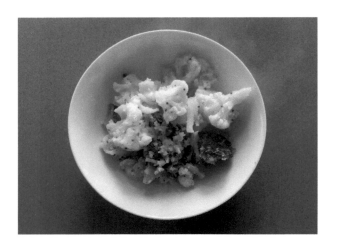

INGREDIENTS
Choose your vegetables. We use the following;

1 head of cauliflower, cut into florets, including stalks
1 head of broccoli, cut into florets, including stalks
2 medium carrots, finely sliced
1 medium onion, finely sliced
¼ red cabbage and ¼ white cabbage, both finely sliced
1 garlic clove, peeled, finely chopped or grated
2 cm cube fresh ginger, peeled, finely chopped or grated
Salt and pepper to taste

METHOD
Prepare all the ingredients as above.
Steam all the vegetables in a large pan, until they are soft then, drain them well.

Whilst the vegetables are steaming, warm the sesame oil in a frying pan on a low heat.

Then add garlic and ginger and, very carefully, cook the garlic and ginger until it is soft but not brown.

Return vegetables to the pan or warmed serving dish, spoon over oil dressing, mixing well.

Note
Dressing can also be made with olive oil or butter and mixed herbs added.

Braised Red Cabbage
Serves 2

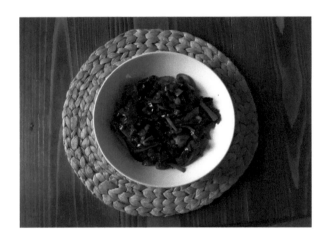

INGREDIENTS
½ medium red cabbage, finely sliced and diced
1 dessertspoon fennel seeds
1 medium onion, finely sliced
1 clove of garlic, peeled, grated or finely chopped
2 medium carrots, cut into thinly sliced batons
6 – 8 mushrooms, thinly sliced
1 tablespoon refined olive oil
1 tablespoon balsamic vinegar

METHOD
Prepare all the ingredients as above.
Place the red cabbage, onion, fennel seeds and carrot into a sauté pan / frying pan, together with the oil onto a medium heat.
Fry gently until onion, carrot and cabbage have softened, (approximately 10 minutes) and are slightly brown.

Add garlic and mushrooms, continue to fry with carrot, cabbage and onion until cooked. Then add a splash (about a tablespoon) of balsamic vinegar. Let it reduce until there is virtually no liquid left and the cabbage is slightly sticky. Serve and enjoy.

Cauliflower Steaks with Cheesy Topping
Serves 2

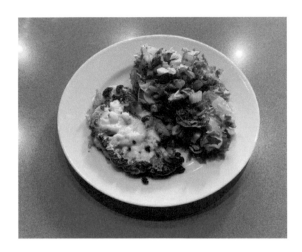

INGREDIENTS

1 large head of cauliflower

50 grams of good strong melting cheese, grated (we use blue cheese because it keeps its flavour when cooked)

2 - 3 tablespoons of refined olive oil

Salt and Pepper to taste

METHOD

Take off all the green outer leaves of the cauliflower, leaving the whole white head of the cauliflower. Don't cut out the central core as this helps to keep the 'steak' together.

Cut the cauliflower in half, down from the top through its central stem/ core. (See photo.) From each half of your cut cauliflower, cut a slice/steak of cauliflower, again from the top through its central stem/core, no more than 2 centimetres thick. (See photos.)

<u>Remember to keep the stem/core intact.</u>

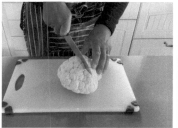 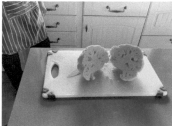 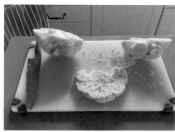 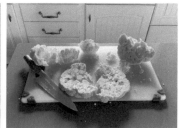

You should now have two cauliflower slices/steaks
Preheat your grill to hot
Place a large frying pan on a high heat. Add the oil and when the oil is hot, place each slice/steak into the hot oil.
Reduce the heat to low - medium and fry the slices/steaks until golden brown.
Carefully turn the slice/steak over in the pan and fry that side until it is also golden brown, approximately 5 minutes each side or until the stem/core is soft.
Season with salt and pepper,

If your frying pan is suitable for placing under your grill, divide the grated cheese of your choice between the two cauliflower slices/steaks and evenly sprinkle over the tops of the two cauliflower slice/steaks.
Place under your preheated grill and grill them until the cheese has melted and started browning.

If your frying pan is not suitable for placing under your grill, carefully transfer the cauliflower slices/steaks onto a baking tray and grill as above.

Serve straight away. We adore these cauliflower steaks with a large salad.

Homemade Sauerkraut

Makes approximately 1.4 litre Jar

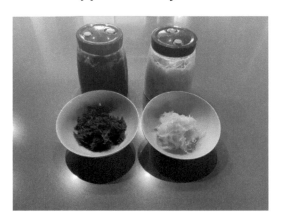

INGREDIENTS

1 large white cabbage, approx 1 kilo
Fine sea salt or cooking salt, approx 25 grams

Tips

We use a clean and dry 1.4 litre Lakeland Fermentation Jar.

We use the glass Pickling Pebbles, or you can use the ramekin method as below. The common white cabbage works well and always choose a large fresh one.

Remember to slice your cabbage as thinly as possible which allows the salt to draw the brine therefore allowing it work quicker. We use our Magimix to slice our cabbage.

Salt ratio is very important to your success, too little and your sauerkraut will not preserve, too much will prevent your sauerkraut's fermentation.

Every 1 kilo of prepared cabbage needs 25 grams fine cooking salt or sea salt. Never use coarse salt or flakes as they take far too long to dissolve.

METHOD

Slice the cabbage into quarters, remove and discard the stalk. Slice each quarter as thinly as possible, transferring the slices to a large glass or stainless steel bowl. Weigh the prepared cabbage and sprinkle over salt. Mix or toss the salt and cabbage together until the cabbage begins to feel damp. Take a handful of your salted cabbage mixture at a time, placing it into the prepared jars, pressing down each layer firmly. Leave a gap at the top big enough for a ramekin, or a pickling pebble - we prefer to use the pickling pebble method.

RAMEKIN METHOD.

Fill a ramekin with ceramic baking beans and wrap with cling film, then place inside the filled jar, on top of the prepared salted cabbage mixture - this helps to keep the cabbage submerged in the brine which is produced.

Put the lid onto the jar, remember to depress the silicone stopper to form an airtight seal - the one way valve in the lid will allow excess gas to escape and stop oxygen getting in. Store in a warm place around 21° / 70° is perfect.

The following day, open the jar, check to see if enough brine has been produced to cover all the cabbage, if not top it up with a little home-made brine. (To make the brine, mix 1 litre of hot water with 1½ tablespoons of salt, leave it to cool before topping up the sauerkraut.)

After 8 days the sauerkraut should be ready. Taste it, and if you prefer a stronger flavour, leave it a further 4 - 5 days. Once it tastes as you like it, store it in the fridge. It should keep for up to a month, but not in our house! Enjoy it, it is beautiful.

Tip: For a change we often use red cabbage instead, it is delicious!

DESSERTS

Baked Vanilla Cheesecake
Serves 8

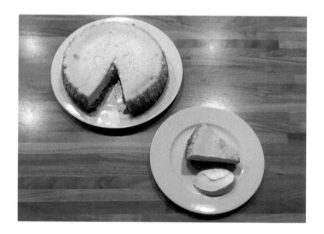

INGREDIENTS

Base
200 grams crushed pecan nuts (pecans can be pulsed in a food processor until roughly crushed, but don't over-process)
75 grams unsalted butter
Pinch of salt

Filling
300 grams full fat cream cheese
50 grams stevia <u>or</u> sweetener of your choice
25 grams coconut flour
350 ml crème fraîche
3 large eggs beaten
1½ tablespoons vanilla extract <u>or</u> vanilla bean paste

METHOD
Preheat the oven 150° / Fan 130° / 300° / Gas 2

For the Base
Place pecans in a food processor and pulse until roughly crushed.
Melt butter in a microwave bowl in microwave on full power 30 seconds at a time, until it has melted.
Add crushed pecans into melted butter, mix thoroughly with a spoon, until all crushed pecans and melted butter are combined.
Place crumb mixture into a prepared lined 18 cm/7 inch quick release cake tin. Make sure to press it down firmly and evenly with the back of a spoon over the base of the tin.
Place in the fridge until base sets.

For the Filling
In a large bowl mix together cream cheese, stevia and coconut flour.
Add in beaten eggs, crème fraîche and vanilla extract or vanilla bean paste, mix thoroughly.
Remove prepared base from the fridge and pour the filling mixture onto biscuit base until it is half full. Place it into the preheated oven on the middle shelf, then top up the cake tin with the rest of the filling mixture.
Bake for 55 minutes until barely coloured, just set at the edges and it is still a bit wobbly in the middle of the cheesecake.
Turn off the oven, <u>leave</u> the cheesecake in the oven until completely cold.
When it is cold remove cheesecake from the cold oven, leave the cheesecake in its tin and place it straight away into the fridge for it to firm up overnight.
Once the cheesecake has set and chilled, remove it from the tin; you can keep it in an airtight container in the fridge for up to 5 days (if you can resist it that long!).

SERVING

Remove the cheesecake from the fridge and take it out of the airtight container. Let the cheesecake come up to room temperature before serving. We serve ours with fresh fruit, e.g. strawberries or raspberries and either whipped double cream, crème fraîche, or Greek yogurt.
It is also delicious on its own.

Julie's Fudgy Dark Chocolate Torte

Serves 12

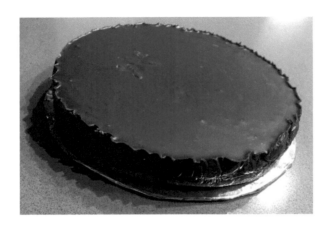

INGREDIENTS

Base
200 grams pecan nuts, blended into a coarse powder
75 grams unsalted butter, softened
Pinch of salt

Filling
150 grams unsweetened dark chocolate, I use 85% cocoa solids 20 grams stevia <u>or</u> sweetener of your choice
225 grams salted butter, thinly sliced
85 ml double cream
2 teaspoons vanilla extract <u>or</u> vanilla bean paste

METHOD

Base
Prepare 20 cm/8 inch round spring form tin by cling-filming the inside and base of the tin. Place the pecans into a food processor and blend to a coarse powder,

then put this powder into a bowl. Pour the softened butter into the bowl with the crumb mixture and add a pinch of salt.

Mix all the ingredients until well combined.

Place all the crumb mixture into the prepared tin on top of the clingfilm, press it down with the back of a spoon, or spatula.

Make sure it is evenly spread over the base of the tin. Place in fridge until base has set.

Filling

Place all the filling ingredients as above into a microwaveable bowl, place in the microwave, on full power, for 30 second intervals until everything has melted. Remove from the microwave, either stir well or give it a quick whisk with a hand whisk, until everything is mixed together and is silky smooth, leave to cool.

Remove the prepared base tin from the fridge and pour the cooled chocolate mixture into the tin on top of the base. Return it to the fridge for one to two hours or until the fudgy chocolate top has set.

Before serving remove the torte from the fridge, let it warm up to room temperature. You can serve it with double cream, crème fraîche, Greek yogurt, by itself or with a few berries of your choice, or a mixture.

If any fudgy chocolate torte is left (<u>NEVER IN OUR HOUSEHOLD!</u>) place it into an airtight box and keep it in the fridge or place in a freezer for up to a month.

Note

For a special occasion dessert, you can decorate the top with swirls of whipped double cream, add berries of your choice on top of the cream then grate some more dark chocolate over the entire top.

'**EXTREMELY** NAUGHTY BUT **EXTREMELY** NICE'

Chocolate Orange Brownie Celebration Cake

Serves 10

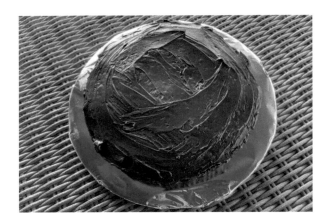

INGREDIENTS

70 grams ground almonds
30 grams almond flour
100 grams unsalted butter, softened
20 grams cacao <u>or</u> cocoa powder
30 grams stevia <u>or</u> sweetener of your choice, to your taste
2 large eggs
1½ teaspoons orange essence
½ teaspoon baking powder

METHOD

Preheat the oven 180° / Fan 160° / 350° / Gas 4
Line the base and sides of a 18cm / 7 inch round cake tin with greaseproof paper or a liner.
In a bowl whisk the softened butter and stevia until light and fluffy, add in the rest of the above ingredients until they are all well combined.

Pour the mixture into the prepared tin and level the top of the cake with a spatula or the back of a spoon.

Place onto the middle shelf in the preheated oven, for 40 - 45 minutes.

Check by inserting a skewer into the middle of the cake, if it comes out clean it is cooked. If not, give it a few more minutes in the oven, repeat with the skewer to make sure it is cooked.

Allow to cool completely in the tin before removing the cake.

Serve with freshly whipped double crème fraîche or Greek yogurt.

VARIATION

This cake can be transformed to a stunning celebration cake by using the Dark Chocolate Ganache (recipe can be found further on in the Dessert section of this book.)

It can be further enhanced by adding a small amount of orange essence to the ganache to your taste.

Coffee and Walnut Cake

Serves 10 - 12

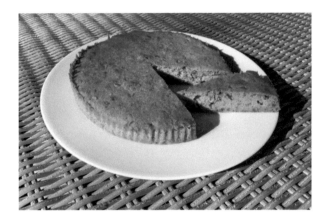

INGREDIENTS

60 grams ground almonds

40 grams almond flour

100 grams unsalted butter, softened

30 grams stevia or sweetener of your choice

2 large eggs

50 grams walnuts, chopped in small pieces

1 teaspoon baking powder

3 tablespoons espresso / strong coffee

1 teaspoon coffee essence

1 - 2 tablespoons milk / water (optional)

METHOD

Preheat the oven 180° / Fan 160° / 350° / Gas 4

Line a 20 cm/8 inch loose bottom cake tin with a liner or greaseproof paper. In a bowl cream the butter and stevia until light and fluffy.

Next add in all the rest of the ingredients and make sure to combine them well.

(At this stage if the mixture feels too thick, you can add 1 to 2 tablespoons of milk or water, combine it well. It should look and feel like a batter).

Pour the batter mixture into the prepared tin, level the top with either a spatula or the back of a spoon.
Place the cake on to the middle shelf of the preheated oven and bake for 30 - 40 minutes, until the top of the cake feels firm to the touch.
Alternatively you can check to see if it is cooked by inserting a skewer into the middle of the cake, if it comes out clean it is cooked. If not leave it in the oven for a few minutes more, then repeat test with the skewer.
Remove from the oven, allow it to cool completely in the tin, before removing it.
Serve on it own or with freshly whipped double cream, crème fraîche or Greek yogurt. This cake can be stored in an airtight container for up to two weeks.
(This never happens in our house!)

Sugar Free Lemon Mug Cake

Serves 2

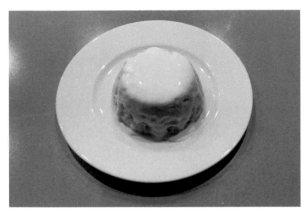 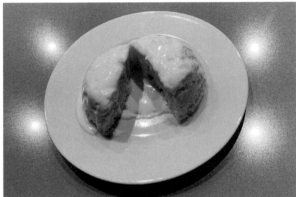

INGREDIENTS

For the Cake
40 grams almond flour
20 ml double cream
15 grams stevia <u>or</u> sweetener of your choice
2 tablespoons, lemon juice
½ teaspoon baking powder
1 egg

Note
If using ground almonds you may need to add 10 - 20 grams more as they are coarser than almond flour.

For the Glaze
12 grams unsalted butter
10 ml double cream

10 grams stevia or sweetener of your choice
Squeeze of lemon juice

METHOD
Grease the inside of 2 mugs or a small microwave bowl with melted butter.

For the Cake
Put all the dry ingredients into a mixing bowl and stir until well combined.
Add all the wet ingredients into this mixture and stir until well combined. If
you feel that the batter is too wet add a little more almond flour, mix well,
repeat if necessary until you get the consistency of the batter right.
Transfer the batter mixture into the prepared mugs or dish and remember to
level the tops.
Place into the microwave, microwave on high for 90 seconds <u>or</u> bake in a
preheated oven, 180° / Fan 160° / 350° / Gas 4 for approximately 15 minutes.
Remove from the microwave or oven, and turn cake upside down on a plate
ready to serve.

For the Glaze
Melt the butter, stir in the lemon juice, stevia and double cream, allow the
glaze to cool slightly, so the glaze thickens, but still pours.
Pour over the cake and serve whilst everything is still warm.

Note
You can also add a dessertspoon of double cream, crème fraîche, Greek yogurt
or sugar free vanilla ice cream to turn it into a proper treat.

Extra Rich Chocolate Mug Cake

Serves 2

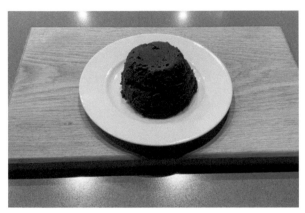 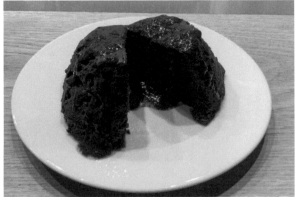

INGREDIENTS

15 grams coconut flour
½ teaspoon baking powder
20 grams cacao powder
20 grams stevia <u>or</u> sweetener of your choice
1 large egg
50 ml double cream
20 grams unsweetened dark chocolate chips
¼ teaspoon vanilla extract or to taste (optional)
1 teaspoon butter - to grease the mugs or small microwave bowl

METHOD

Prepare 2 mugs or a small microwave bowl by placing ½ teaspoon of butter into each mug, or dish, melt the butter. (I do this by placing them in the microwave, on full power for 20 - 30 seconds).

Remove from the microwave, grease the inside of the mugs or dish with the melted butter, this helps to turn the cake out beautifully.

Place all the dry ingredients in a microwaveable bowl, combine them so there are no lumps.

Next add in the wet ingredients, mix well, so they are thoroughly combined.

Divide the prepared cake mixture evenly between the 2 mugs or dish, levelling the tops. Place them into the microwave on high for 1½ minutes - <u>no</u> longer or they will become too dry.

Alternatively, they can be baked in a preheated oven, 180° / Fan 160° / 350° / Gas 4 for approximately 15 minutes.

Enjoy straight from the mugs or dish, or you can turn them out onto a plate. Serve with ice cream, double cream, crème fraîche or Greek yogurt.

For a special treat you could make the following:

Optional Chocolate Sauce

Melt 20 grams sugar free chocolate, broken into small pieces, with 10 grams of unsalted butter in the microwave on full power for 20 - 30 seconds or until melted. Mix well.

When mixture has cooled slightly, I then add 30 ml of double cream (optional), stir in well then and pour chocolate sauce over each of your chocolate mug cakes.

This is one of my family favourites and is truly delicious! Enjoy.

Shortbread Biscuits

Serves 12 - 14

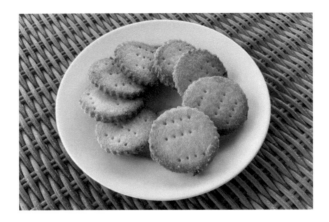

INGREDIENTS

250 grams ground almonds
70 grams salted butter
30 grams stevia <u>or</u> sweetener of your choice
2 teaspoons of vanilla extract <u>or</u> bean paste to taste

METHOD

Place all the above ingredients into a medium bowl and mix well until they are all combined.

Using your hands make the mixture into a dough ball, cover it with clingfilm and place it into the fridge for 15 minutes to firm up.

While the dough is in the fridge, preheat the oven to 180° / Fan 160° / 350° / Gas 4.

Cover a baking tray with greaseproof paper.

Take the cooled dough out of the fridge, roll it out to form an even layer and, using a medium sized cutter, cut out the biscuit shapes.

Place biscuits onto the lined baking sheet.

Put the baking tray into the oven on the middle shelf and bake for approximately 12 - 14 minutes, keep an eye on them to ensure they do not burn, as everyone's oven temperature can vary slightly.
Remove from oven and allow to cool completely.

Can be kept in an airtight container for up to a week - if they last that long!

Dark Chocolate Sugar Free Mini Fudge Bars

Makes 36 bite sized bars

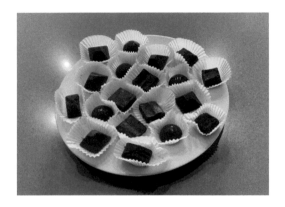

INGREDIENTS

150 grams unsweetened dark chocolate - I use 85% cocoa

50 grams stevia <u>or</u> sweetener of your choice

225 grams salted butter sliced

85 ml double cream

2 teaspoons vanilla extract <u>or</u> vanilla bean paste

METHOD

Line a 20 cm x 20 cm/8" x 8" square tin with either foil or greaseproof paper.

Place all the ingredients into a microwaveable bowl, place into microwave on full heat for 30 second intervals until everything has just melted.

Remove from the microwave, either stir well or give it a quick whisk with a hand whisk, until everything is mixed together and is silky smooth.

Allow mixture to cool slightly, then pour it into the prepared tin.

Place in the fridge for approximately 1 - 2 hours or until the fudge has set.

Remove fudge from tin using the liner as it stops the fudge breaking.

Cut into 36 bite sized bars - I like to serve them cold. These can be stored in an airtight container in the fridge.

Note
I have frozen them, but make sure they are not touching each other. I do this by popping them into mini muffin cases, then placing them in an airtight box in to the freezer.
To be really honest they do not stay around very long, whether in the fridge or the freezer.

Martin's 'Notella' Chocolate and Hazelnut Spread

Makes 500 grams

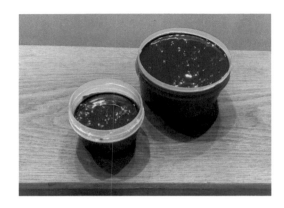

INGREDIENTS

500 grams of skinned hazelnuts (You can buy these already skinned and roasted at Grape Tree)

1½ tablespoons vanilla bean paste or vanilla extract <u>NOT</u> vanilla essence

Small pinch of salt

75 grams of 85% cocoa dark chocolate, broken up into pieces

METHOD

Preheat the oven 200° / Fan 180° / 400° / Gas 6

If the nuts are <u>not roasted</u>, spread out the hazelnuts onto a baking tray and roast them in a preheated oven for 10 minutes.

<u>DON'T</u> let them burn, <u>remember</u> to turn them over halfway during the 10 minutes roasting time.

Leave the nuts to cool.

When they are cold, add all the nuts to a Magimix or blender.

Blend the nuts until they start to form nut butter consistency, about 4 - 5 minutes. Add the pinch of salt, vanilla and chocolate pieces.

Blend again for a couple of minutes, don't worry if all the chocolate has not blended in, as the little chunks are a nice surprise!

Note
We store our nut butter in an airtight container in the fridge, this stops it melting. It is delicious on ice cream, with Greek yogurt, or on flaxseed crackers, to name but a few!

Dark Chocolate Walnut Fat Bombs

Makes 20 - 25

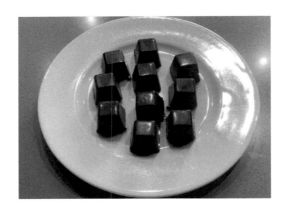

INGREDIENTS
   100 grams 85% cocoa dark chocolate, broken up into small pieces 55 grams coconut oil
   50 grams walnuts, chopped into small pieces
   1 teaspoon cinnamon
   ¼ teaspoon stevia <u>or</u> sweetener of your choice
   1 teaspoon vanilla extract <u>or</u> vanilla bean paste (optional)

METHOD
Prepared all the ingredients as above.

Tip: I chop my walnuts up on a board with a knife - it saves washing my food processor for such a small amount. Remember to save a few of the larger pieces to decorate the tops of your fat bombs.

In a microwaveable bowl, place the chocolate and coconut oil and place in microwave on full power for bursts of 30 seconds at a time, it usually takes 4 bursts.

Next add the walnuts, cinnamon and stevia to the melted chocolate/coconut mixture and, if you are using vanilla extract or bean paste, add this as well. Combine all the ingredients thoroughly.

I use mini ice cube trays and using a spoon I divide the mixture into the individual cubes of the trays. (You can use silicone sweet or chocolate moulds, but I prefer these as there is no arguing in the family about who had the biggest one!)

Place the filled ice cube trays into your freezer for 5 minutes, until the tops have just set. Remove the ice cube trays from your freezer and (if using) place the larger pieces of chopped walnuts which have been saved on the top of the mixture in your ice-cube trays.

Place them in the fridge for approximately 20 minutes or until they have fully set.

Eat and enjoy, they are extremely yummy!

Quick and Easy Brownie Cake

Serves 12

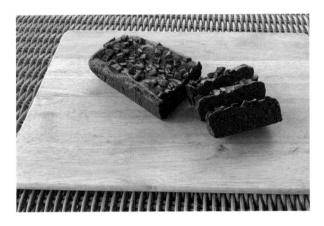

INGREDIENTS

200 grams almond flour

30 grams stevia <u>or</u> sweetener of your choice

30 grams unsweetened cocoa powder

60 grams unsalted butter, melted

30 grams unsweetened chocolate chips 85% cocoa

3 large eggs

1 - 2 tablespoons milk if needed

METHOD

Preheat the oven to 180° / Fan 160° / 350° / Gas 4

Line a 2 lb loaf tin with greaseproof paper or a liner.

Mix all the ingredients, except the chocolate chips in a mixing bowl.

Tip: If the mixture feels too thick, you can add in 1 - 2 tablespoons of milk to loosen its consistency.

Pour mixture into the prepared tin. Sprinkle the chocolate chips on top. Bake for 30 minutes or until a skewer when inserted in centre of the cake comes out almost clean.
Place the cake, still in the loaf tin, onto a cooling rack and leave it to cool. Once it's almost cold remove from the loaf tin.

Slice, serve and enjoy.

Dark Chocolate Ganache

Covers an 18 cm/7 inch sponge cake

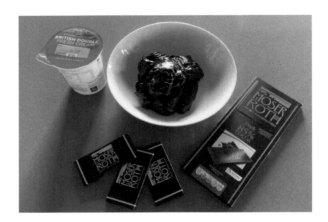

INGREDIENTS

250 ml double cream
170 grams dark chocolate, minimum of 75% cocoa broken up into small pieces

METHOD

Prepare the above ingredients.
Put the cream into a medium size pan and place the pan on a medium heat, until it starts to simmer.
As soon as it starts to simmer remove from the heat!
Stir in all the broken pieces of chocolate, until chocolate has melted and the mixture is nice and smooth.
Allow to cool for a few minutes, stir again, if necessary, until it is nice and smooth. Leave to cool at room temperature prior to using it.
Any leftovers can be stored in an airtight box with a lid either in the fridge for a few days or longer in the freezer.

Almond and Coconut Crumble Mixture
Serves 8

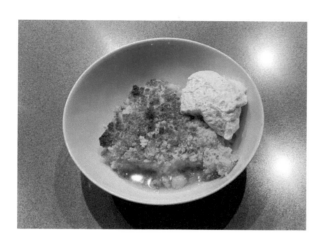

INGREDIENTS

Crumble Mixture
113 grams ground almonds
113 grams coconut flour
1 level teaspoon baking powder
30 grams stevia <u>or</u> sweetener of your choice to taste
150 grams unsalted butter, softened
Pinch of salt

Plus Filling of Your Choice
2 large Bramley apples, peeled, cored, cut into wedges, or
3 'in season' Comice pears, peeled, cored, cut into wedges, or
10 - 12 sticks 'in season' rhubarb, depending on its size, cut into wedges
20 grams stevia <u>or</u> sweetener of your choice to taste

Optional

¼ teaspoon cinnamon can be added to either the Bramley apples / Comice pears, <u>or</u> ¼ teaspoon dried powdered ginger to rhubarb

METHOD

Preheat the oven 180° / Fan 160° / 350° / Gas 4

Base

In a large mixing bowl, mix all the above dry ingredients together.
Add in softened butter, using your fingers to mix all your ingredients until they form a crumbly mixture.

Filling

This can be anything of your choice that falls in line with the fruits found in our 'YES' list. We tend to use Bramley apples, Comice pears, or our home-grown rhubarb when in season.
With the exception of the Comice pears which can be peeled and sliced, we soften the Bramley apples and rhubarb plus some stevia, in the microwave on full heat. We taste when cool for sweetness, you can always add a little more stevia <u>BUT</u> you cannot take it out.
The prepared filling is placed into an ovenproof dish and crumble mixture is loosely spread over the top.

<u>Remember</u>

If you are planning to use this crumble mixture straight away, make sure you have prepared the ovenproof dish by greasing it and putting in your prepared filling before putting on the crumble topping. Level off the crumble topping with the back of a spoon or spatula, but don't press down too hard. Place the dish onto the middle shelf of the preheated oven for 30 - 35 minutes.

Note

If the crumble topping looks like it is starting to burn, cover it with foil, remove the foil in the last 5 minutes of baking, so crumble topping is nice and golden brown.

Serve with double cream, Greek yogurt, crème fraîche or sugar free ice-cream. Enjoy.

WEEKLY ESSENTIALS

Julie's Pastry

Covers top and base of an 18cm/ 7 inch pie dish

<u>Baked pie crusts</u> are ideal for quiches, meat pies, vegetable pies and fruit pies.
Remember this pastry is gluten free, low carb and sugar free.

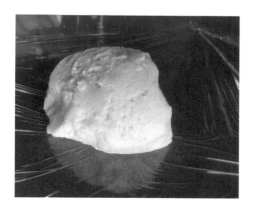 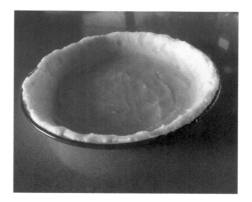

INGREDIENTS
130 grams ground almonds
20 grams almond flour <u>or</u> coconut flour
75 grams melted butter
10 grams stevia

Note
¼ teaspoon of salt instead of stevia if making savoury pies.

METHOD
Preheat the oven 180° / Fan 160° / 350° / Gas 4
Place all the ingredients in a bowl, mix together until everything is combined.
Do not grease the pie dish because as the pie cooks, the natural oils from the almonds will grease the pie dish for you.

Use a third of the pastry mixture for the pie top. Roll it out first between two sheets of clingfilm and return the trimmed off pieces to the remaining mixture to use for the pie base.

Press the remaining dough into the bottom and sides of the pie dish using the palm of your hand.

Using a fork, prick the bottom of the pie dish several times so that the crust can vent whilst cooking, it keeps the crust from bubbling up.

Fill the pastry dish with the filling of your choice.

Place the prepared pie lid on top of the filled pie and press to seal the top of pie to its sides.

Make a couple of slits in the pie top to let the steam out whilst it is cooking.

Cover the edges of the pie crust in foil, to prevent it from burning.

Place the pie on an oven tray.

Place the pie on the middle shelf of the preheated oven for 40 - 50 minutes, or until the pie top is golden brown.

If the centre of the pie starts to burn cover it with more foil.

Remove from the oven, place it on a cooling tray, leave for 20 - 30 minutes to cool before serving.

Note

Sometimes the oil from the ground almonds runs out of the pastry, this is normal and the oven tray prevents it from going all over the oven.

Tip: These pie crusts can be frozen for up to 12 months

All savoury fillings should be precooked and left to cool before using them in your prepared pie dish, this ensures that any meat, chicken or fish are properly cooked.

Sugar Free Lemon Curd

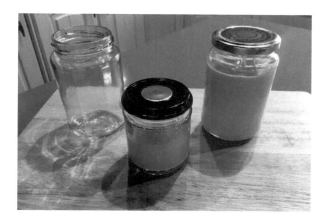

INGREDIENTS

120 grams butter, salted or unsalted
4 lemons, these give approximately 120 ml lemon juice
6 large egg yolks
60 grams stevia or sweetener of your choice / taste

METHOD

To sterilise your jam jars
Preheat the oven to its lowest temperature.
Place the jam jars, plus their lids into the preheated oven on the middle shelf for 20 minutes.

PREPARE THE INGREDIENTS
Place the egg yolks, stevia, and lemon juice in a bowl, whisk until combined and leave on one side.
In a medium sized saucepan, melt the butter over a low heat. Once it has melted remove from the heat, away from the stove.

Pour the egg, stevia and lemon mixture from the bowl into the saucepan, give it a quick whisk and return it to the stove on a low heat.

WHISK the mixture CONTINUOUSLY for a few minutes until it thickens.

Remove from heat and pour the curd mixture into the sterilised jam jars. Put their lids on and leave to cool completely.

Label the jars and store in the fridge.

Once opened it should be kept in the fridge and used within 10 days.

Sugar Free Vanilla Ice Cream

Serves 8

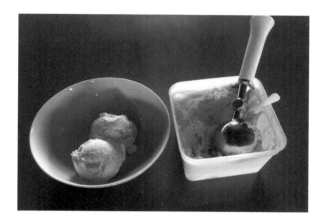

INGREDIENTS

600 ml double cream
2 teaspoons vanilla extract <u>or</u> vanilla bean paste
20 grams stevia <u>or</u> sweetener of your choice to taste

METHOD

Using an ice cream maker

Place all the above ingredients into a large jug and using an electric hand whisk, whisk the ingredients until everything has combined and the mixture is not quite at the soft peak stage.

Pour the mixture from the jug into the ice cream maker, following the manufacturer's instructions.

We like ours on a medium setting so it makes a lovely whipped ice cream. Serve immediately and enjoy.

If there is any ice cream left (<u>NOT</u> in our house ever!), place it in an airtight container and store in the freezer for up to 3 months.

Without an ice cream maker

Make it in exactly the same way, <u>but</u> instead of pouring the mixture into an ice cream maker, pour it into a 1 litre freezer box with a lid. Put the lid on the box and place it into the freezer for approximately 45 minutes. As it begins to freeze around the edges, remove from the freezer and stir it vigorously with either a fork or spatula. Return it to the freezer.

Continue to check the mixture every 30 minutes, stirring vigorously as it is freezing. Repeat this process for 2 to 3 hours or until frozen.

Tip: If you have a hand held mixer, you could use this.

Variations

Swap the double cream for full fat Greek yogurt, using exactly the same quantities. This is absolutely delicious and you can always add in berries and chocolate chips. Experiment to find your own favourite additions and flavours.

Note

Remember to take the ice cream out of the freezer at least an hour before you wish to serve it so it reaches room temperature.

Serve and enjoy.

Martin's Tandoori Spice Paste/Marinade

Serves 4 - 6

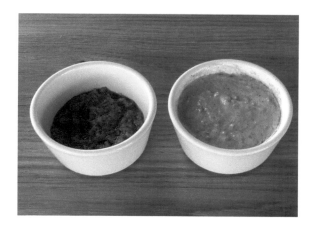

INGREDIENTS

4 large garlic cloves, peeled, crushed <u>or</u> grated
2 tablespoons lemon juice
15 grams fresh ginger, peeled and grated
½ - ¾ teaspoon red chilli powder
½ teaspoon sweet paprika
1 heaped teaspoon ground cumin
1 heaped teaspoon garam masala
1 teaspoon salt
1 tablespoon refined olive oil
¼ teaspoon ground turmeric
1 tablespoon ground coriander

METHOD

Place all the ingredients from the list above into a medium sized bowl. Using a spoon mix all these ingredients until they are all well combined.

To save time, all the above ingredients can be placed into a mini food processor and blitzed until smooth, however, we like the coarser consistency resulting from doing it manually.

Note
At this stage the tandoori paste can be kept in an airtight jar in the fridge indefinitely.

Tip: We use this paste to rub into raw chicken and other meats prior to roasting them in the oven.

Marinade for Tandoori Chicken, Meat, Fish or Vegetables.

Serves 4 - 6

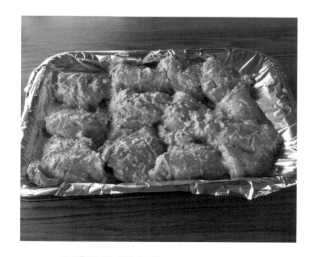 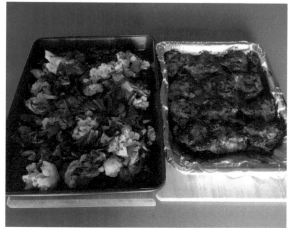

INGREDIENTS

120 grams full fat Greek set yogurt
Martin's Tandoori Spice Paste as shown above

METHOD

If making the marinade straight away, add the yogurt to the prepared tandoori spice paste in a medium bowl and mix well with a spoon until well combined. Add skinned chicken, meat, fish or vegetables to the marinade, cover the bowl with clingfilm and put in the fridge until required. Try and leave the bone in any meat used as this adds flavour to the meat.

Cook as per Tandoori Chicken recipe that can be found in the 'Dinners Section' of this book.

Kebab Dressing/Marinade

Serves 2

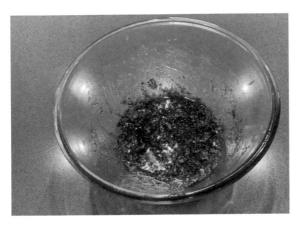 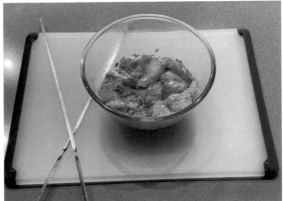

INGREDIENTS

2 tablespoons extra virgin olive oil
I teaspoon cumin
I teaspoon dried thyme
¼ teaspoon cinnamon
I clove garlic, peeled and crushed Juice of ½ lemon
Salt and pepper to taste

METHOD

Mix all the above ingredients in a bowl.
This can be used straight away or stored in the fridge until later, remember to stir it again before use.
The mixture can be used as a marinade for meat, fish or vegetables, or just brushed on them during the cooking process.

Cook as per Chicken Kebabs recipe that can be found in the 'Dinners Section' of this book.

Salad Oil Dressing

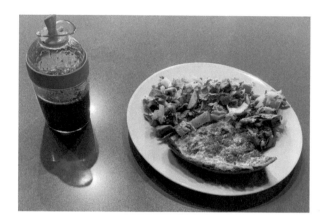

INGREDIENTS

75 ml extra virgin olive oil

75 ml balsamic vinegar or cider vinegar or white or red wine vinegar, or any vinegar of your choice, except pickling or malt vinegar

The above two ingredients can be doubled up in equal parts, 50% oil, 50% vinegar, in order to make larger quantities and the remaining ingredients (as below) can then be increased or adjusted, but not necessarily doubled up, according to your own individual tastes.

I teaspoon English mustard powder

I teaspoon mixed dried herbs or dried herbs of your choice e.g. oregano, thyme, etc. Fresh herbs can be used, but they need chopping up very small before adding to the salad dressing container.

½ - I teaspoon stevia or sweetener of your choice

Salt and pepper to taste.

OPTIONAL
Juice of ½ lemon

METHOD
We use an 'Oxo good grip' mini or large salad shaker, to mix our dressings but you can use any bottle or container that has an air tight lid.

(Otherwise you can combine all the ingredients in a measuring jug, then use a mini whisk to combine all the ingredients thoroughly.)

Mix together all the above ingredients, whisk/shake them thoroughly depending which method you prefer to use, until they are all well combined, emulsified and the vinegar and oil are no longer separated.

Note
If the salad dressing is not used straight away, the oil and vinegar will separate, it will need whisking/shaking again before using it.

Drizzle on salads, steamed or sautéed vegetables.

The salad dressing can be stored in the fridge until it has all been used up.

Tahini Dressing

Makes 250 millilitres

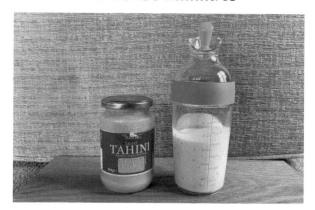

INGREDIENTS

65 grams tahini
Juice of a lemon
2 tablespoons extra virgin olive oil
1 small clove garlic, peeled and crushed/grated
Pinch of salt
Water

METHOD

Place all the above ingredients, except the water, in a small mixing bowl and mix them together until everything is well combined.

Add the water a little at a time and continue mixing until it forms a paste/dressing of the required consistency.

Note

This dressing can be enjoyed with crudities, or used to dress salads, or drizzled over cooked vegetables.

If you want to use it as a dip for veggies etc. add less water.

It can be stored for up to 2 weeks in an airtight container in the fridge. This is one of our favourite dressings as it is so versatile and tasty.

Chapter 20:
Recipe Successes and Disasters!

Over the last two and half years, whilst completely changing our lifestyles and eating habits, we've constantly been trying to come up with new recipes that include the foods we now eat. This is in order to prove that food can still be really healthy, but also really tasty as well. It is possible to still eat plenty of the right sort of food and lose weight as well.

We often comment that what we are eating now really doesn't feel like any type of 'restricted' diet. That was one of the reasons that inspired us to write 'Losing It' and include pictures of our meals. Along the way we've tried to adapt 'traditional' recipes, but using only ingredients from our compliant foods. Some of these recipes have been great successes, others have been total disasters.

Thanks to Julie's skills in the baking department, our cake, dessert and treat recipes have been enormous successes with everyone. They have all been adapted from the use of traditional flours, sugar and normal baking ingredients, to fit in with our programme.

Likewise, the main course dishes have been adapted by myself, omitting starchy carbs, thickeners, sugar and again, only contain ingredients from our 'Yes' list of foods.

We've tried to adapt recipes like pizza, jams, and marmalade and although they have worked to an extent, they either haven't been very good adaptations or the end results weren't worth the initial effort.

Our latest idea was to come up with a recipe for a compliant bread, however, because we haven't eaten a slice of bread for two and a half years, we thought it was probably not worth the effort. We don't eat meals that we feel would benefit from the addition of bread any more. We do have some recipes worked out for bread, but haven't included them in this book.

Our message here though, is, experiment with the foods you can eat. Use your imagination to come up with your own concoctions. One of the things we have found out is, if you use food from our 'Yes' list, most of the results are edible, even if they don't look particularly appetising!!

Don't be afraid to contact us via our Website and Social Media Pages for advice and to share your own success stories regarding recipes. If you've got this far with us, you'll know that we are in the same boat as everyone else and any advice, opinions and suggestions are greatly welcomed by us and the others involved with us.

Chapter 21:
Daily Diary Example

Below is a template of our daily food diary. Please feel free to photocopy this to complete yourselves, or alternatively, make and complete your own.

Also below is an excerpt from our diary. It has been absolutely essential for us to be able to refer back to it over the past two and a half years.

It's reminded us to keep on track and has also been great for looking back in order to eliminate any foods that have had a negative or bad reaction on our progress. We're sure you will all find yours helpful as well.

Incidentally, we have kept ours even whilst on holiday. 'A bit over the top' I hear you say, but no, it really isn't. It's been both essential and a godsend.

Make sure you include the weights of your protein, i.e.: meat, fish and cheese. Endeavour to keep within your protein limits. Remember, only 25 grams of cheese a day and 100 grams of meat or fish at any one serving. Depending how big your hands are, a handful of mixed nuts is between 30-50 grams, so keep an eye on how much you grab for your snacks.

Daily Diary example

Day and Date	
Breakfast	
Lunch	
Snack	
Dinner (including dessert)	
Treats*	

* (We would include our 1 oz of dark chocolate here.)

Additional information, notes and observations from that day.

Example of an entry in our diary.

Breakfast	Fasted
Lunch	50 grams home made Greek yogurt 20 grams home made nut butter 30 grams mixed toasted nuts 10 grams 85% dark chocolate chips
Snack	1oz 85% dark chocolate
Dinner (including dessert)	Quarter of home made cheese and onion pie Celeriac chips Sautéed asparagus and mushrooms
Treats	None

Observations.

We've been experimenting with some new recipes for a couple of months now and found our weight had gone up a couple of pounds, so back to basics for a while to get back on track.

We look through our diary on a regular basis to check we are keeping on track with our weight. We never want to go back to being overweight and unhealthy again. It's just like checking your bank balance really. You need to keep checking that you're in credit and not overdrawn. It is the same with your weight and health. Keep it in credit at all times and regularly review your status and be ready to make a few small adjustments. Keeping the diary makes it so much easier to do this.

One of the things we have recently noticed is, two and a half years ago we could eat certain foods and they would make no noticeable difference to our 'gut', bodies or weight. Two and a half years down the line and that situation appears to have changed somewhat.

We definitely can't eat anywhere near as much as we used to and if we do have a period of eating a bit too much, our weight does seem to slowly creep back on again.

Certain foods don't seem to suit us anymore. I have already mentioned beef and lamb! This is why it's important to keep a diary. Because we each eat the same every day and we pretty much have the same reactions to the food we eat, we just keep one between us, or at least Julie does!

If you and your partner, friend, child or whoever you're doing your programme with is eating differently, then it's important to keep your own diary. Make sure it's accurate and honest. It is no good keeping one that isn't a true record of everything you've eaten.

Just make sure you supply your gut with the best food you can, what suits you best and what makes you feel good.

Chapter 22:
Our Vision for the Future

Our vision for the future is actually, first and foremost, to ensure we stay slim and continue with **our** healthy lives. We want to be able to live the rest of our lives carefree and not tied down by being overweight, unhealthy and forever at the doctor's surgery with weight-related illnesses and ailments. We want to enjoy the rest of our lives, debt free, stress free, healthy and slim.

Well, we are actually there now! Obviously we are realistic to the fact that problems can crop up at any time and place, however, we are now in a place where those sort of situations and problems feel very much easier to deal with.

We are hoping that our books will inspire and help others achieve the same healthy lifestyles and outlook that we both now have.

We want to help people via our Social Media Sites and Website and we welcome interaction from those people who have been kind enough to purchase our books.

We are not authors or experts in nutrition, but just two ordinary people who, through a little self-determination, have completely changed their lives by making a few little everyday changes.

You can do this yourselves if you really want the same results.

In the future we are aiming to set up 'workshops' around the country where we can share our experiences and experiments with other people who have found themselves in the same situation we found ourselves in. These 'workshops' will not only consist of a talk/discussion with us, but also include food tasting using recipes from our books.

The 'workshops' will not be like the usual 'slimming clubs' where there is a membership fee etc. Our vision is that we can help and inspire you to lose your weight, become healthy and then continue like that without having to become lifelong members of those clubs who, in our opinion, are the only ones who benefit.

Chapter 23:
Our Final Parting Words for Now!

Our Final Parting Words

IF YOU HAVE GOT THIS FAR THEN YOU HAVE READ ALL ABOUT OUR INCREDIBLE JOURNEY AND CONTINUING HEALTHY LIFESTYLE

We hope you have tried some of our recipes as well as experimented with a few of your own favourite family versions. Remember to share your recipes and experiments with us and everyone else via our Social Media and Websites.

By now you will feel like us: "A Million Dollars". Although that is probably an understatement.

<u>**Definitely**</u> healthier, loads more energy, less stressed, sleeping better, toned up, younger looking!

Wouldn't it be great if we could bottle these feelings and SPRINKLE them onto our loved ones, friends and doubting Thomas's, so they all could experience the same benefits we now enjoy!

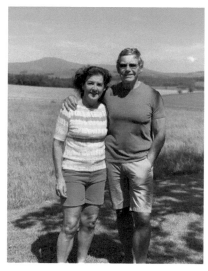

Julie and Martin Carrick.
June 2020

KEEP UP THE GOOD WORK and ENJOY <u>**YOUR**</u> LIFE, IT IS REALLY WORTH IT!!

REMEMBER IT'S NOT WHAT YOU EAT **BUT** WHAT YOU **DON'T** EAT THAT MATTERS!

Acknowledgments and Thanks

We would like to thank Apple, and in particular their store in Leeds, for giving us the advice, confidence and inspiration to begin, continue and finish our first book. Without Ross, Ian, Rachel and Dan, we would still be just playing solitaire on our iPads, never mind writing this, our second book. They are truly very knowledgeable about the products they sell and how they can be used to their full potential. We found them very inspirational.

A big thank you to Booths Supermarkets and Grape Tree health food stores. Firstly because of their valiant services provided during the recent Covid-19 pandemic.

Absolutely outstanding.

Likewise to Lakeland, who continued to provide an excellent online service throughout the pandemic. Secondly for their support, and permission allowing us to promote our book on their premises.

Another thank you to us for our patience and understanding with each other, which at times was testing, especially during the pandemic lockdown when DIY jobs and taking advantage of the lovely weather got the better of writing this book!

Thanks to all our friends who again spurred us on to writing a sequel to our first book. These thanks are also for the Doubting Thomas's who told us we were wasting our time.

Thanks again to Catherine and her team at 2QT, Settle, for her patience and understanding.

Finally, a huge thank you to Kitty, our social media advisor!

Where would we have been without her patience with two oldies who are really only just getting to grips with texting!

Here we are now making videos, writing blogs and hashtags!

Thanks also to her Mum and Dad for allowing her to give us all the time she gave us and for being our main Guinea pigs.

About the Authors

Julie and Martin Carrick are down to earth Yorkshire people. They are both originally from Sheffield and now reside in the Yorkshire Dales near Settle. They have two grown up boys, who are both married.

Julie and Martin are both former Police Officers and are now retired.

Neither of them are writers, authors or experts on nutrition. They are just ordinary folk who have a passion for life and an even greater passion for food and cooking.

They are both keen motorcyclists and can be often found on the roads around the Dales and the Lake District, as well as venturing across the water into other parts of Europe, usually in search of some sun! Talking of sun, they travel a fair bit and enjoy trying the local food wherever they find themselves.

This book shares their journey on a completely different eating experience than they were accustomed to previously, in an effort to lose weight and become healthier.

They've certainly achieved great success and believe that other people will be very interested in achieving and sharing that same success!

Now is the time for you to join them on their journey to better health and longevity.

Index for Recipes

Side Dishes and Accompaniments

Dessert

THE
FLOWER
GARDEN

LAURENCE KING

Published in 2019 by
Laurence King Publishing Ltd
361–373 City Road
London
EC1V 1LR
United Kingdom
T + 44 (0)20 7841 6900
F + 44 (0)20 7841 6910
enquiries@laurenceking.com
www.laurenceking.com

A catalogue record for this book is available
from the British Library.

ISBN: 978-1-78627-409-0

Printed in China

Front cover: Cosmos and *Ammi* in a meadow
Back cover: Cosmos, zinnias, dill and California
poppies
Page 10: The columbine *Aquilegia* x *hybrida*
'MacKana Giant'
Page 164: Lupin seeds four days after germination
Page 180: Zinnias and marigolds in a cutting garden

THE
FLOWER
GARDEN

How to grow
flowers from seed

Clare Foster & Sabina Rüber

Laurence King Publishing

Contents

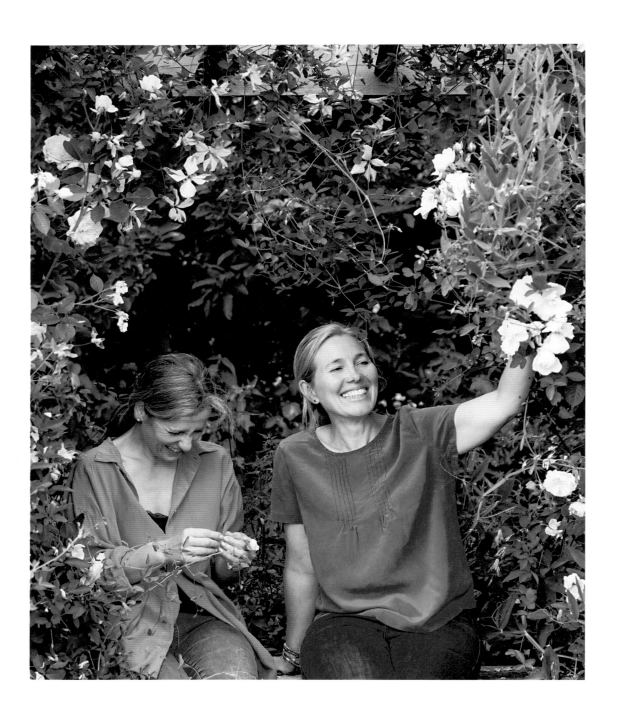

Introduction

In 2012 photographer Sabina and I started a project: to grow as many annual flowers from seed as we could. We soon realized that there was an enormous and exciting range of plants that were cheap, quick and often amazingly easy to grow in this way – not only annual flowers, but also perennials, ornamental grasses and herbs. That first year, though initially full of hope and excitement, was – quite literally – a wash-out, as it was the wettest spring for decades. I was growing flowers on my allotment and most of my seedlings were washed away, then re-sown, only to be deluged once again. The following year I moved house and was in transition for a while. That meant no growing for me, but Sabina was forging ahead with our plan.

I wasn't ready to give up, however, and I was inspired by all the beautiful photographs Sabina was taking of her home-grown flowers. In 2013 I inherited a greenhouse. Suddenly I was able to grow much more, including the half-hardy and more exotic flowers that needed extra protection in spring. That same year I made a new cutting patch, which I filled almost entirely with plants I had raised from seed. Rather than buying expensive perennials at £7 a pop, or trays of bedding plants, I had spent a few pounds on packets of seed that would produce many plants almost for free.

I was hooked, and as soon as you start growing flowers from seed, you'll feel the same. There is nothing more satisfying than planting a tiny seed in spring and watching it emerge and grow. As you become more experienced, you'll find that it isn't as daunting as you might have once thought. Yes, the weather and other challenges such as slugs, snails and mice will make you despair at times, but when it boils down to it, most seeds want to grow for you – that is what they're programmed to do. Sabina and I have found that there is usually no exact science for growing from seed and that trial and error is the best way of learning. One person's method for germinating larkspur might not work for someone else, who has a different set of conditions to work with, since weather, temperature, compost quality, seed freshness and a host of other circumstances will affect both germination and how that particular seedling grows. Once you accept this, you can have a huge amount of fun experimenting. Most of the plants in this book are annuals, which flower later in the year they are sown, or perennials that should also flower in the first year. We want instant gratification and a flower border or cut-flower patch that will look full and glorious by mid to late summer.

In this book, we have divided the flowers according to type or purpose. First come the traditional Cottage Garden Favourites, from airy love-in-a-mist to statuesque hollyhocks. The group most often associated with flowers grown from seed, these relaxed, informal plants give the garden a soft, romantic feel, and many will self-seed and reappear year after year like old friends.

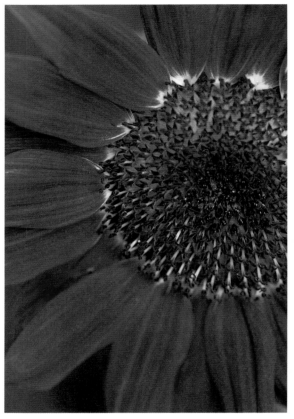

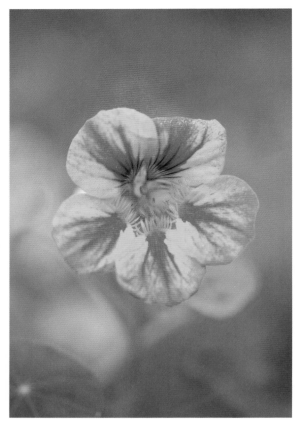

Helianthus annuus 'Chocolate'

Tropaeolum majus

In 'Filigree Fillers' we suggest some understated filler plants to enhance a summer border, colonizing unsightly bare patches to give the garden a more fluid look. Typically these filler plants have small white flowers, often in the cow parsley family, but they also come in subtle, pretty pastel shades.

The next section, 'Bold and Beautiful', contains many plants that provide a hit of summer colour, quickly producing an astonishing kaleidoscope of hues to bring a smile to your face.

Flowers and plants should appeal to all the senses, and no garden is complete without a few deliciously scented flowers, as described in the fourth section, 'Sweetly Scented'. Plant some

in pots around your back door, so the perfume wafts in as you enter the house.

'Exotic Beauties' contains plants that add glamour to the garden, their brightly coloured blooms and lush foliage giving an opulent feel. Since most of these plants are tender, it will help if you have a greenhouse or conservatory to start them off in.

In the sixth section we suggest some herbs, as well as edible flowers, which are becoming increasingly popular; they add subtle flavour and a Michelin-starred look to both sweet and savoury dishes and drinks.

Finally – but perhaps most importantly – we feature some species to help in the

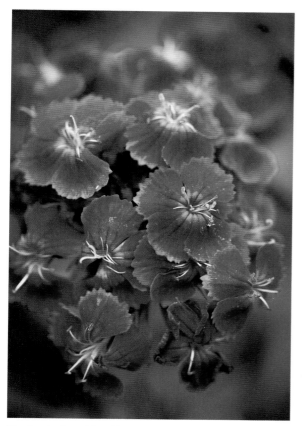

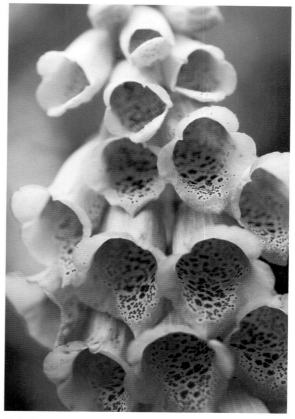

Dianthus barbatus 'Oeschberg'

Digitalis purpurea

attempt to reverse the sad decline of bees and other beneficial insects in our gardens. Most of the flowers grown from seed appeal to bees, especially single, nectar-rich blooms, but here we select a few that will attract them in droves.

If you're new to this game, stick to the easiest plants, marked with ✻ throughout the book. Generally these are the hardiest, toughest, quickest-to-grow flowers, and you won't need a greenhouse for them. If you want to get into growing the half-hardies, such as cosmos and zinnias, you may need to invest in a mini-greenhouse or cold frame, since they will need added protection in the spring before it's warm enough to plant them out. But whatever your aspirations, we hope you'll give it

a go. We want to demystify the process of growing from seed and open your eyes to the range and sheer beauty of the plants you can grow in this way.

Throughout the book we use both common names (such as poppy or sunflower) and botanical Latin names. The Latin names are made up of the genus or family name (*Helianthus*); the species, which appears after the genus (*Helianthus annuus*); and if appropriate the cultivar or variety name, which comes last (*Helianthus annuus* 'Chocolate'). The cultivar names are often the distinguishing note of each plant, and if you are searching for them online or in a catalogue, this is the name you'll need.

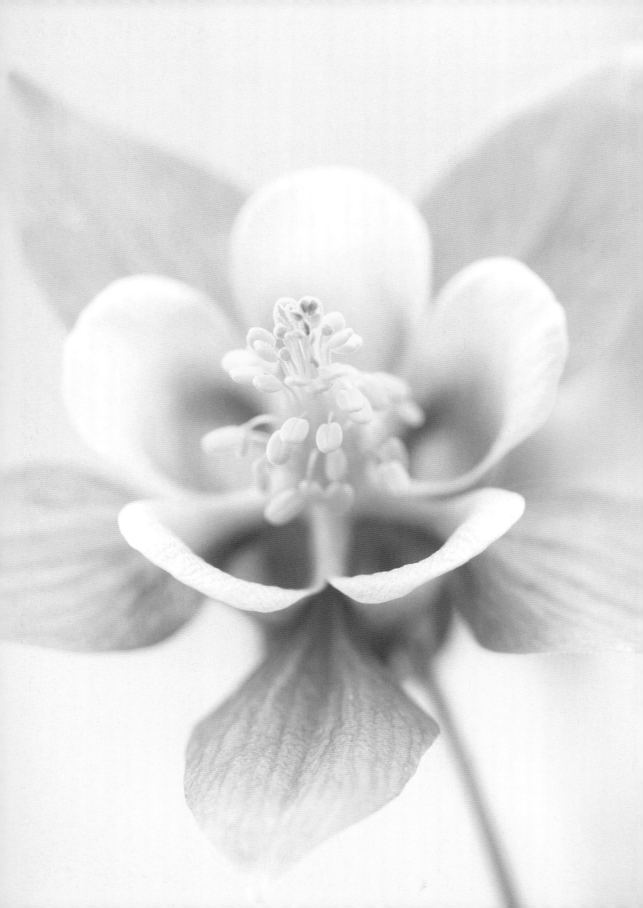

Part I

Choosing your flowers

Cottage Garden Favourites, Filigree Fillers, Bold and Beautiful,
Sweetly Scented, Exotic Beauties, Edible Flowers and Herbs,
Bee-Friendly Flowers

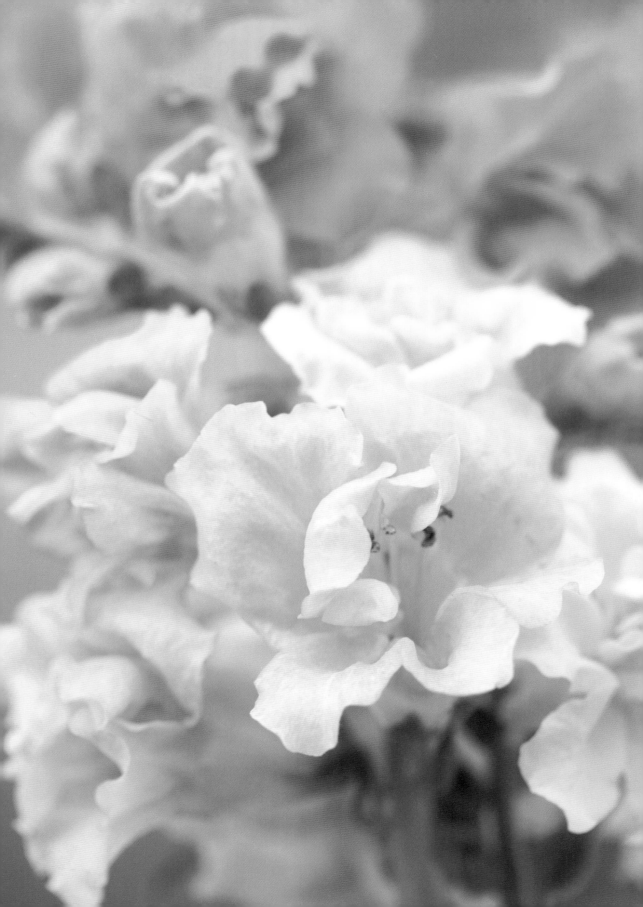

Cottage Garden Favourites

Hollyhock (*Alcea rosea*)

Snapdragon (*Antirrhinum*)

Columbine (*Aquilegia*)

Larkspur (*Consolida*)

Sweet william, carnation and pinks (*Dianthus*)

Foxglove (*Digitalis*)

Wallflower (*Erysimum*)

Honesty (*Lunaria annua*)

Lupin (*Lupinus*)

Love-in-a-mist (*Nigella*)

Poppy (*Papaver*)

Annual phlox (*Phlox drummondii*)

Scabious (*Scabiosa atropurpurea*)

Antirrhinum majus
'Madame Butterfly'

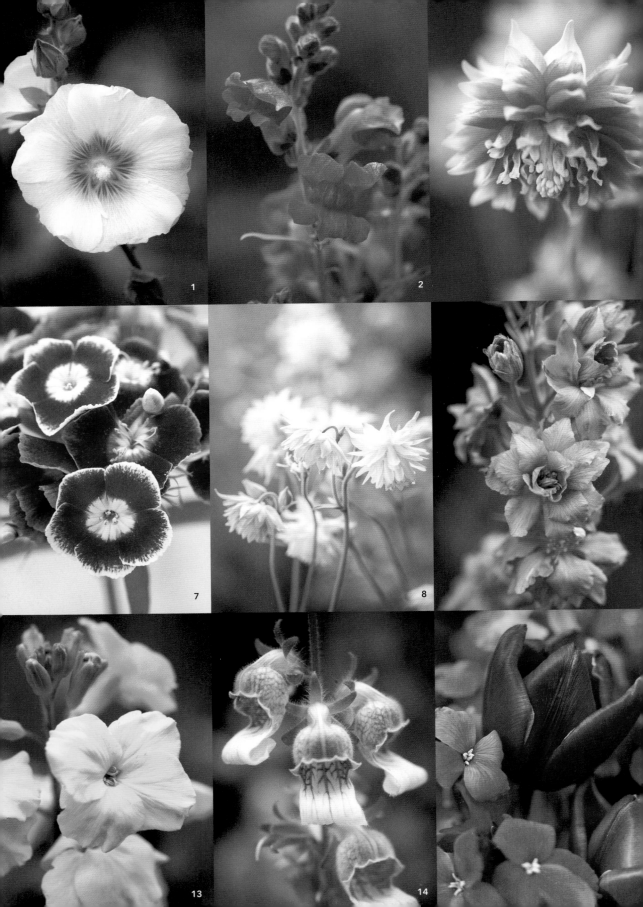

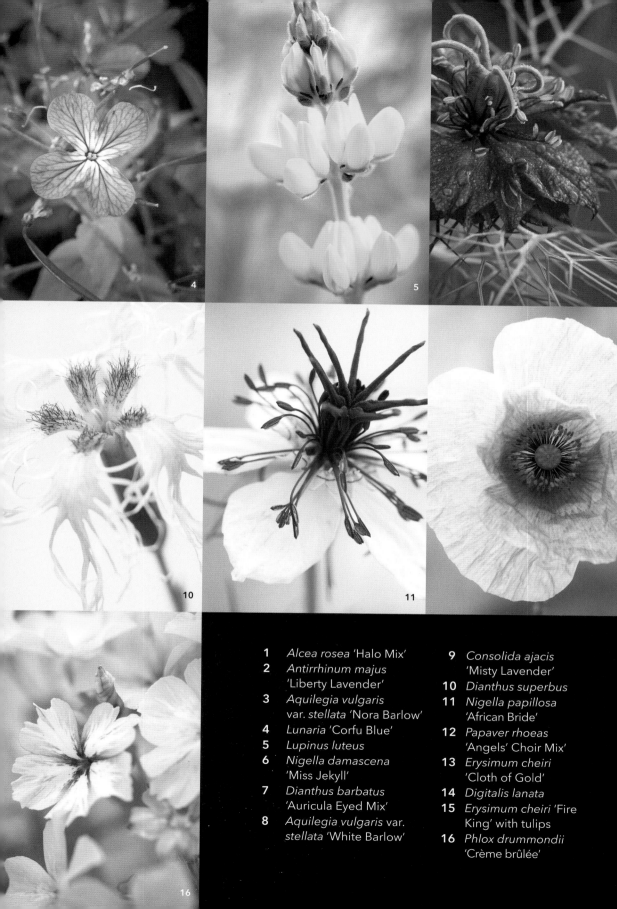

1 *Alcea rosea* 'Halo Mix'
2 *Antirrhinum majus* 'Liberty Lavender'
3 *Aquilegia vulgaris* var. *stellata* 'Nora Barlow'
4 *Lunaria* 'Corfu Blue'
5 *Lupinus luteus*
6 *Nigella damascena* 'Miss Jekyll'
7 *Dianthus barbatus* 'Auricula Eyed Mix'
8 *Aquilegia vulgaris* var. *stellata* 'White Barlow'
9 *Consolida ajacis* 'Misty Lavender'
10 *Dianthus superbus*
11 *Nigella papillosa* 'African Bride'
12 *Papaver rhoeas* 'Angels' Choir Mix'
13 *Erysimum cheiri* 'Cloth of Gold'
14 *Digitalis lanata*
15 *Erysimum cheiri* 'Fire King' with tulips
16 *Phlox drummondii* 'Crème brûlée'

Hollyhock (*Alcea rosea*)

- Short-lived perennial
- Height: 1.5–2.5 m
- Sow: under cover in spring or direct in late summer or early autumn
- Site: sun, well-drained soil
- Flowers: mid to late summer

No cottage garden is complete without a bright, blowsy hollyhock or two – but you may be surprised to learn that this quintessentially 'English' plant has exotic origins. It has been popular in British gardens since being introduced from Turkey and the Middle East in the sixteenth century, and is easily grown from seed to produce the sturdy, statuesque plants that peep over many a garden wall in summer. There are hollyhocks to suit every colour scheme, from darkest plummy purple to lemon yellow and creamy white, and the flowers can be single or double – although, as with many flowers, the doubles aren't as good for attracting pollinating insects, since they contain less pollen.

If you're sowing in spring, sow the large seeds into individual modules of compost, germinating them at 16–18°C before potting them on throughout the growing season. You can plant them out in the summer (knowing that they probably won't flower that year) or keep potting them on, over-wintering them in a cold frame before planting them out in spring. They are generally unfussy about the soil they grow in, as long as it is well-drained, and they often seed themselves in the most unpromising places, in cracks between paving or at the base of a wall. The only downside to growing hollyhocks is that they are prone to fungal rust, which appears as raised, reddish spots on the leaves (see page 179).

Varieties
The 'Halo' seed mixtures are lovely, with single flowers in a range of pastel colours with a darker eye, and they are also available in single colours. 'Black Knight' is a favourite, with glossy, almost black flowers, while 'Crème de Cassis' is similarly dark, with single and semi-double flowers on the same stem. The fig-leaf hollyhock, *Alcea ficifolia*, and related seed mixes such as 'Antwerp Mix' are also worth growing.

Sowing and growing
Sow hollyhock seed under cover in spring, or direct in late summer or early autumn. Whichever you choose, be aware that, like a biennial, the plant is unlikely to flower strongly, if at all, in the first year.

Hollyhocks need an open, sunny spot where they can stretch up towards the light.

1 'Halo Mix'
2 'Black Knight'
3 'Crème de Cassis'
4 'Antwerp Mix'

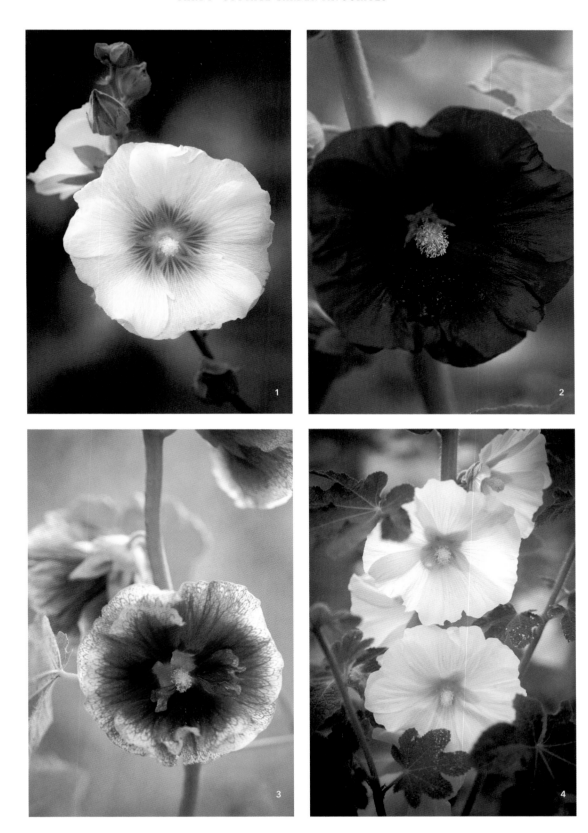

Snapdragon (*Antirrhinum*)

- Half-hardy annual
- Height: 30–100 cm
- Sow: under cover in mid spring
- Site: sun, any soil
- Flowers: late summer to autumn

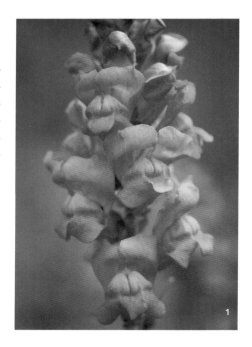

Snapdragons bring cheerful colour to the garden in late summer. The botanical name derives from the Greek *anti* (like) and *rhinum* (snout), and it's easy to see why from the individual blooms. These southern European flowers have been grown in Britain since Roman times and were especially popular with Victorian gardeners, who developed gaudy stripy and bi-coloured forms, some of which have recently been resurrected. For some, this brashness is just too much, and if subtlety is required, the single-colour strains, which form graceful spires, are worth tracking down. They are good candidates for containers, and are excellent for cutting, lasting for well over a week in the vase.

Varieties

You can't go wrong with the plain-but-beautiful F1 varieties 'Liberty Crimson', 'Liberty Lavender' and 'Admiral White', all of which grow to about 1 m. Older cultivars recently reintroduced include the luscious 'Crimson Velvet', antique pink 'The Rose' and pink and apricot 'Appleblossom', and all have good old-fashioned charm. For flower-arranging, the 'Potomac' series is very good, with tall, strong stems and multiple flowers in a range of colours. If you want shorter flower heads, for a container perhaps, choose a variety such as the velvety-purple 'Black Prince' or 'Night and Day', which has deep red-purple flowers with white throats. Both grow to about 45 cm.

The emerging seedlings are prone to damping off, so don't overwater them in the early stages of their life.

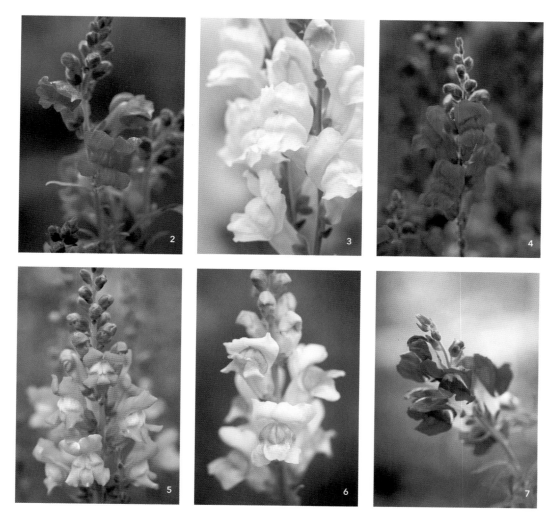

Sowing and growing

Snapdragons are half-hardy annuals, so they should be sown under cover in mid spring. The tiny seeds are best sown in a small seed tray. Start them off on a warm windowsill at 20–23°C, where they will germinate readily within days, and prick them out into modules or 7 cm pots when the seedlings are big enough to handle. You may need to pot them on as they grow, and it's best to keep them under cover until it is warm enough to start hardening them off, before planting them out in early summer.

1 'Potomac Orange'
2 'Liberty Lavender'
3 'Admiral White'
4 'Crimson Velvet'
5 'The Rose'
6 'Appleblossom'
7 'Night and Day'

Columbine (*Aquilegia*)

- Short-lived perennial/biennial
- Height: 50–80 cm
- Sow: under cover in spring or direct in early summer
- Site: any reasonable soil in dappled shade
- Flowers: late spring to early summer

These characterful spring flowers bloom at a time when other flowers are in short supply. Strictly short-lived perennials, they flower the second year, so can be treated as biennials. The botanical name comes from the Latin *aquila* (eagle), as the flowers' spur-shaped petals were thought to resemble eagle's claws. In the UK, *Aquilegia vulgaris* is the species from which most plants derive, but the family is diverse, and there are many different species across the globe. In North America, species include the white and mauve *A. caerulea*, the official state flower of Colorado, and *A. canadensis,* which has quirky red-and-yellow flowers.

Varieties

The many forms of *A. vulgaris* cross-fertilize readily to produce weird and wonderful crosses, so if you want the purity of a single strain, make sure you plant one type only. Of the *A. vulgaris* relatives, 'Nora Barlow', named after Charles Darwin's granddaughter, is one of the best-loved, with double, spurless blooms in deep pink with creamy tips. In the same series, you can find black, pink, blue and white Barlows, while the cultivar 'Greenapples' has similar nodding, double flowers that emerge lime green, open to pale apple green and fade to white. *A. viridiflora* is more unusual, a beautiful Asian species with delicate, bell-like greenish-brown flowers.

1 *A. viridiflora*

Aquilegias need light to germinate, so sow the seeds on the top of the compost or cover them very lightly with vermiculite.

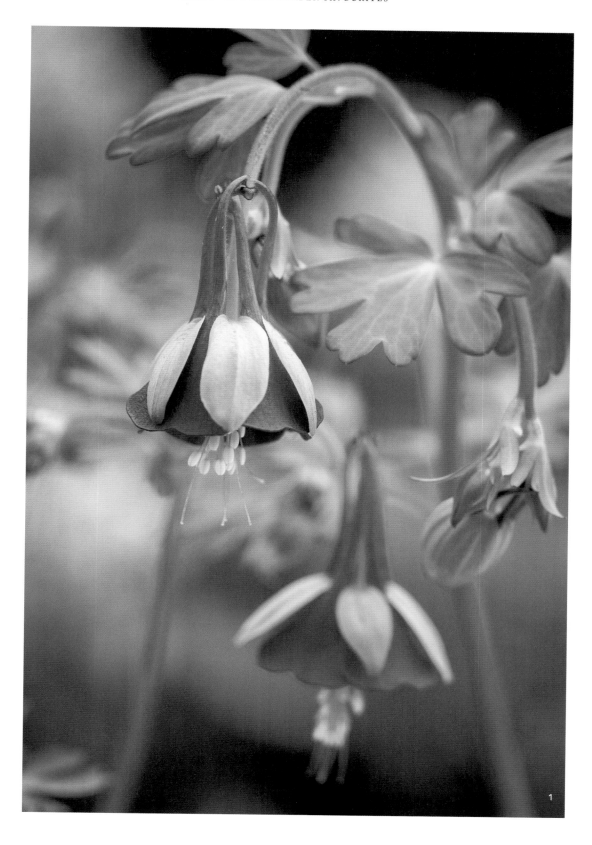

1

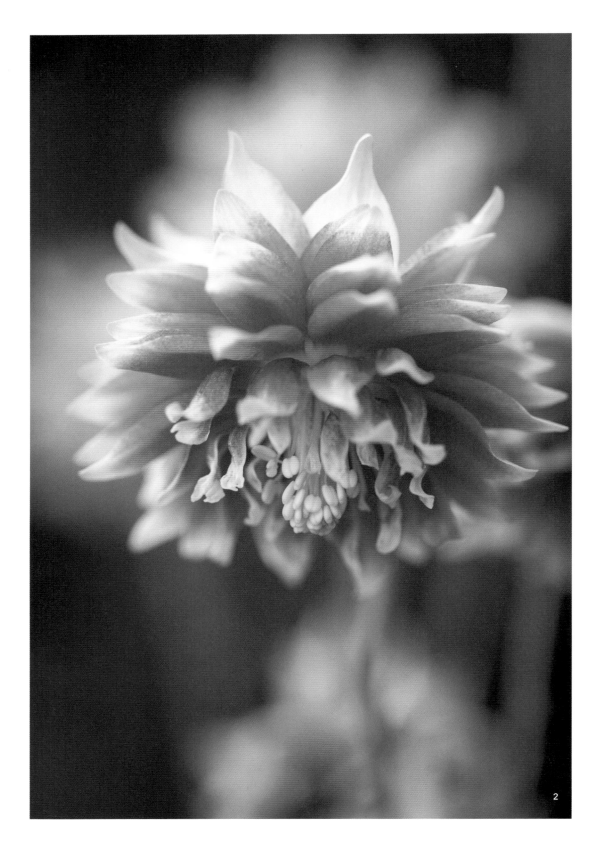

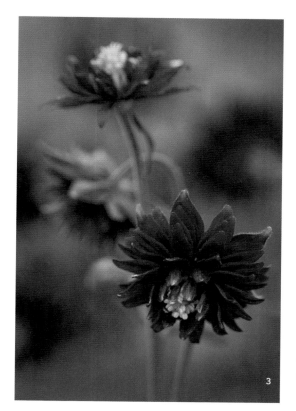

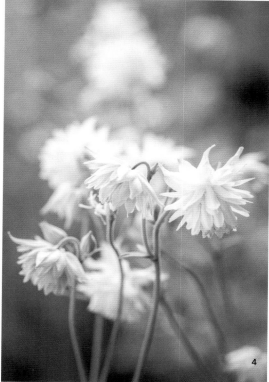

Sowing and growing

Most *aquilegias* grow best in dappled shade in a good loamy soil. Despite self-seeding with abandon once established, they can be oddly temperamental to grow from seed, especially if the seed isn't fresh, and sometimes need a period of cold before they germinate. Once rooted, though, most are unfussy and easy-going. Perhaps the best way to sow the seed is when it is fresh in late spring or early summer, direct into the soil; it will germinate the following spring and flower later that year. You can also sow under cover in spring: sow thinly on top of moist compost in seed trays at 18–20°C, moving to a cooler place once it has germinated. Grow the plants on throughout the summer and plant out in September to flower the following year.

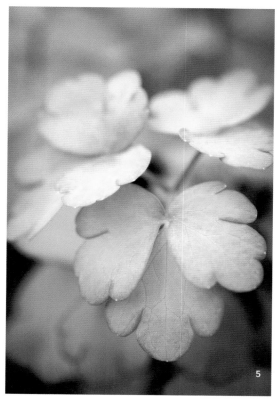

2 'Nora Barlow'
3 'Black Barlow'
4 'White Barlow'
5 'Sunburst Ruby'

Larkspur (*Consolida*)

- Hardy annual
- Height: 60–100 cm
- Sow: direct in late summer or under cover in early spring
- Site: full sun and rich, fertile soil
- Flowers: midsummer to autumn

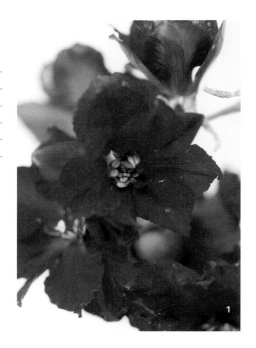

Larkspur is a widely used common name that covers the perennial *Delphinium* as well as the annual *Consolida* family, and it is the latter that we cover here, as they are easily grown from seed to flower in the same year. Representing fickleness in Victorian times, larkspurs are wonderful, willowy plants in colours that range from sky blue and rose pink to pure white, slightly more relaxed and delicate than their *Delphinium* cousins.

Varieties

For cut flowers, choose the more traditional, densely flowered types of *C. ajacis* (also known as *C. ambigua*) in the 'Giant Imperial' group, which have rather stiff spikes of double flowers, and are available in seed mixes with a range of colours. If you like to know exactly what colours you are growing, single varieties such as 'White King' and 'Dark Blue' are available. Moving away from these traditional *Delphinium* colours, 'Misty Lavender' has flowers in a dusky, antique pinky-grey. Even more delicate are forms of *C. regalis*, branching, bushy plants with graceful single flowers that float in the breeze. 'Blue Cloud' and 'Snow Cloud' are most widely available, and, as their names suggest, they grow into billowing clouds with which other plants can mingle.

Sowing and growing

In our experience, larkspurs aren't the easiest plants to raise from seed, and germination can be hit-and-miss. The easiest way is to sow them direct in late summer, leaving the seeds to their own devices to overwinter and germinate in spring. But if you prefer to sow them under cover, give the seeds a couple of weeks in the fridge before sowing them in a seed tray in early spring. Sow on the surface of the compost and cover lightly with vermiculite, germinating them in a cool greenhouse at 16–18°C. Plant out into soil that has been well prepared in advance with well-rotted compost or manure.

1 'Dark Blue'
2 'White King'
3 'Misty Lavender'
4 'Blue Cloud'
5 'Snow Cloud'

Larkspurs are cool-climate plants that will benefit from a period of cold if they are to germinate.

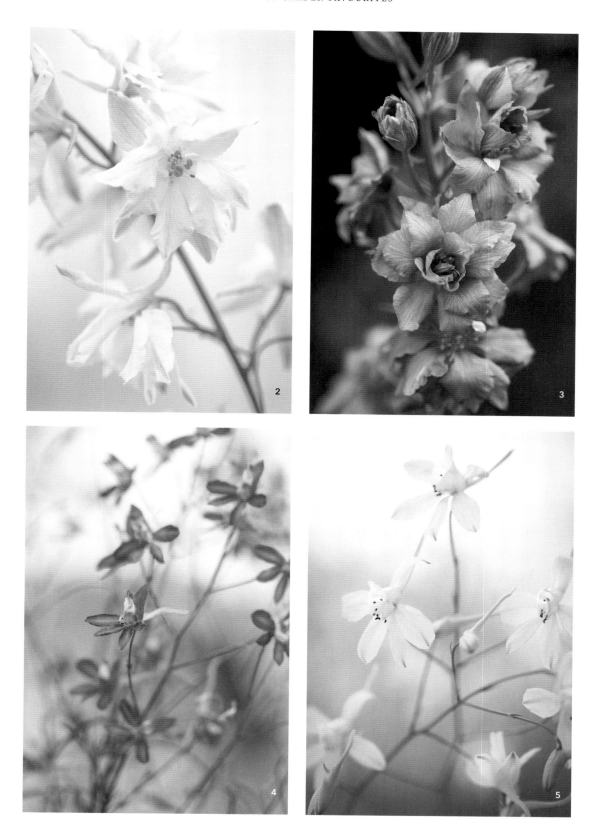

Sweet william, carnation & pinks (*Dianthus*)

- Short-lived perennial/biennial
- Height: 30-70 cm
- Sow: direct or under cover in late spring or early summer (sweet williams); under cover in late winter (other species)
- Site: full sun, gravel or well-drained soil
- Flowers: sweet williams late spring, other species early to midsummer

With a name that means 'divine flower', *Dianthus* is a group that includes old-fashioned carnations (*D. caryophyllus*) and pinks (*D. plumarius*) as well as sweet williams (*D. barbatus*). There are many hundreds, if not thousands of varieties of carnation and pinks and, although both are easy to grow from seed, it is probably easier to buy them as plants, since they are widely and cheaply available from nurseries and garden centres. Growing sweet williams from seed, however, is more satisfying, as they are useful for both borders and containers, and the range available from seed is superior to that found in garden centres. The other group worth growing from seed – and just as easy – contains some of the species themselves, such as *D. carthusianorum* and *D. superbus*, which have grown in popularity in the last few years.

year if you sow it in early spring, it is incredibly easy to grow from seed, and perfect for a gravel garden. Growing to about 50 cm, it produces sprays of small, intensely coloured magenta flowers in little clusters of six or seven that float above tussocks of grassy leaves on strong stems. Finally, *D. superbus* has delicate, wispy flowers that belie its incredible toughness. The species itself is sugar-pink, but there is also a white form, 'Alba', and a seed mix called 'Spooky', with flowers in shades of lilac, rose and white.

Varieties

There are dozens of cultivars of sweet william, but 'Auricula Eyed Mix' is one of our favourites, as well as 'Sooty', which has red stems, dark leaves and blooms as near to black as flowers can be. Sweet williams are excellent for cutting, lasting well in water, and their petals are also edible, perfect for pepping up salads or desserts. Of the other *Dianthus* species, *D. carthusianorum* gets our top vote. A perennial plant that flowers the same

1 'Auricula Eyed Mix'

All Dianthus hate being wet, so ensure that they are planted in a free-draining area of the garden and don't overwater them, or stem rot will cause their demise. They are perfect for gravel gardens.

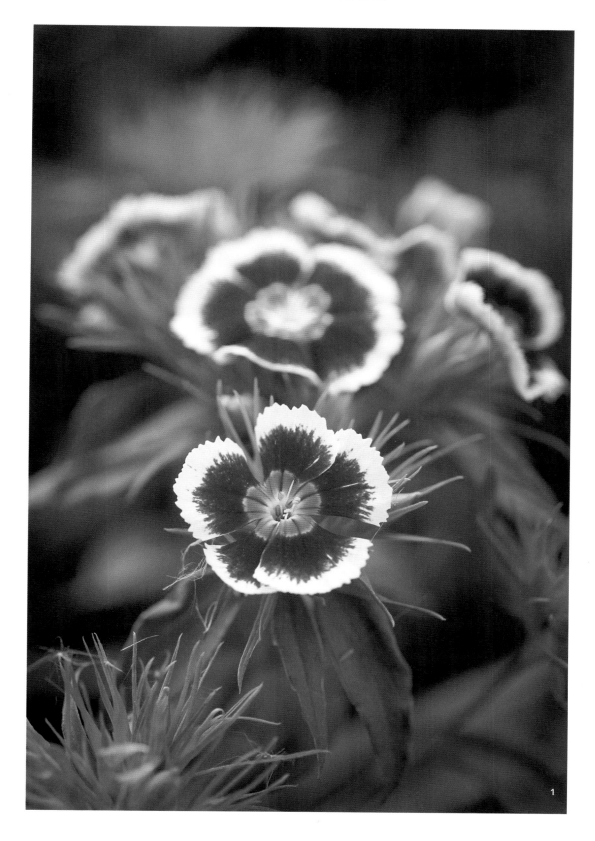

1

Sowing and growing

Sweet williams are short-lived perennials that are often grown as biennials, to be sown in late spring or early summer and overwintered outside before flowering the following spring. They can be sown direct in the garden or under cover, but either way they need a period of cold to initiate the flower buds, so if you are sowing them in modules, germinate them in a cold frame rather than giving them too much heat, and then plant them out in the garden in autumn so they can spend the winter outside. Perennial species such as *D. carthusianorum* and *D. superbus* will flower the same year if you sow them in late winter under cover. The seeds are big enough to plant in individual modules, on the surface of the compost or covered lightly with vermiculite because they need light to germinate. Keep them warm at 18–21°C until they germinate, and then move to a cooler place, planting them out in the garden as soon as all danger of frost has passed.

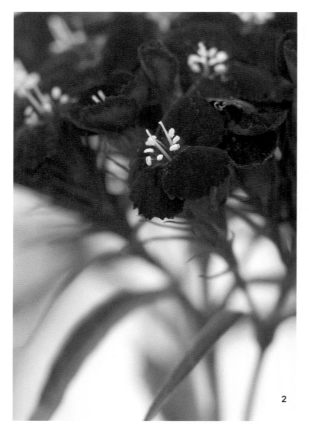

2

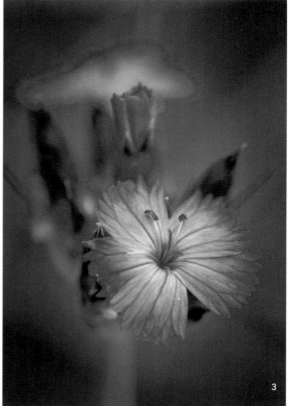

3

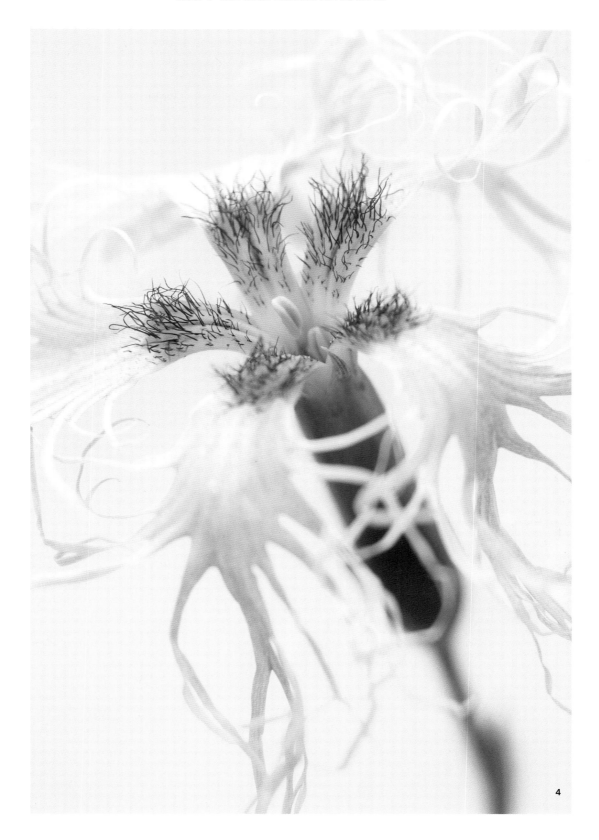

4

Foxglove (*Digitalis*)

- Biennial/short-lived perennial
- Height: 60–150 cm
- Sow: direct or under cover in summer or early spring
- Site: dappled shade, well-drained, humus-rich soil
- Flowers: late spring to early summer

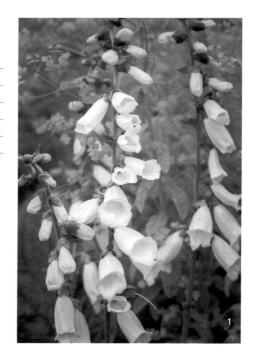

1

We all know and love foxgloves, but have you tried growing them from seed? Most are remarkably easy, and germinate readily. The foxglove is deeply rooted in myth, history and medicine as the source of a horribly potent poison, and indeed all parts of the plant are poisonous if ingested, causing abnormal heart rhythm and even death. So keep a healthy distance from these plants, and if you choose to have them in your garden, educate children and adults alike to steer clear. Having said that, you can't be poisoned simply by touching them or by breathing in the pollen, so it's perfectly safe to handle the plants or seeds, or cut the blooms to put in a vase – but it's prudent to wash your hands afterwards.

Varieties

The white form of the biennial British foxglove, *D. purpurea* 'Alba' (also known as *D. purpurea* f. *albiflora*), is lovely with ferns, anemones and other plants that also enjoy light shade. Two foxgloves that are equally easy to grow from seed are the pretty *D. lutea* and its cousin *D. grandiflora*, both of which have buttery-yellow flowers. Both are native to southern Europe, so will tolerate more sun than the British foxglove, and both are reliably perennial, coming back to flower for several years before dying back. They look fabulous with almost anything, from orange *Geums* to purple *Salvias*. Another species that has risen in the popularity stakes recently is the copper-brown *D. ferruginea*, known as the rusty foxglove, which produces spikes of closely packed flowers that taper to a point; it is elegant and unusual. Some of the hybrid foxgloves have brought in fabulous colours, including the strawberries-and-cream pink of *D.* x *mertonensis*, a cross between *D. grandiflora* and *D. purpurea*, and the exquisite peachy-pink of 'Sutton's Apricot'.

1 *D. purpurea* 'Alba'
2 *D. purpurea*

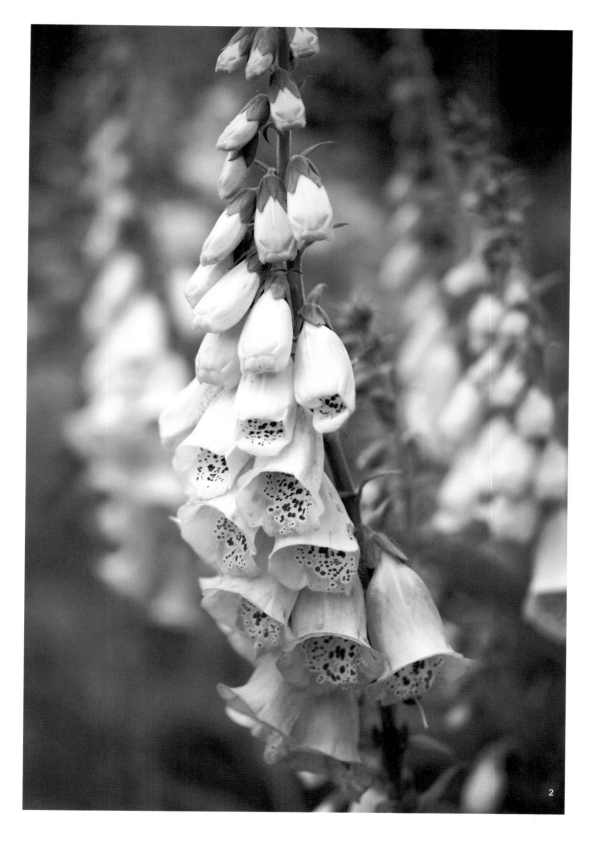

2

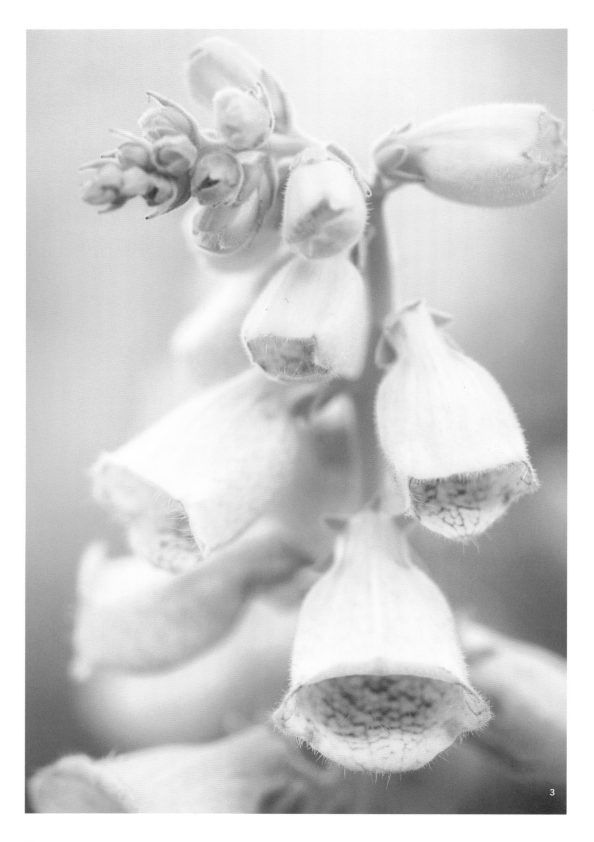

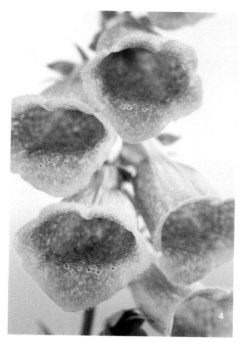

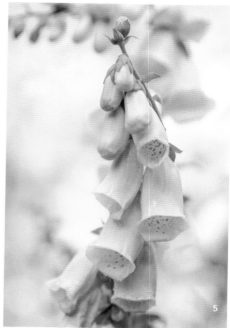

Sowing and growing

The seed germinates best if sown fresh, so if you are collecting your own seed after the plants have flowered in the summer, sow immediately onto good seed compost in a seed tray. Leave them in a greenhouse or cold frame until they have sprouted, pricking out the seedlings when they are large enough to handle. You can also sow direct, by simply scattering the seed and hoping for the best. Seed can also be sown in early spring, when the weather is colder; germinate them at 15–18°C and plant the seedlings out as soon as the soil warms up in late spring. The British foxglove, *D. purpurea*, is a biennial, flowering in its second year, so to ensure you have a display every year you will need to sow a second batch the following season. Most foxgloves need a position in dappled shade, in a good humus-rich soil, but the yellow foxgloves mentioned above, as well as *D. ferruginea*, will tolerate a sunnier spot.

Foxglove seeds are tiny and need light to germinate, so if you're sowing them under cover, press them very lightly into the surface of damp compost and water from below by placing the seed tray in a gravel tray half filled with water.

3 *D. grandiflora*
4 *D.* x *mertonensis*
5 'Sutton's Apricot'

Wallflower (*Erysimum*)

- Biennial
- Height: 35–50 cm
- Sow: direct or under cover in late spring or early summer
- Site: rocky, poor soil, in the cracks between paving stones or by a wall
- Flowers: late spring to early summer

Wallflowers are part of the cabbage family – the brassicas – although you wouldn't know it from their bright, sweetly scented flowers. In France they are known as *giroflée*, meaning clove-scented, and they have been grown for centuries. Appreciated for their strong colours in early spring, a time of year when many other flowers are more subdued, they provide a great foil for tulips in particular, balancing the bulbs' poker-straight stems with softer, hummocky flowers. They also bridge the gap between early spring bulbs and summer annuals.

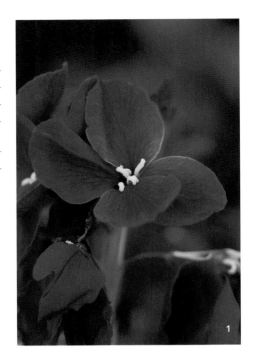

Varieties

Most of the wallflowers mentioned here are forms of the biennial *Erysimum cheiri*, the English wallflower. These grow best from seed, as opposed to perennial wallflowers such as 'Bowles' Mauve', which are propagated from cuttings and usually bought as plugs or potted plants. Some of the best varieties are the oldest, including the delightful 'Vulcan', with its warm-scented flowers in a kind of orange-tinged rusty crimson, dark and velvety. Growing to about 35 cm, it is shorter and bushier than other wallflowers, the perfect skirt to a swathe of willowy tulips such as orange *T.* 'Ballerina' or dusky 'Ronaldo'. *E. cheiri* 'Fire King' is a lighter, brighter orange that glows in a border, while 'Giant Pink' is raspberry pink, a good foil for 'Orange Emperor' tulips if you are feeling brave. More subtle shades are also available, including 'Aurora', with dusky, pinky-apricot flowers.

Sowing and growing

Wallflowers are easy to grow from seed, and the best time to sow is late spring or early summer. The small seeds are best sown thinly in seed trays, covered with a fine layer of compost. Germinate at 16–20°C, and prick out the seedlings into individual pots when they are big enough to handle. Grow them on until late summer or early autumn, then plant them out in their final growing positions, in a sunny spot in well-drained soil, giving them time to get their roots going before the weather turns cold. They can also be grown in containers.

1 'Vulcan'
2 'Aurora'
3 'Primrose Bedder'
4 'Giant Pink'

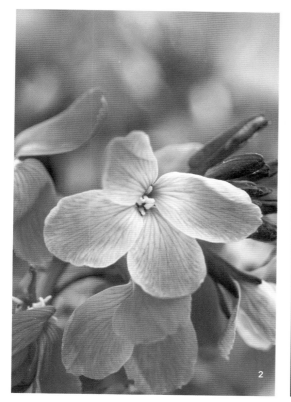

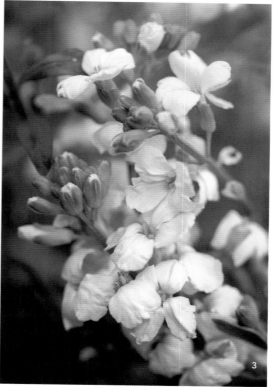

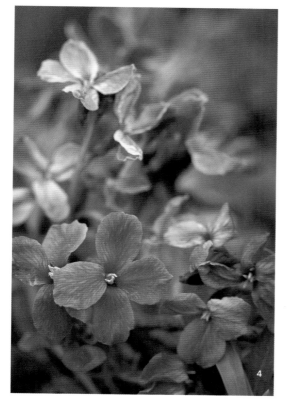

*Grow wallflowers in large
drifts for extra visual impact.*

Honesty (*Lunaria annua*)

- Biennial
- Height: 50–100 cm
- Sow: direct or under cover in late spring
- Site: sun or partial shade, any soil
- Flowers: early to late spring

Honesty is very useful for early spring, an easy companion for tulips and *Euphorbias* with its loose sprays of magenta, purple or white flowers. But it is best-known for its seed pods (see p.166), those translucent papery discs that shimmer silver in the sun and can be cut for the house in the same way as the flowers. Most forms are biennial, flowering in their second year, but they self-seed freely to weave their way around other plants, creating a natural look.

Varieties

The common honesty, *Lunaria annua*, has flowers of variable colour, ranging from purple through magenta to a slightly paler pink, with coarse, dark-green leaves. There is also a dark form, with purplish leaves and magenta-pink flowers, which is sometimes sold as 'Chedglow'. The white-flowered *L. annua* var. *albiflora* is lovely, but even more useful is its variegated form, 'Alba Variegata'. In its first year its leaves appear to be a uniform green, but in the second it produces silvery-white leaves and delicate white flowers that light up dark corners of the garden. One of the most recent additions to the family is *L. annua* 'Corfu Blue', with purple-blue flowers and dark-flushed stems. I have been growing it for several years and it self-seeds magnificently, producing strong plants that flower very early in the year – and go on and on. Last year mine flowered from the end of February right into the summer.

Sowing and growing

Collecting and sowing your own honesty seed is one of life's pleasures. The large discs can be cut from the plant and dried on paper to sow the following year. Hidden within the papery layers of the pod are the seeds, usually three, large and flat and easy to handle. Since they are biennials, the best time to sow them is in late spring or early summer, direct or in modular trays. Leave them in their modules until the end of the summer, when they should be planted out to form strong root systems and leaves over the autumn and winter, before flowering the following spring.

Don't keep the young plants in pots for too long or they will form long tap roots that will become restricted.

1 *L. annua* var. *albiflora*
2 'Alba Variegata'
3 *L. annua*
4 'Corfu Blue'

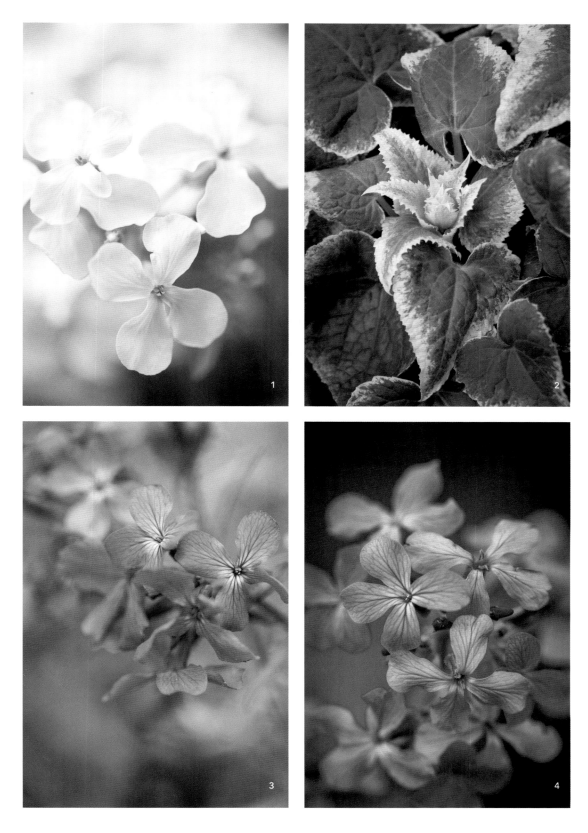

Lupin (*Lupinus*)

- Hardy perennial/annual
- Height: 45–120 cm
- Sow: direct or under cover in early spring or early autumn
- Site: open, sunny position, well-drained soil
- Flowers: early summer

Statuesque and colourful, this cottage-garden favourite is easy to grow from seed, but if you are collecting your own seed, bear in mind that named varieties will not come true (the seedling's flowers will not be the same as those of the parent). As ornamental plants, lupins came to Europe in the nineteenth century. They enjoyed a massive surge of popularity in the 1930s and 1940s, after the English gardener George Russell exhibited his new range of hybrids at the Chelsea Flower Show in 1938 and took the gardening world by storm.

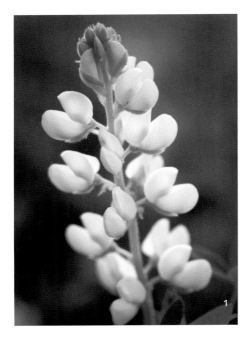

Varieties

Because lupins don't come true from seed, named cultivars that you may have fallen in love with are not available as seeds. However, bright and cheerful seed mixes with names such as 'Tutti Frutti' can be found, as well as a range of more recently developed annual lupins, smaller and more relaxed in habit. It is these that we would suggest growing from seed, because they are easy to germinate and flower quickly in one season. *Lupinus cruickshankii* (also known as *L. mutabilis* 'Sunrise' and 'Blue Javelin') is tall and branching, with scented white, gold and *Delphinium*-blue flowers rising in tiers above the leaves. Other annual lupins include dwarf types such as *L. elegans* 'Pink Fairy' (60 cm) and *L. nanus* 'Snow Pixie' (45 cm), ideal for pots or the front of a border.

Sowing and growing

Lupins' big, pea-like seeds are easy to handle and can be sown individually in modular trays or small pots, or you can sow five or seven seeds around the edge of a deep pot. Sow in early autumn or early spring and keep at 20–23°C, to be planted out in mid spring as soon as the soil starts warming up. Once you've planted them out, be wary of slugs. Plant the seedlings in a sunny position in any well-drained soil, as long as it's not very chalky.

Soaking lupin seeds for a few hours before sowing can help them to germinate more readily.

1 'Snow Pixie'
2 'Sunrise'

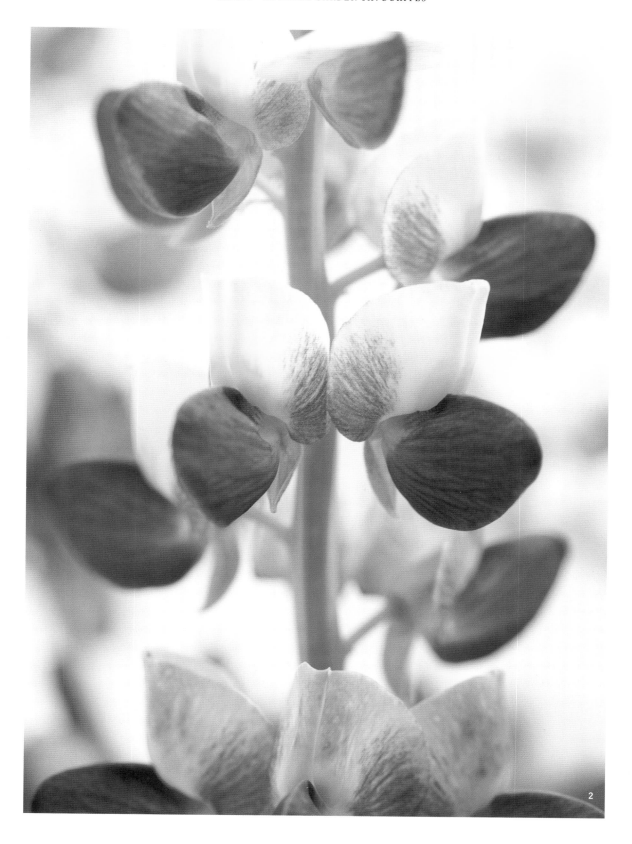

2

Love-in-a-mist (*Nigella*)*

- Hardy annual
- Height: 30–60 cm
- Sow: direct in mid spring or late summer
- Site: full sun and well-drained soil
- Flowers: early to midsummer

Easy to grow from seed, love-in-a-mist is a classic cottage garden flower grown for its delicate blue, pink and white flowers and clouds of fine, ferny foliage – the clue to its name. The flowers are worth a close look: each is a miniature work of art, with layers of coloured sepals, stamens and spiky horns in the centre. These horns are retained when the flower fades, leaving a wonderfully architectural seed pod.

Varieties

There are various cultivars of the well-loved *N. damascena*, and you can't go wrong with the pale-blue 'Miss Jekyll', named after the redoubtable Victorian gardener Gertrude Jekyll, or its white counterpart, 'Miss Jekyll Alba'. A 'Miss Jekyll' seed mix is also now available with blue, pink and white flowers. Also from this species comes 'Albion Green Pod', which has fresh white flowers with a boss of green stamens in the middle, followed by a fantastic green seed pod. 'Albion Black Pod' is similar, with darker green stamens and a dark purple-black seed pod. Another species of *Nigella*, *N. papillosa* (also known as *N. hispanica*), has risen in popularity recently; it is slightly taller than *N. damascena* and has larger, more substantial flowers. *N. papillosa* 'African Bride' has showy white flowers with contrasting stamens of deepest purple rising dramatically from the centre of the flower, while *N. papillosa* 'Midnight' has stunning grey-blue flowers with blue-black stamens. Both have ornamental, spidery seed pods.

1 *N. damascena* 'Miss Jekyll'

Nigella is one of the easiest flowers to grow from seed, so it is an excellent choice for a beginner. Always leave some of the flowers to go to seed: not only are the seed pods attractive, but also the plant will self-seed to provide more for the following year.

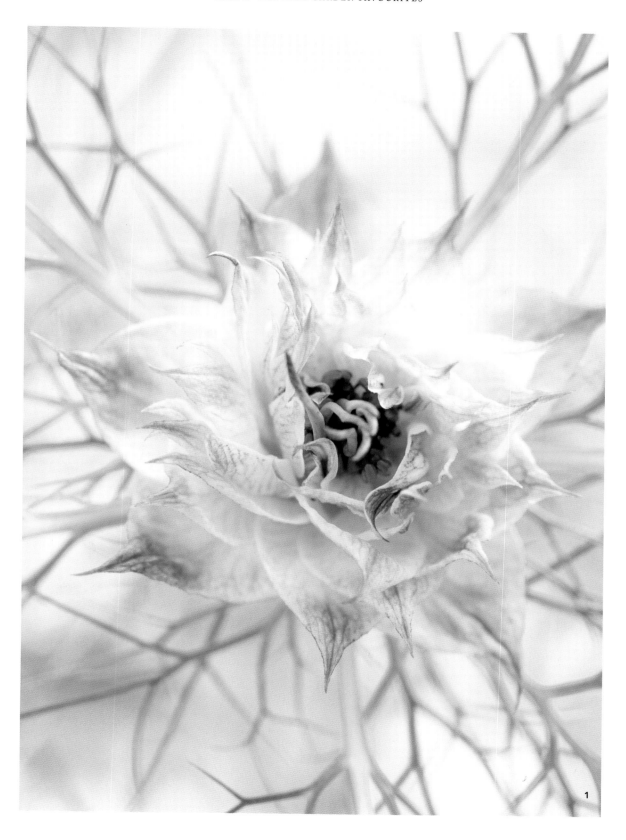

1

Sowing and growing

All *Nigella* are best sown direct, in mid spring or late summer. Sow in drills, or simply scatter the seed where you want the plants to flower, in full sun or part shade, and rake it in. Easy-going and eager to please, these pretty flowers will grow in most soils but do best in a fairly moist, well-drained spot. They will flower from early to mid summer.

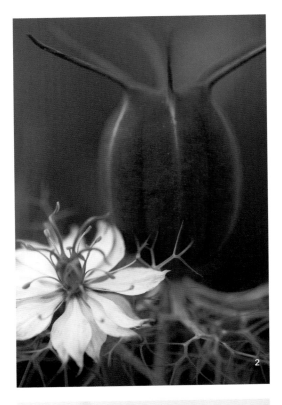

2 'Albion Black Pod'
3 'African Bride'
4 'Albion Green Pod'
5 'Midnight'

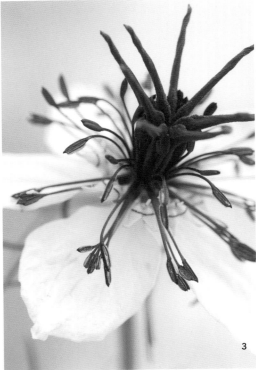

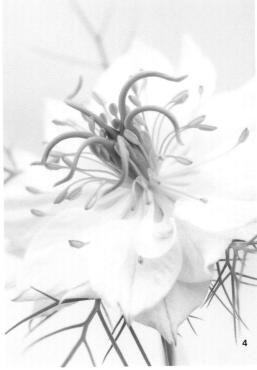

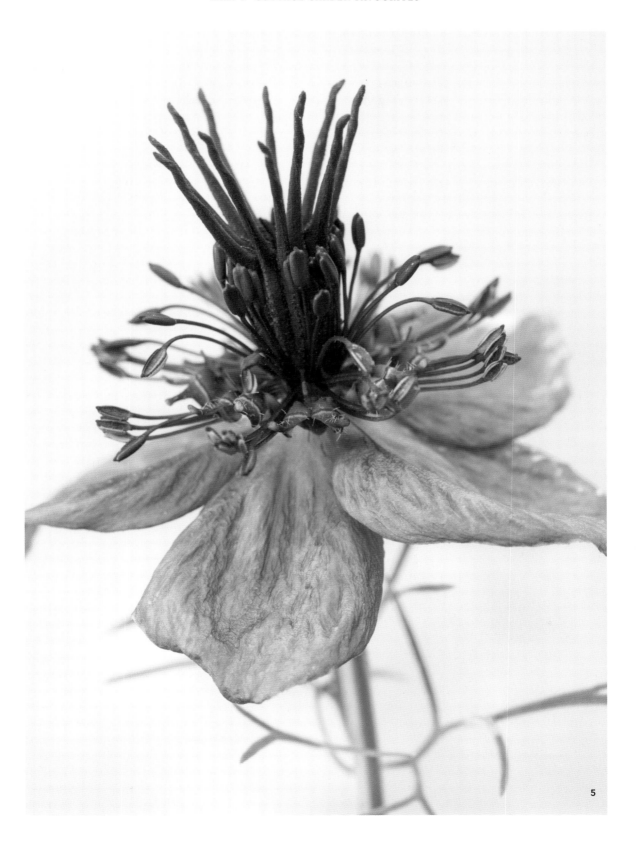

5

Poppy (*Papaver*) ☀

- Hardy annual/biennial
- Height: 45–100 cm
- Sow: direct in mid spring or late summer (annuals); direct or under cover in late spring or early summer (biennials)
- Site: full sun and poor soil
- Flowers: early to midsummer

With their crushed-silk flowers in rainbow colours, poppies are one of the joys of early summer. Their flowers may last only a week or so, but such ephemerality is worth it for the jewel-like beauty they bring to the garden. The northern European field poppy, *Papaver rhoeas*, is the well-known and evocative symbol of World War I. The blood-red blooms were once a common sight in cornfields, but modern pesticides and farming methods have contributed to the poppy's demise, all the more reason to grow them in our gardens.

Varieties

The annual *P. rhoeas* is easy to grow from seed in borders and wild-flower meadows. Related forms include 'Mother of Pearl' (singles and doubles in pinks, creams and silvery greys) and 'Angels' Choir Mix' (doubles in various colours). A new strain, 'Pandora', has also caught our attention, with double flowers in a range of unusual dusky shades from deepest purple-crimson to silvery grey-mauve. More sophisticated in form and colour are the opium poppies, *P. somniferum*, which come in both single and double flowers in a wide range of colours from deepest velvety purple to pale grey-mauve and creamy white. The seed pods are beautiful, too, especially the peony types, with their opulent flowers, including 'Peony Flowered Mix'. The other group of poppies to try from seed are the biennial Icelandic poppies, *P. nudicaule*, which – unlike most poppies – are useful for cutting. Mixes come in subtle shades ('Meadow Pastels') or brighter reds and oranges ('Champagne Bubbles' Group).

1 'Mother of Pearl'
2 'Angels' Choir Mix'
3 'Pandora'
4 *P. somniferum*

All annual poppies resent root disturbance, so they should be sown direct where you want them to flower.

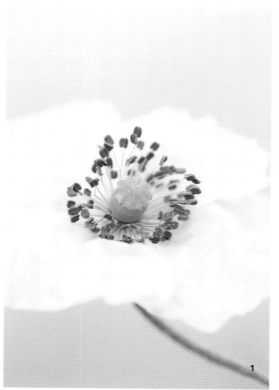

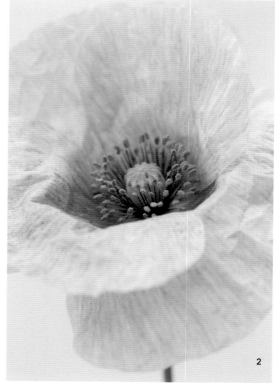

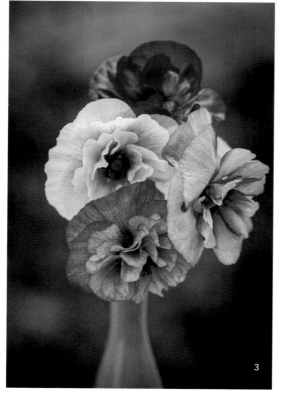

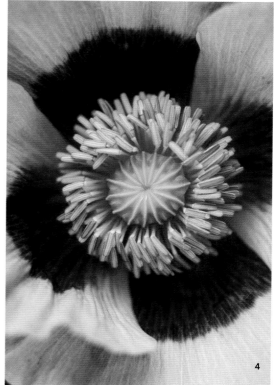

Sowing and growing

Sow annual poppies thinly, either broadcasting or in drills, into finely raked soil in mid spring or early autumn, and keep well watered. Thin out the seedlings when they have emerged and are big enough to handle, remembering that the plants will grow quite large. Once they are established, they will self-seed and reappear year after year. Sow biennial poppies in late spring or early summer, to flower the following year. Unlike other poppies, they can be transplanted, so they can be sown direct or in seed trays, and planted out in late summer or early autumn.

5 'Candy Floss'
6 *P. somniferum* seed pod
7 'Black Peony'
8 'Meadow Pastel'

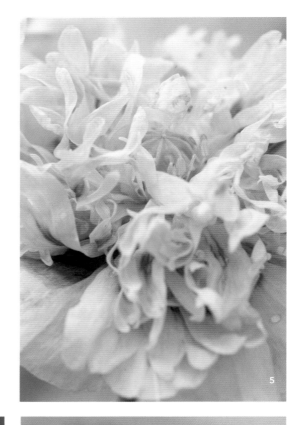

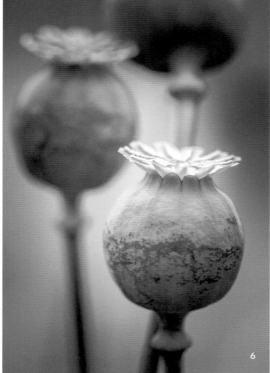

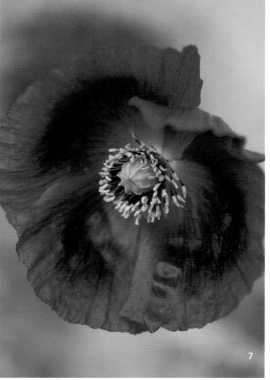

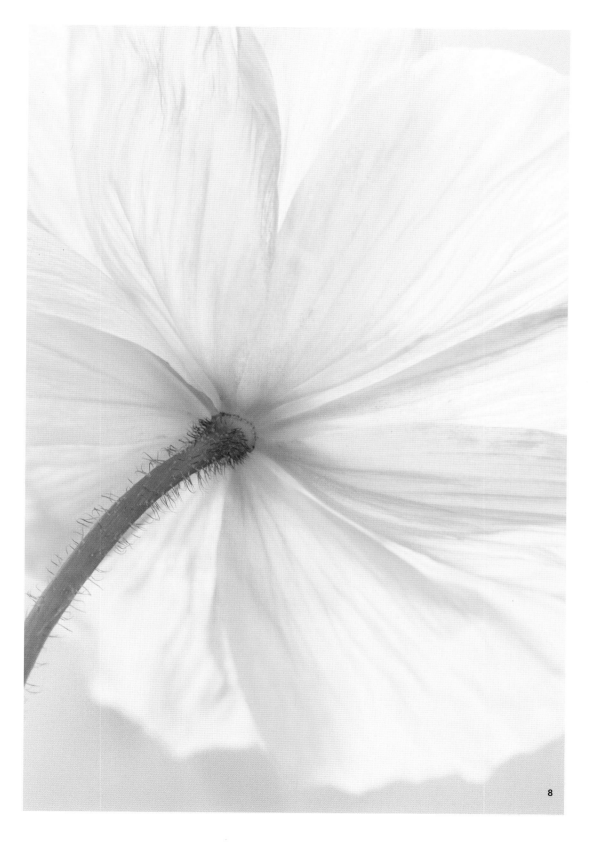

Annual phlox
(*Phlox drummondii*)

- Half-hardy annual
- Height: 30–50 cm
- Sow: under cover in early to mid spring
- Site: sun or partial shade in moist but well-drained soil
- Flowers: mid to late summer

Phlox has been grown in Europe since the seventeenth century, when the perennial *Phlox paniculata* was brought over from the American colonies. The family contains some 60 species, but we focus on just one here, the annual *P. drummondii* from Texas. It is the quickest to flower from seed and excellent for containers, producing generous clusters of flowers. Popular as a swift-growing bedding plant, annual phlox is subject to the breeders' tendency to favour the brightest, brashest colours, but don't be put off. If you pick carefully through what is available, you'll find strains that are subtle and beautiful.

Varieties

Our favourite phlox is 'Crème Brûlée', which has pale coffee-and-cream flowers with darker stars in the centre. The different tones in each flower pick up other colours, whether in the border or in the vase, and it is an excellent cut flower. 'Cherry Caramel' is similar, with caramel-coloured flowers and a more prominent rose-pink centre, while 'Phlox of Sheep' comes in a range of pastel shades and bi-colours – cream, orange, yellow, pink and white. In the US, and becoming more widely available in the UK, are the excellent '21st Century' phloxes: neat, mounded plants with flowers that keep going all summer. For something a little different, try 'Twinkling Beauty' or 'Twinkle Star Mix', which has complex starry flowers with pointed petals. Colours are a lottery, ranging from pale pink to vibrant purple, and some flowers have white centres and edging, others darker centres. They are not for the faint-hearted!

Sowing and growing

Sow in mid spring under cover in a modular seed tray, several seeds to a module. Germinate at 18–20°C and grow on in a greenhouse or cold frame. Harden the seedlings off as they grow and plant them out in early summer, in sun or partial shade and a fertile, moist but well-drained soil. Don't let them dry out in hot, sunny weather, especially if you're growing them in containers.

1 'Crème Brûlée'
2 'Cherry Caramel'
3 'Phlox of Sheep'
4 'Twinkling Beauty'

Annual phlox is easy to grow from seed and ideal for containers. As a half-hardy, it should be sown under cover in early to mid spring.

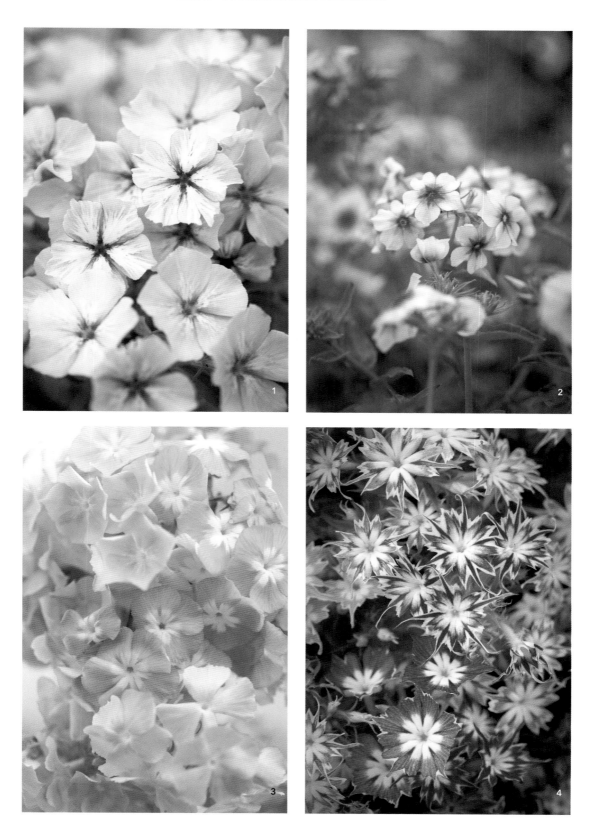

Scabious (*Scabiosa atropurpurea*)

- Hardy annual
- Height: 50–80 cm
- Sow: direct in mid spring or under cover in early spring or autumn
- Site: full sun, poor soil
- Flowers: mid to late summer

Also known as the pincushion flower, *Scabiosa atropurpurea* is a relaxed, willowy flower on tall stems, closely related to the field scabious, *Knautia arvensis*. It is relaxed and unfussy, as content in a meadow as in a border, and will flower all summer and well into autumn, its fragrant, bee-friendly blooms continuing to appear if they are cut regularly. Native to the Mediterranean, it was one of the first scabious species to be introduced into cultivation in the sixteenth century, when it was used to treat a range of skin complaints.

Varieties

Cultivars of *S. atropurpurea* vary from white to deepest purple-black. The simplest option is to choose a colour mix such as 'Tall Double Mix', especially if you are growing it in a cut-flower patch and want a range of hues. If you prefer the control of a single colour, there are plenty of options. One of the most sultry and sophisticated is 'Black Knight', its velvety dark-purple flowers scattered with white stigmas. 'Fata Morgana' is a delightful clotted-cream colour, while 'Snowmaiden' is pure lacy white. 'Salmon Queen' is a very good pink, and *S.* 'Butterfly Blue' is the perfect shorter variety for pots. If you're looking for a cut-flower curiosity, try *S. stellata* 'Ping Pong' (sometimes known as 'Sternkugel' or 'Drumstick'). This has pale-blue flowers, but it is the seed heads that provide the spectacle, a collection of papery bracts that form a perfect drumstick sphere.

Keep picking or deadheading the flowers over the summer and your plants will bloom for months.

1 'Tall Double Mix'

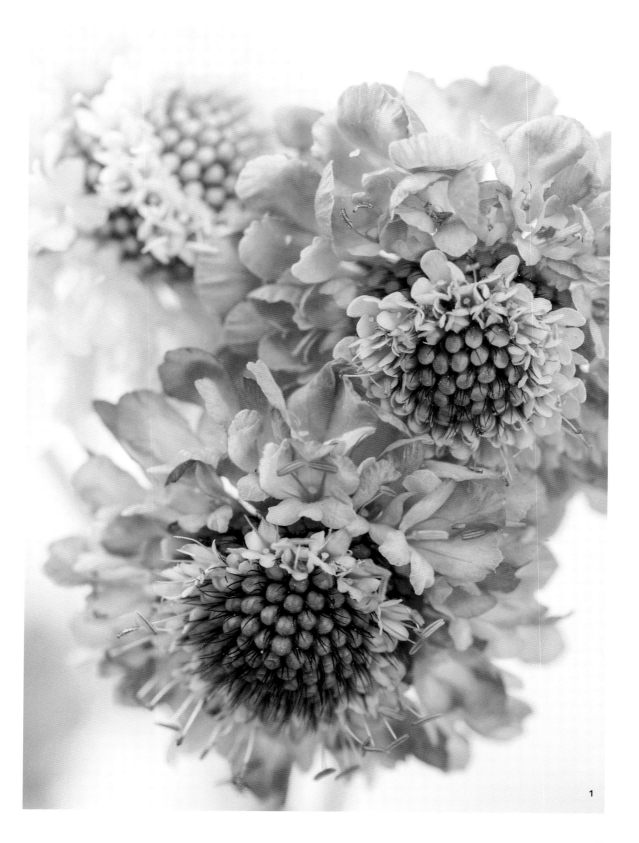

1

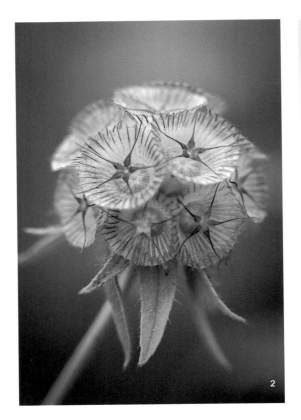

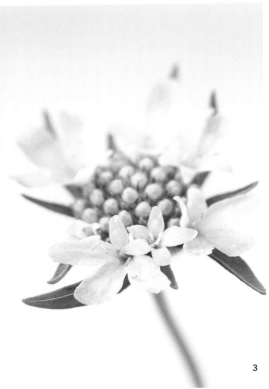

2

3

Sowing and growing

If you choose to sow under cover, sow in early autumn or early spring in modular trays, several seeds to a cell, and cover with a very fine layer of sieved compost. Germinate at 15-20°C. If the weather is warm enough, plant the seedlings straight out from the modules, but if you prefer to wait, grow them on in 7 cm pots. Give them a sunny spot in a border, cutting garden or meadow planting, remembering that they do best in poor soil, so there is no need to add large amounts of compost or give them fertilizer as they grow. If sowing direct, wait until the soil warms up sufficiently in mid to late spring.

2 'Ping Pong' seed head
3 'Ping Pong'
4 'Snowmaiden'
5 'Fata Morgana'
6 'Black Knight'
7 'Salmon Queen'

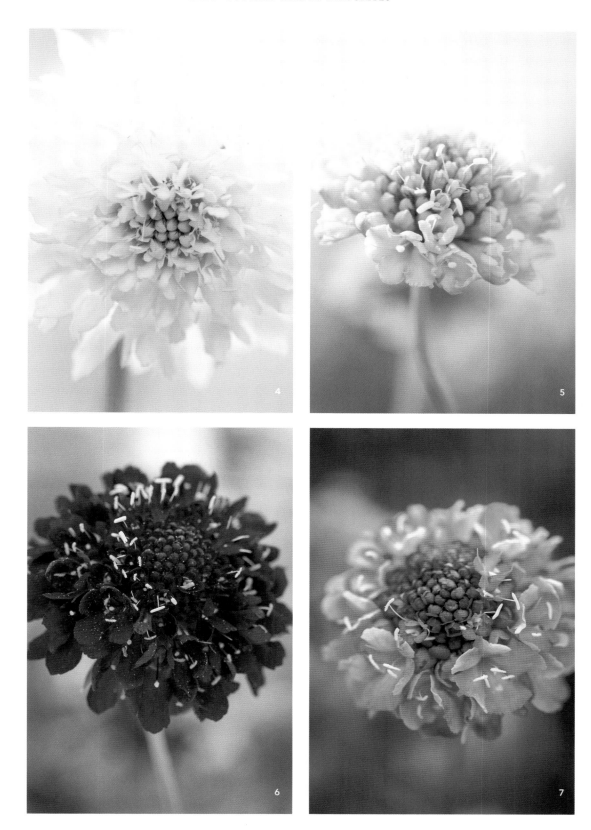

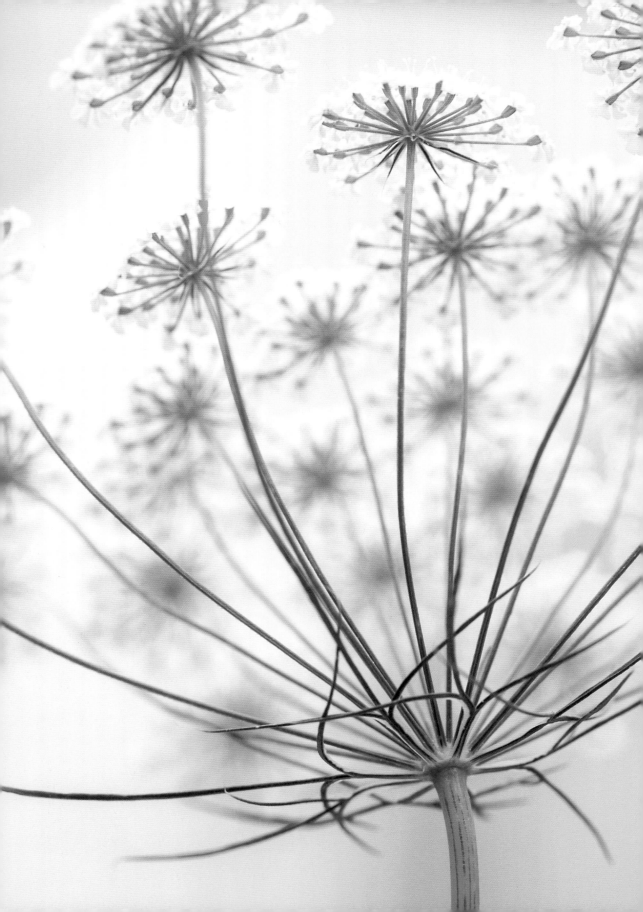

Filigree Fillers

Bishop's flower (*Ammi*)

Quaking grass (*Briza maxima*)

Hare's ear (*Bupleurum rotundifolium*)

Baby's breath (*Gypsophila*)

Rabbit's tail grass (*Lagurus ovatus*)

Venus's navelwort (*Omphalodes linifolia*)

White lace flower (*Orlaya grandiflora*)

Switch grass (*Panicum* 'Frosted Explosion')

Mexican feather grass (*Stipa tenuissima*)

Ammi majus

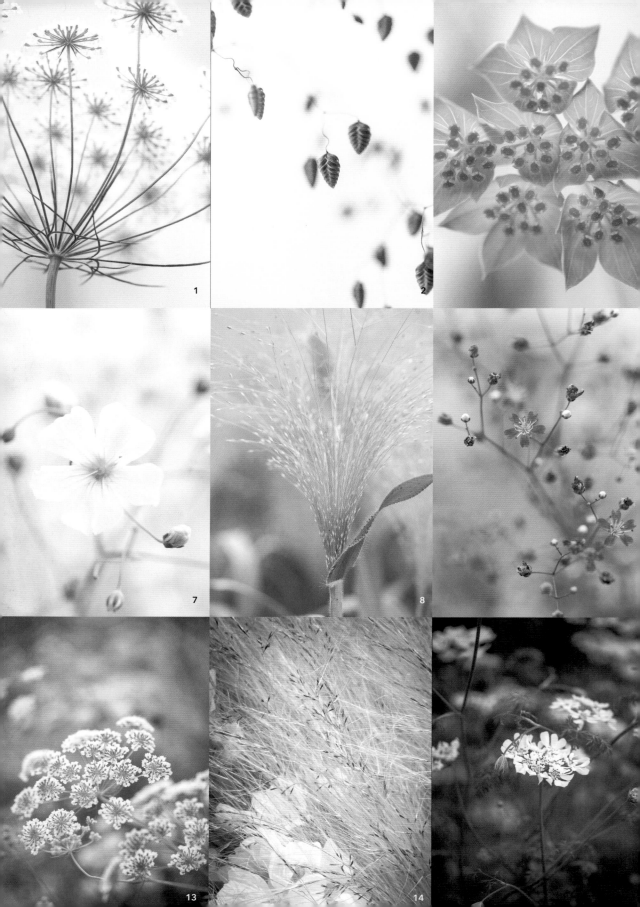

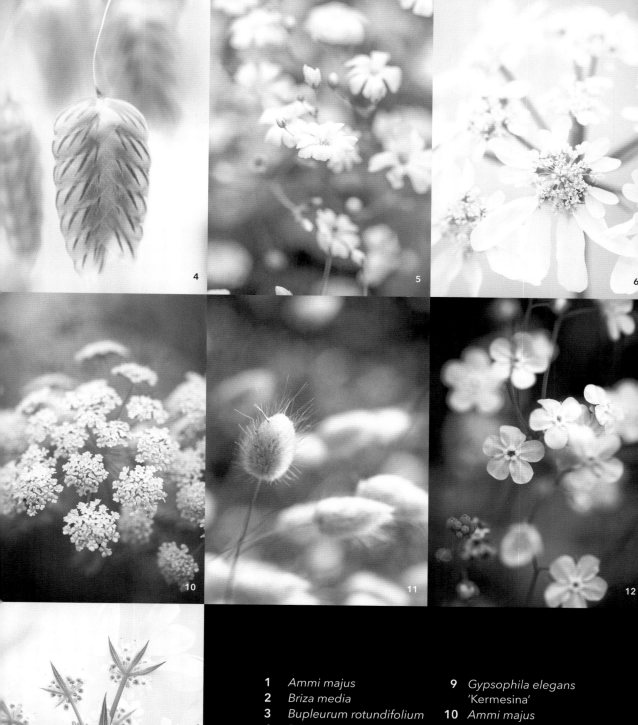

Bishop's flower (*Ammi*)

- Hardy annual
- Height: 1 m
- Sow: direct in late summer or under cover in spring
- Site: sun or partial shade, moisture-rich soil
- Flowers: early to midsummer

Ammi majus is one of the most useful annuals, and a plant that has leapt into fashion with the recent swing to a more natural style of gardening. It is a subtler form of the common cow parsley, with delicate white flowers that appear to float in weightless clouds above bulbs and other lower-storey plants, or weave effortlessly among taller perennials as a linking plant. The small clusters of tiny blooms explode from their narrow stalks; look at the flower head upside down and marvel at the way nature has constructed it. It is pleasingly tall (particularly if sown in late summer) and has fresh green, feathery foliage and long, statuesque stems.

Either sow Ammi under cover in spring, or direct in late summer, which will produce taller, sturdier plants. Alternatively sow at both times of year for successional flowers.

1 *A. majus*
2 *A. majus*
3 *A. visnaga*
4 'Green Mist'

Varieties

Various cultivars are available, including 'Graceland', 'Snowflake' and 'Queen of Africa', but generally there is very little difference between them. The lesser-known *A. visnaga* has more densely clustered and domed flower heads, like those of angelica, and therefore offers slightly more visual interest from a distance. It also flowers a little later than *A. majus* and, although it grows to about the same height, feels more substantial – less frothy lace and more architecture. The cultivar 'Green Mist' has a green tinge to its flowers and looks wonderful with purple or blue larkspur.

Sowing and growing

Both *A. majus* and *A. visnaga* are easy to germinate at 18–20°C and can be sown in modules under cover or direct into the ground. Once planted, they need little attention other than regular watering if the weather is dry. Both are favoured by flower-arrangers, but don't pick all your blooms: leave a few to go to seed and they will self-seed happily, so you won't have to plant more the following year.

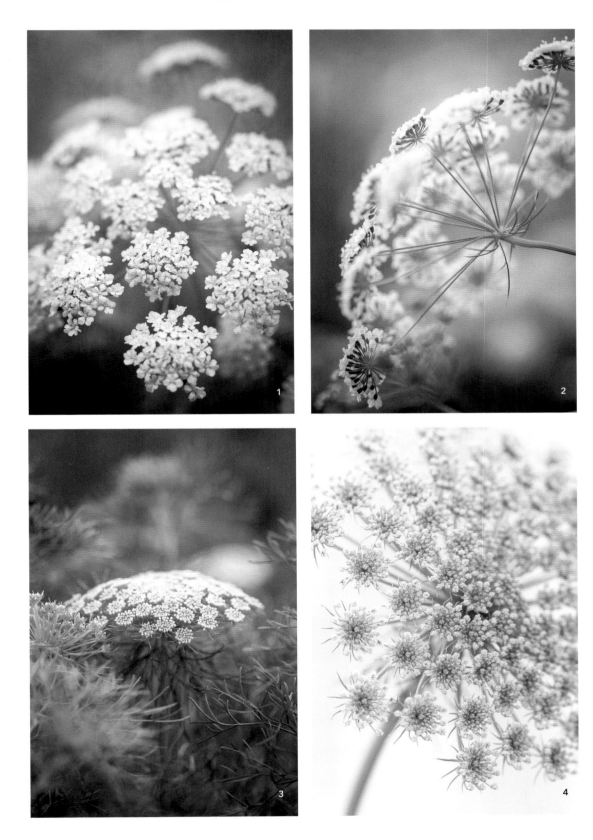

Quaking grass (*Briza maxima*)

- Hardy annual
- Height: 45–60 cm
- Sow: direct or under cover in spring
- Site: full sun, well-drained soil
- Flowers: mid to late summer

Briza maxima is a delightful annual grass that produces lots of hanging flowers like little pendants throughout the summer. Palest green and layered like fish scales when they first appear, they turn silvery gold as they age, shimmering in the light and rustling in the breeze. *Briza* is an easy addition to the front of a border, where it will weave in and out of other herbaceous plants, giving a soft, natural look, and self-seeding to make its own way around the garden the following year. It also makes an excellent cut flower that can be dried as well as used fresh. Try spraying the seed heads silver or gold for a lovely Christmas decoration.

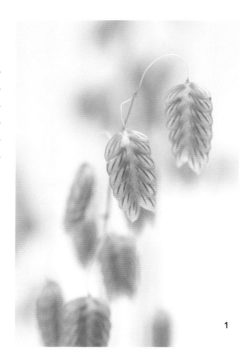

1

Sowing and growing

Preferring a spot in full sun and well-drained soil, *Briza* is an easy-going plant that can be sown under cover in mid spring or direct as soon as the soil has warmed up. Sow in modules and germinate at 18–20°C. When sowing direct, thin the plants out to at least 30 cm apart, or move the seedlings around within the border to create a naturalistic look.

1 *B. maxima*

Briza can be sown direct or under cover, but sowing in modules gives you more control.

Hare's ear (*Bupleurum rotundifolium*)

- Hardy annual
- Height: 50-90 cm
- Sow: direct in autumn or early spring
- Site: an open, sunny position in moist, well-drained soil
- Flowers: early to late summer

Bupleurum rotundifolium is one of those useful foliage plants that, once you have it, you feel you can't be without. In fact, happily, you won't need to be, since it self-seeds everywhere from year to year if it is given a space it likes in full sun with well-drained soil. It's like a loose-flowering *Euphorbia* without the irritating white sap, and has umbels of acid-green flowers and rounded leaves through which the stem grows. It's not a classic 'flowery' flower, but is incredibly useful for cutting, and lightens a dense border with an injection of fresh green. *Bupleurum* is brilliant for knitting together a flower arrangement, its lime-green flowers uniting the brightest, most clashing colours.

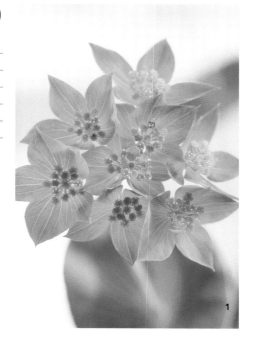

1

Sowing and growing

Growing *Bupleurum* couldn't be easier in moist, well-drained soil. The wild form – now quite rare – was once an arable weed on chalk or limestone. It is best sown direct, but if you want backup, sow a few seeds in modules in autumn or early spring so that the plugs can be planted out when large enough without disturbing the roots. Being fairly tall, it has a tendency to flop like a gawky teenager, and it needs a home among other mid height perennials or grasses to give it some framework and support. It looks particularly good with dark-blue salvias, perhaps with a grass or two thrown in – *Stipa tenuissima* or *Pennisetum alopecuroides* 'Hameln'.

1 'Griffithii'

Bupleurum is very hardy, so it can be sown in early spring direct into the soil where you want it to flower; or, for larger plants the following year, sow in autumn.

Baby's breath (*Gypsophila*)

- Perennial/annual
- Height: 45–100 cm
- Sow: under cover in autumn or early spring, or direct in mid spring
- Site: full sun, well-drained soil
- Flowers: early to midsummer

Gypsophila has become something of a cliché for florists, who favour it as an easy foil for more colourful blooms. But as a garden plant it is both useful and beautiful, forming rounded domes with wiry stems clothed in a mist of tiny white flowers in late spring or early summer.

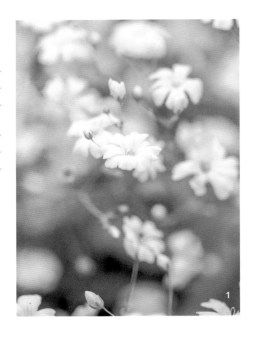

Varieties

The traditional flower-arranger's *Gypsophila* is the perennial form, *G. paniculata*, which can look lovely with other cottage-garden favourites, such as carnations and pinks. There are several cultivars, including the double-flowered 'Schneeflocke' ('Snowflake') and the pale-pink 'Flamingo', both of which produce dense clouds of flowers on tangled stems. However, it is the annual form, *G. elegans*, that has risen in popularity. With tiny single flowers that don't smother the plant so completely, it is less wedding-cake frills than traditional baby's breath, and much more elegant as a result. Growing to about 45 cm, the cultivar 'Covent Garden' is the most widely available. More unusual but equally desirable is the deep-pink 'Kermesina'.

Sowing and growing

Annual *Gypsophila* can be sown in spring, for flowers in early summer, or in autumn, for earlier flowering. Sow it under cover or direct in later spring, once the soil has warmed up. If you are sowing under cover, use a small seed tray or pot, and leave to germinate at 18–20°C. Prick out the seedlings and grow on in small pots, to be hardened off and planted out in late spring or early summer. The perennial variety is best sown under cover in early spring.

Gypsophila needs a sunny spot in the garden in extremely well-drained soil that isn't too rich.

1 'Covent Garden'
2 'Kermesina'

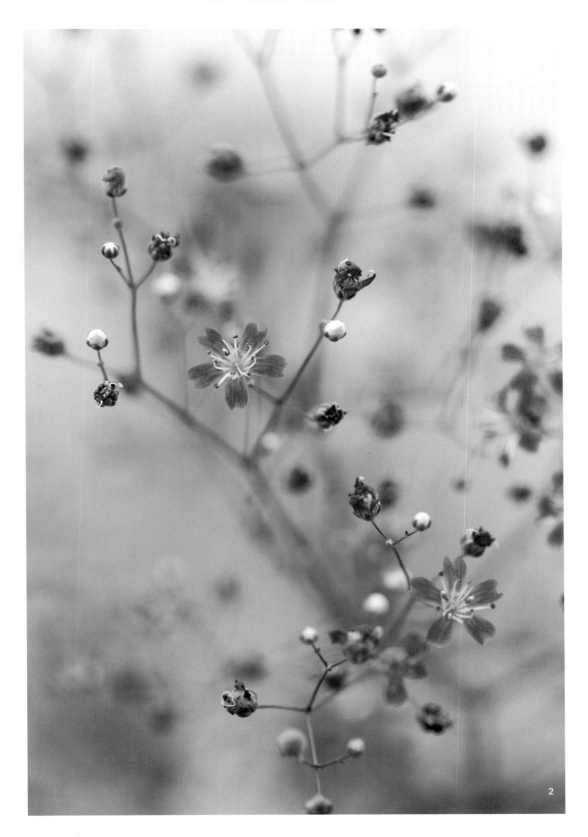

2

Rabbit's tail grass (*Lagurus ovatus*)

- Hardy annual
- Height: 30–50 cm
- Sow: under cover in early spring or direct in early autumn or mid spring
- Site: full sun, well-drained sandy soil
- Flowers: mid to late summer

Lagurus ovatus is one of a handful of annual grasses that can be grown easily from seed to pad out borders and provide material for the cutting garden. Its appealing fluffy flowers grow on arching, wiry stems, silvery and soft, and light enough to move in the slightest breeze. Towards the end of the summer, the flowers turn golden brown and dry beautifully on the plant. The flowers can be cut for summer flower arrangements, and as a result the plant will produce more buds in a cut-and-come-again way.

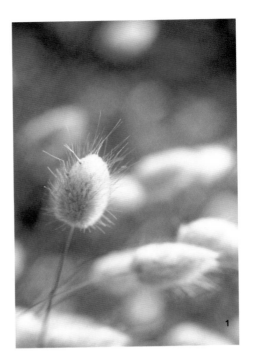

Sowing and growing

Lagurus can be sown direct in mid spring or early autumn, or in modules under cover in early spring. As always, sowing in modules will give you more control and increase your chances of raising more plants successfully. Sow in early spring at 18–20°C and plant out the seedlings in late spring or early summer, in a sunny spot. Since this is a grass that grows naturally near the sea in sand dunes and coastal grassland, it does best in a light, sandy soil that drains freely. Recreate these conditions as much as you can by adding sand or grit to your garden soil.

The seed heads dry to an attractive burnished brown, lasting well into autumn and winter on the plant.

1 *L. ovatus*

Venus's navelwort (*Omphalodes linifolia*)

- Hardy annual
- Height: 25–45 cm
- Sow: under cover in early spring or early autumn
- Site: full sun, will tolerate dry conditions
- Flowers: mid spring to early summer

Omphalodes linifolia is not widely grown, but we love it for its delicately fragrant white spring flowers and its grey-green foliage. Native to the dry, stony grasslands of the Mediterranean, it is drought-tolerant and will self-seed gently to weave its way around the garden, providing clouds of tiny, white forget-me-not flowers that form cushions at the front of a border or rock garden.

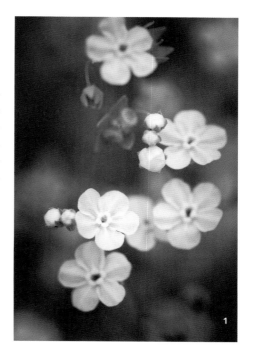

Varieties
Perennial species of *Omphalodes*, such as *O. cappadocica* and *O. verna*, are more widely grown, but not generally available from seed. Although there are other annual species, *O. linifolia* is the only one in general cultivation in the UK and US.

Sowing and growing
Since *Omphalodes* flowers in late spring and early summer it must be sown inside or in a propagator at 20–23°C in early spring, and grown on in a cooler greenhouse or cold frame before being planted out in mid spring. Sow in modules so you can plant them out without having to pot them on. It should self-seed profusely the following year, and you can collect the seed if you want to spread it elsewhere in the garden or grow it in pots.

The flowers are tiny so group the plants in threes, fives or sevens when planting out for extra impact.

1 *O. linifolia*

White lace flower
(*Orlaya grandiflora*)

- Hardy annual
- Height: 50–70 cm
- Sow: direct or under cover in mid spring or late summer
- Site: full sun in well-drained soil
- Flowers: early to late summer

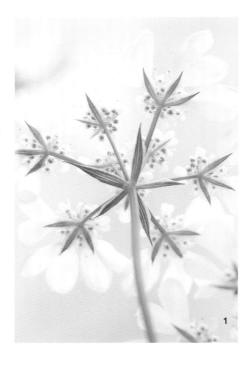

1

Orlaya **is the darling of British cut-flower growers, and perfect for bringing a natural look to both borders and bouquets. Growing wild in the olive groves and vineyards of the Mediterranean, it is surprisingly hardy and, like other hardy annuals, can be sown in late summer, giving you sturdier, earlier-flowering plants the following year. It is similar in nature to** *Ammi majus*, **but has more substantial, complex flowers, with larger outer petals on each floret, creating greater impact from a distance. The snow-white flowers dance on wiry stems above ferny foliage, mixing easily with other annuals or when dotted around in a herbaceous border.**

in modules and remove all but the strongest seedling, you can plant them out straight from the cell to minimize root disturbance, and the plants should grow on successfully if you handle them gently. Sow in early spring and plant out in mid to late spring, or – for bigger, earlier-flowering plants – sow in late summer and keep in a cold frame or greenhouse over the winter. *Orlaya* can also be used in containers.

Varieties
The species itself, *O. grandiflora*, does not need improving, and although there are a couple of cultivars ('White Finch' and 'Minoan Lace'), these are likely to be slightly more romantic names for the same plant.

Sowing and growing
Like other tap-rooted annuals, *Orlaya* must be handled with care, and some people would advise only planting direct. However, it is one of those 'choice' annuals where you never get many seeds in a packet so, to eliminate the haphazardness of sowing direct and to have more control over germination, we think it's best to sow under cover. If you sow the seeds

Give the plants a spot in full sun. They will grow in most soils, but prefer a reasonably fertile, well-drained soil.

1 and **2** *O. grandiflora*

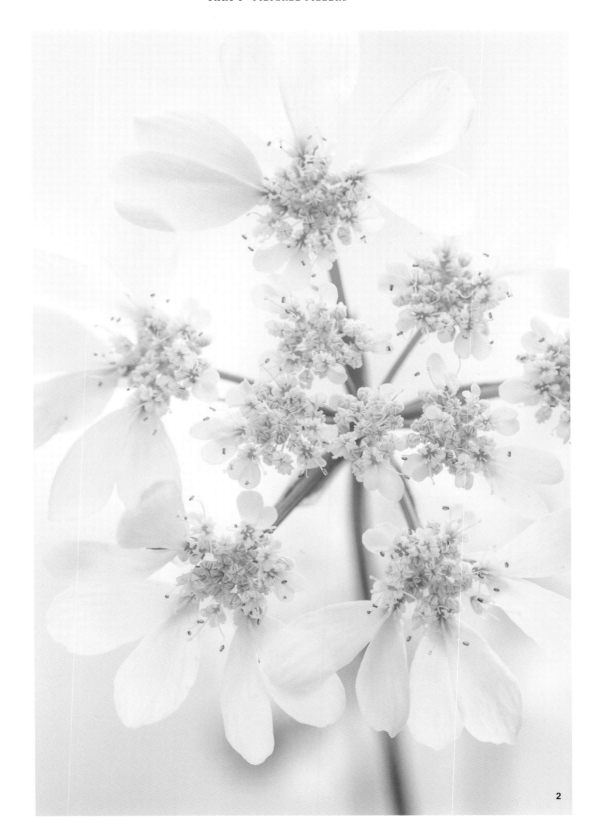

2

Switch grass
(*Panicum* 'Frosted Explosion')

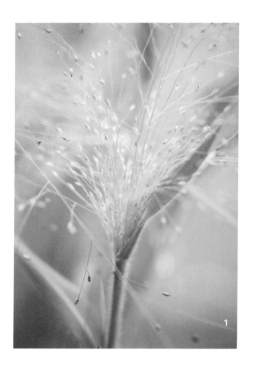

- Hardy annual
- Height: 45–60 cm
- Sow: direct or under cover in spring
- Site: full sun, well-drained soil
- Flowers: mid to late summer

Panicum 'Frosted Explosion' works well as a filler in the border, its airy fronds exploding in puffs of pale silvery-green. Each frond has a tiny seed on the tip that catches the light, sparkling and dancing in the wind, and the overall effect is one of movement and light to balance the more static plants in a border. It is also a fantastic bouquet-filler, and is useful for large pots and containers.

Sowing and growing
Sow the seed under cover in early to mid spring in a modular seed tray, several seeds to a module. Cover lightly with a fine layer of compost or vermiculite and germinate at 18–21°C. Move to a cooler place after germination and pot on if necessary before hardening off and planting out after all danger of frost has passed. The plants will be happiest in full sun but will tolerate a little shade.

Use this grass as a filler in the border, weaving it around other plants, or as a contrast plant in a large pot or container, where it will balance more colourful flowers.

1 'Frosted Explosion'

Mexican feather grass (*Stipa tenuissima*)

- Short-lived perennial
- Height: 40–60 cm
- Sow: under cover in early spring
- Site: full sun, well-drained soil
- Flowers: mid to late summer

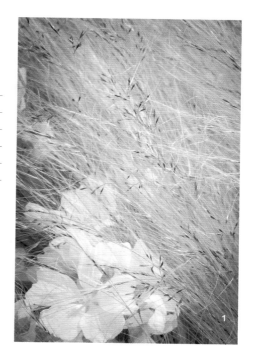

Also known as *Nassella tenuissima*, this is a very useful, easily grown ornamental grass that makes an excellent filler for a border, bringing movement and fluidity to a planting design. In the spring its filament-thin fronds are fresh green, while in the summer the fluffy flower heads are silver-blond, soft and tactile. It self-seeds gently around, so the seedlings can be grown on in pots and used to replace older specimens. It can also be used successfully in containers, to balance more flowery plants.

Varieties

Sometimes cultivar names are used, including 'Pony Tails' and 'Angel Hair', but they are no different from the basic species. An alternative – equally easy to grow from seed but much less widely available – is *S. lessingiana*, which is very similar in looks to *S. tenuissima* but slightly taller and fuller, growing to 1.2 m. It is also said to be hardier and longer-lasting than *S. tenuissima*, so it is definitely worth trying if you can find it.

Sowing and growing

Sow *S. tenuissima* and *S. lessingiana* in modules in early spring, two or three seeds to a module, scattering the finest layer of sieved compost over them. Germinate the seeds at about 20°C – this can take two or more weeks – and either grow the seedlings on in 7 cm pots until you need them, or plant them straight out from the modules in late spring or early summer.

If you overcrowd them, they won't thrive; and in any case they look much better dotted around a border than in a large, unwieldy clump. Alternatively, use one in a container to provide textured contrast to colourful flowers.

These light, flowing grasses revel in sunny spots and need well-drained soil; if their roots stay soggy in winter they will die.

1 *S. tenuissima*

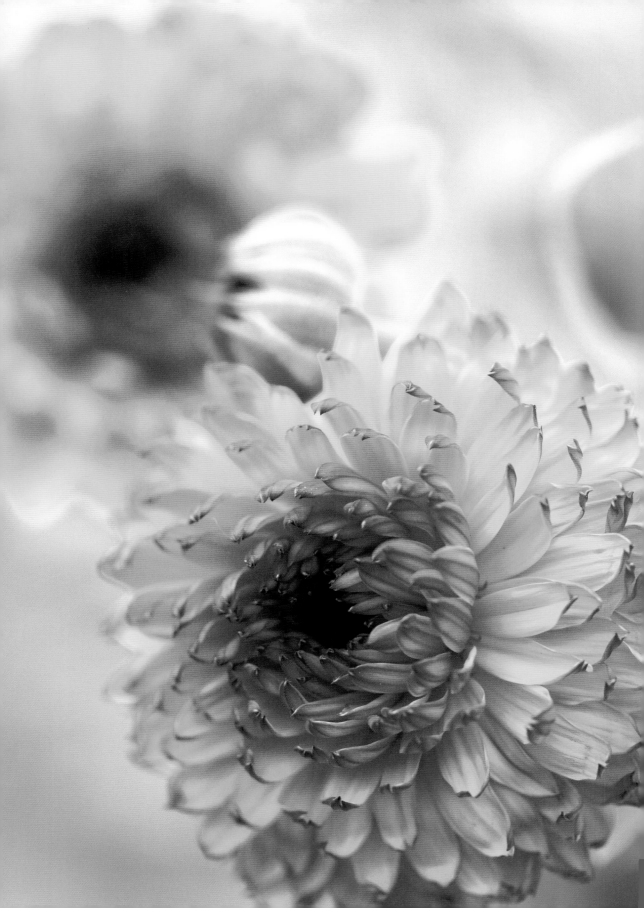

Bold and Beautiful

Pot marigold (*Calendula officinalis*)

Cosmos (*Cosmos bipinnatus*)

California poppy (*Eschscholzia californica*)

Sunflower (*Helianthus*)

Mallow wort (*Malope trifida*)

Black-eyed susan (*Rudbeckia*)

Mexican sunflower (*Tithonia rotundifolia*)

Zinnia (*Zinnia elegans*)

*Calendula
officinalis* 'Neon'

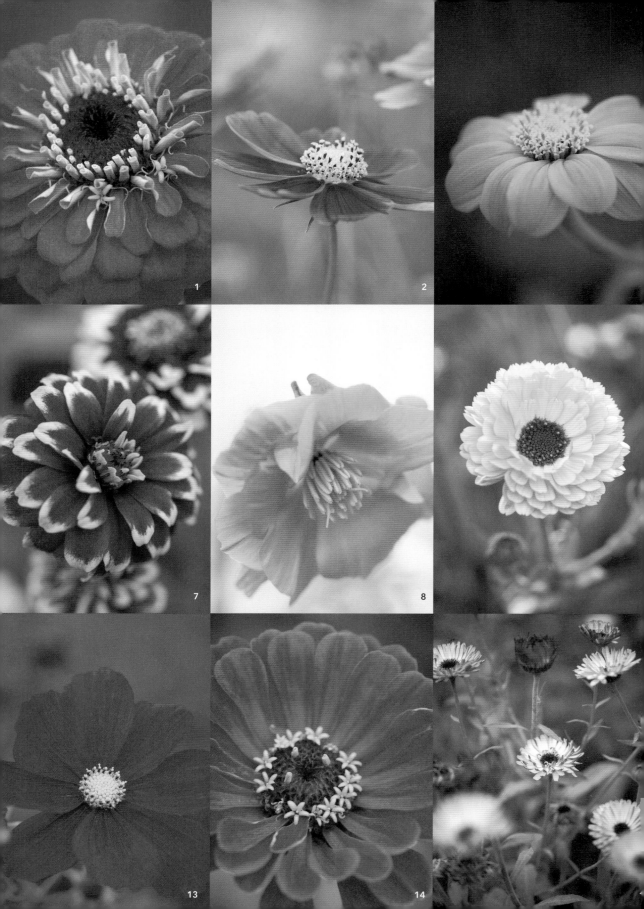

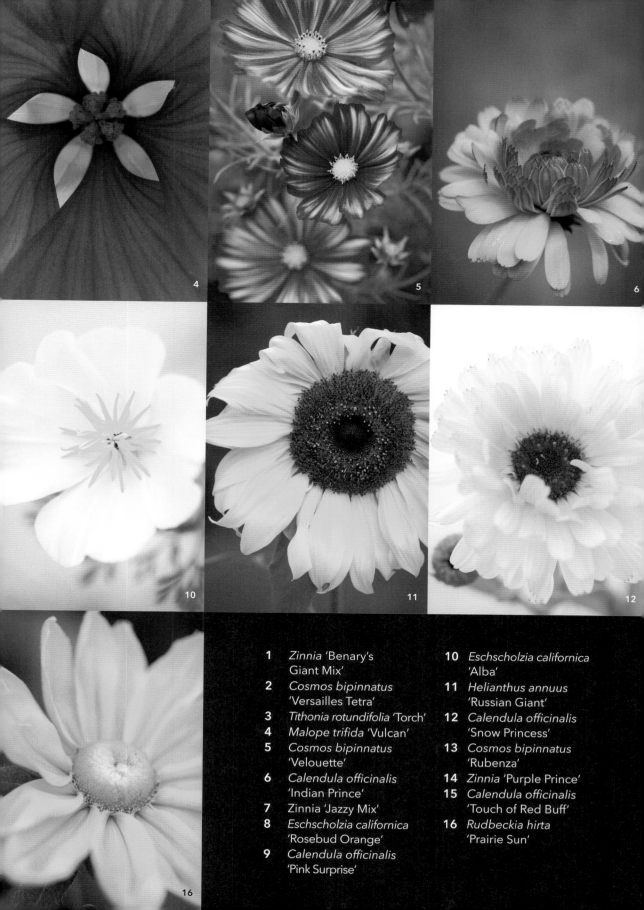

Pot marigold (*Calendula officinalis*)

- Hardy annual
- Height: 30–60 cm
- Sow: direct or under cover in early autumn or spring
- Site: sun or semi-shade, any well-drained soil
- Flowers: early to late summer

Marigolds are an easy, no-fail flower to grow if you want instant satisfaction – a good choice for children or anyone coming to gardening for the first time. Easy to germinate, swift-growing and happy in almost any soil, they provide hot splashes of colour to fill gaps in the border or around the edge of a vegetable plot, and happily adapt to containers. They are good for cutting and, as with many annuals, the more you cut, the more the flowers keep coming. They attract bees, hoverflies and other beneficial insects that help to control aphids and other pests. The petals themselves are edible, with a light, peppery taste.

Sowing and growing

Sow indoors in modular trays from early spring, germinating the seeds at 18–20°C, or outdoors in mid spring when the soil has warmed up. You can also sow direct in early autumn for earlier flowers. Marigolds aren't fussy about soil; they will also grow in full sun or partial shade and be happy in a container. They need very little attention other than the odd watering if the weather is very dry. When they start to bloom, pick or deadhead the flowers constantly and they will bloom for months, even until the first frosts.

Varieties

Tangerine-orange *Calendula officinalis*, the common marigold, is all you need if you want to fill your garden with bright, cheerful colour, but more subtle hues are available, from deep reds to pale yellows. 'Indian Prince' has rich, velvety-orange flowers with a deep rusty-red eye, and the darker colour is echoed on the reverse of the petals. The pale and interesting 'Snow Princess' has creamy-white petals with pale yellow undersides, and a chocolate-brown centre. For something a little different, 'Touch of Red Buff' has bi-coloured petals in a lovely buff pink with brown tips, giving an almost stripy effect. If you want a mix of colours all in one, look no further than the 'Pacific Beauty Mix', with flowers in lemon-yellow, apricot and darker orange.

1 'Indian Prince'
2 'Snow Princess'
3 'Touch of Red Buff'
4 'Pacific Beauty Mix'

Calendula is one of the easiest flowers to grow from seed. The seeds seem to want to germinate, whether sown direct in the ground or in modular trays.

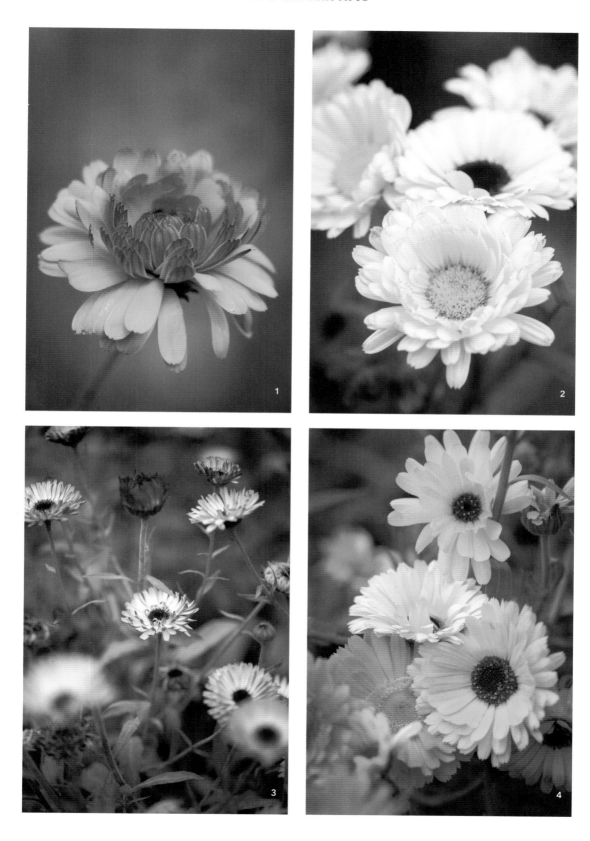

Cosmos (*Cosmos bipinnatus*)

- Half-hardy annual
- Height: 75–120 cm
- Sow: under cover in mid spring
- Site: full sun
- Flowers: midsummer to autumn

Cosmos is immensely satisfying to grow, with fresh-green ferny seedlings that develop over a matter of weeks into substantial plants, some of which can be very tall. Originating in South America, they are tender plants that baulk at the slightest frost – but by the time the cold weather arrives, they will have more than earned their keep, flowering continuously if you keep cutting them. The blooms last longer than a week in a vase, and look great on their own or combined with other flowers. Cosmos can of course be bought as plants in the garden centre, but you'll soon discover that the range of colours and varieties is much wider when grown from seed.

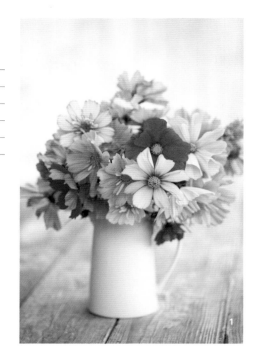

Varieties

The easiest and most elegant cosmos for a border is *C. bipinnatus* 'Purity', with snow-white single flowers on tall, willowy stems. Of the darker varieties, 'Rubenza' has the most striking flowers, wine-red in the centre, lightening to carmine-pink on the edges of the petals, with a central gold boss. 'Sea Shells Mix' has flowers in shades of pink, with petals that emerge furled up or quilled, gradually flattening as they age, while the deep-red 'Pied Piper' has similarly quilled petals. 'Psyche Mix' has delicate semi-double flowers in shades of raspberry, sugar-pink and white. New cultivars pop up all the time; one of the most recent is an interesting pale-yellow form called 'Xanthos', which at a slightly shorter 60 cm is ideal for a pot.

1 'Psyche', 'Dazzler', 'Picotee' and 'Sweet Sixteen' arrangement
2 'Psyche Mix'

Cosmos is a breeze to sow because the seeds are long and thin and easy to handle; they also germinate readily, usually within a week.

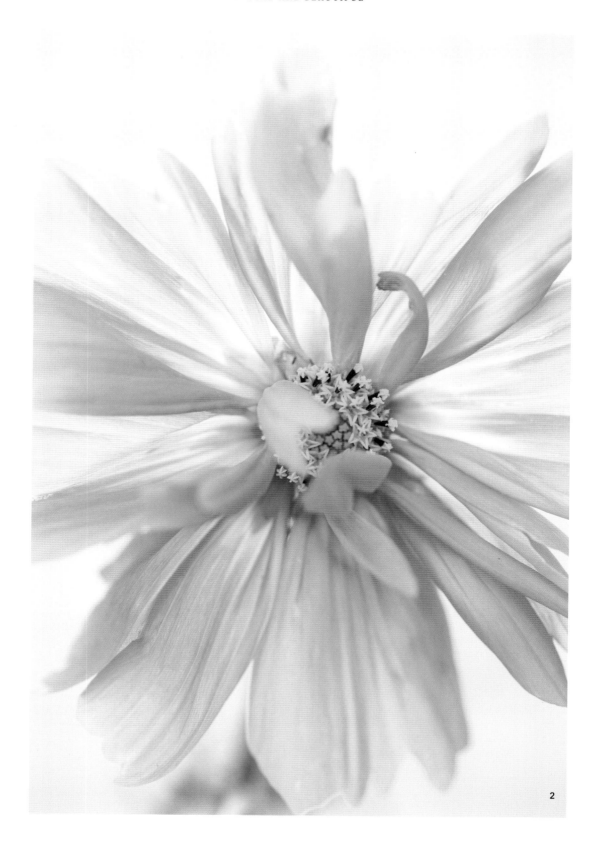

2

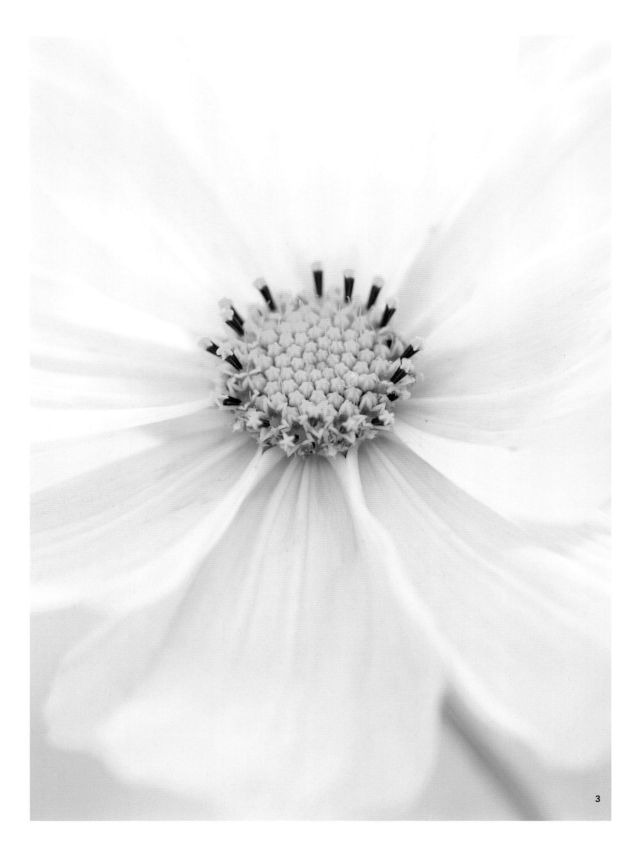

3

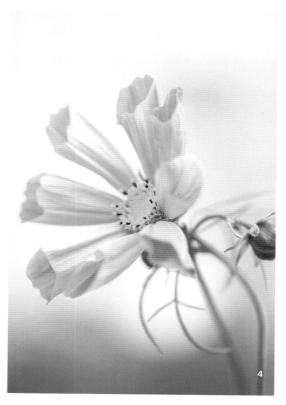

Sowing and growing

Sow under cover in April, two seeds to a module, and germinate at 18–21°C. Remove the weaker seedling of each pair and let the stronger one grow on, pinching out the growing tips if they get too tall and rangy (this causes a branching effect, making bushier, sturdier plants). There is no need to pot them on unless the plants grow very tall. Keep them in a cold frame until the weather warms up, then harden them off by leaving them outside for a week or two before planting out in mid to late May, in a sunny, well-drained spot.

3 'Purity'
4 'Sea Shells Mix'
5 'Rubenza'
6 'Xanthos'

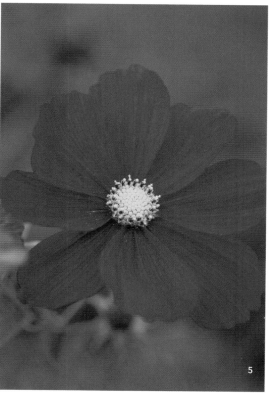

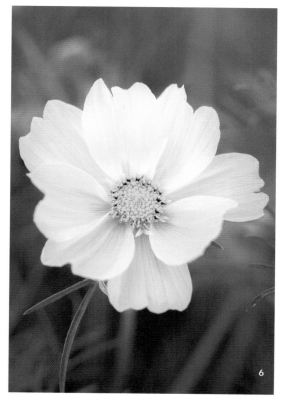

California poppy
(*Eschscholzia californica*) ☀

- Short-lived perennial, grown as an annual
- Height: 45 cm
- Sow: direct in mid spring or late summer
- Site: full sun, poor soil
- Flowers: early to late summer

The first year I had an allotment, I scattered California poppy seed around the edges of my plot. Every year after that they came back, wonderful drifts of tangerine-orange flowers with ferny foliage that were guaranteed to lift the spirits or raise a comment from passers-by. Native to California, where they are the state flower, these brightly coloured blooms are wonderfully simple to grow: simply scatter the seed and they will do their stuff, and the stonier or poorer the soil the better. Their flowers unfurl from buds like little parasols, and even when fully open, they will close again at the fading of the light in the evening, opening once more at the touch of the sun the next day. After blooming, they form long seed pods that crack audibly as they split open to expel the seeds that will grow the following year.

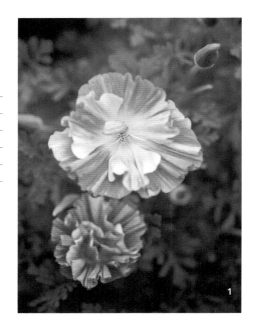

1

Sowing and growing

Sow as soon as the ground has warmed up in mid spring, or in late summer, when seed would be scattered naturally by existing plants. Prepare the ground by digging it over and raking it to a fine tilth, then mix the seed with sand and broadcast it in drifts or clumps throughout a border, or on any empty patch of land. The seeds should germinate with little trouble, and the plants will need watering only in times of extreme drought.

Varieties

For a patch of empty ground, or in a wild-flower meadow, you can't beat the species itself in that cheerful orange – or the slightly larger-flowered 'Orange King' – but if you find the orange hue too much, there are cultivars in more mellow colours. The white 'Alba' is for minimalists, pure white with contrasting golden anthers in the centre, or you could try 'Peach Sorbet', which has blooms of palest apricot. 'Rosebud Orange' is a double form in very dark orange, while 'Pink Bush' has both single and double flowers in pastel pink.

1 'Pink Bush'
2 'Alba'
3 'Peach Sorbet'
4 'Rosebud Orange'
5 *E. californica*

California poppies have tap roots that resent being disturbed, so it is always better to sow them direct.

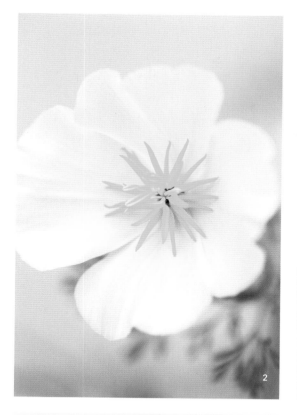

2

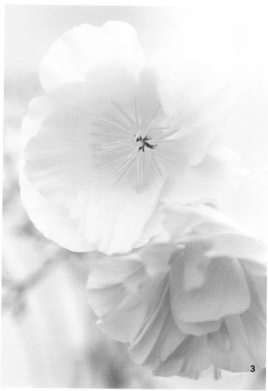

3

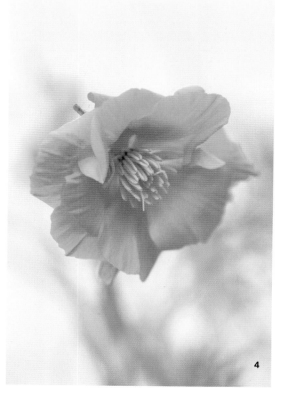

4

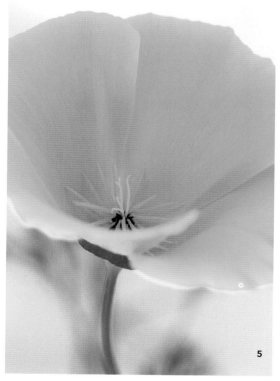

5

Sunflower (*Helianthus*)

- Half-hardy annual
- Height: 0.75–3 m
- Sow: under cover in early to mid spring or direct in late spring
- Site: full sun, rich, well-drained soil
- Flowers: mid to late summer

Sunflowers have a very basic, sensual appeal. Visualize a field of golden flowers in Provence, or a jugful on the kitchen table, and you just know the sight will make you happy. This North American native has been cultivated for thousands of years for its seeds, which are still ground for flour and oil. For our purposes, though, sunflowers are ornamental – with the bonus that they provide a wonderful source of food for birds at the end of the season.

Varieties

Towering single-stem sunflowers are the most popular with children, who compete to grow the tallest. Of these, *Helianthus annuus* 'Russian Giant' is a classic, and will grow 3 m tall if you give it rich soil. Another single-stem variety is 'Summer Breeze', which has slightly paler yellow flowers and an unusual green centre. There is a huge range of sunflowers for cutting, many of which produce much smaller blooms on branching plants, and in a wider range of colours, from deep rusty red to pale yellow and even white. 'Red Sun' has lovely velvety-dark flowers, and, at the other end of the colour spectrum, *H. debilis* subsp. *cucumerifolius* 'Italian White' and *H. debilis* 'Vanilla Ice' have pale-yellow blooms. Somewhere in the middle is *H. annuus* 'Valentine', a beautiful primrose yellow with a dark centre.

1 'Russian Giant'
2 'Red Sun'
3 'Italian White'
4 'Valentine'

Sowing and growing

Helianthus can be sown either under cover in modules or small pots in early to mid spring (in the warmth at 18–21°C) or directly into the soil in later spring. Simply put the seed in the ground, water and wait for it to shoot up, which it will do at an incredible rate, growing almost visibly day by day. Watch out for slugs if you are planting direct: the sunflowers' newly emerging leaves will be open targets for all sorts of molluscs.

Sunflowers are easy to grow in most well-drained soils in full sun, but they will grow even taller and stronger if they have a rich soil, so it pays to add plenty of well-rotted compost or manure to the ground before planting.

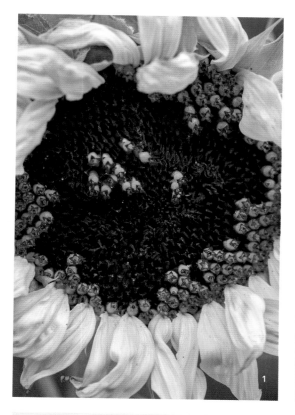

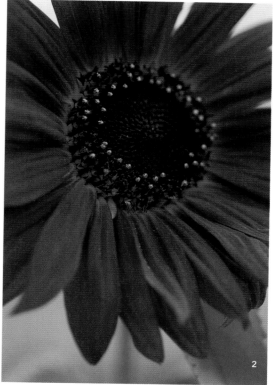

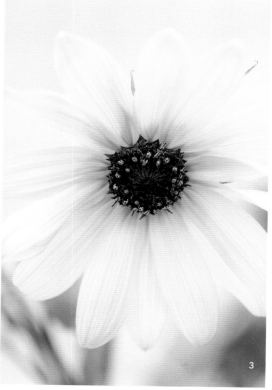

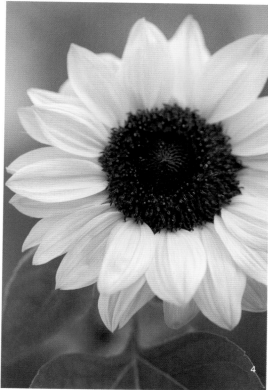

Mallow wort (*Malope trifida*)

- Hardy annual
- Height: 50–100 cm
- Sow: under cover in early spring or early autumn
- Site: full sun or semi-shade in moist but well-drained soil
- Flowers: early to late summer

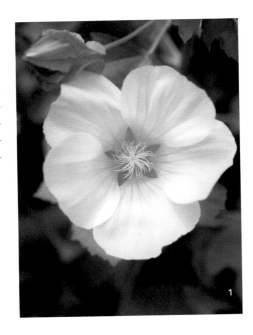

A member of the *Malvaceae* (mallow family), *Malope* is the more glamorous cousin of *Lavatera* and *Malva*, and almost as show-stopping as its other warm-climate cousin, hibiscus. Its large, glossy, trumpet-shaped flowers make quite a statement throughout the summer and into autumn, and are excellent for cutting.

Varieties
Malope trifida 'Vulcan' is the most widely grown variety at time of writing. Its silky, magenta-pink flowers are finely veined with a lime-green star in the centre, its petals voluptuously rounded. 'Alba' is a pure-white form, its snowy flowers contrasting with dazzling green foliage for a fresh, zingy look, while the mixture 'Strawberries and Cream' has both dark- and light-pink flowers, as well as white.

Sowing and growing
Germinate in the warmth at 20–23°C, either in early spring or early autumn, and move the seeds to a cooler place to grow on. Pot on as necessary before hardening off the plants and planting them out once all danger of frost has passed. In the garden they need an open, sunny spot and a fertile, moist but not waterlogged soil. They will start blooming in early summer, and will continue profusely for many weeks if you keep cutting the flowers.

1 'Alba'
2 'Vulcan'

Malope is a swift-growing plant that is best sown in modular trays in early spring, to be planted out in late May once the soil has warmed up.

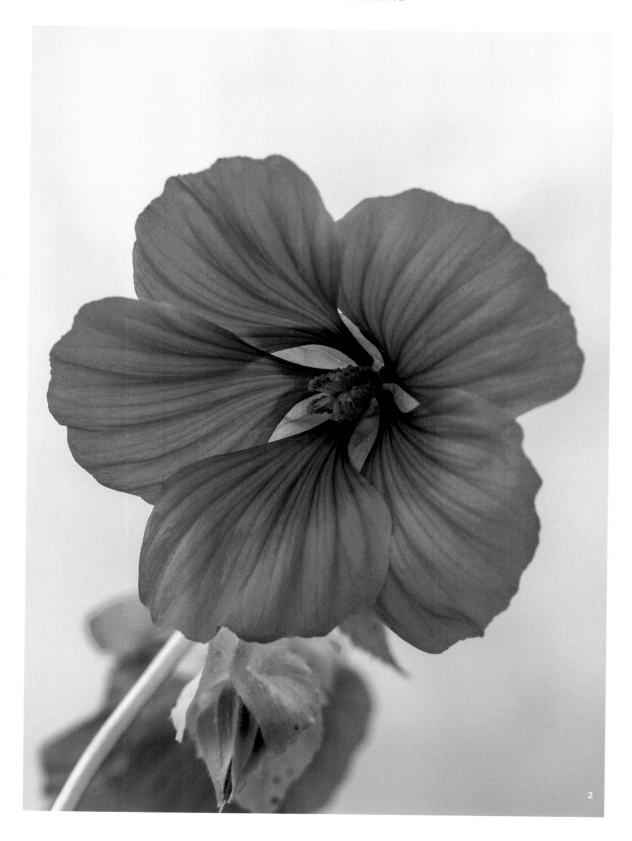

2

Black-eyed susan (*Rudbeckia*)

- Half-hardy annual/perennial
- Height: 50–100 cm
- Sow: under cover in late winter or early spring
- Site: full sun, moist but well-drained soil
- Flowers: midsummer to autumn

Rudbeckias are cheerful, sunny prairie plants from North America, with large, daisy-like flowers that bring a splash of colour to the late-summer flower garden. Many species and cultivars are grown as herbaceous plants, but some can also be grown from seed, mainly forms of *R. hirta*. These short-lived perennials or biennials are often grown as annuals, and they grow quickly enough to flower in the first season. Typically reaching about 60 cm tall, and forming bushy plants that flower well into the autumn, they are especially good for pots and containers, or for a cut-flower patch, blooming prolifically until the first frosts.

Annual Rudbeckias are warm-season plants, so make sure you wait until the weather is pleasantly summery before planting them outside in a sheltered, sunny spot.

1 'Prairie Glow'
2 'Goldilocks'
3 'Cherry Brandy'
4 'Sahara'

Varieties
R. hirta has been bred extensively, so a good range of colours is available, from butter yellow to rusty brown, as well as double and more decorative varieties. In classic yellow, you can't beat 'Prairie Sun', which has a pale-green centre and large golden flowers, while *R. triloba* 'Prairie Glow' has small, dark-orange flowers with pale-yellow tips. *R. hirta* 'Goldilocks' has double orange-yellow flowers, while, towards the darker end of the spectrum, 'Cherry Brandy' has amazing rusty-crimson single flowers. If you're growing the flowers for cutting, you might consider a seed mix such as 'Sahara', which has showy double flowers in dark, sultry shades of amber, copper and deep burnt rose.

Sowing and growing
Rudbeckia is best sown under cover in late winter or early spring. The seeds are small, but I still find it easier to sow them in modules, several to a compartment, and pinch out the weaker seedlings. Sow on the surface of the compost, because the seeds need light, and germinate them in warm conditions, 18–21°C. Once the seedlings have filled the modules, pot them on into 7 cm pots to continue growing until early summer, when you can plant them out in the garden or in containers. Give the plants plenty of water until they are well established.

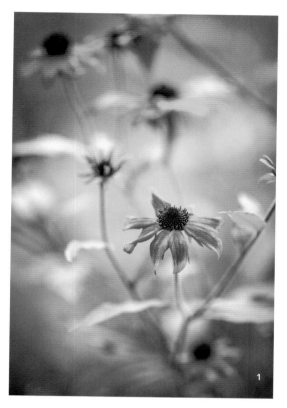

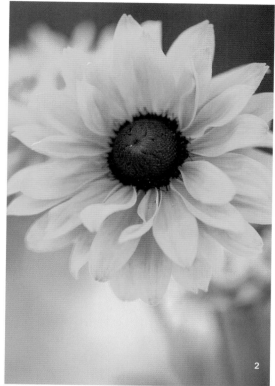

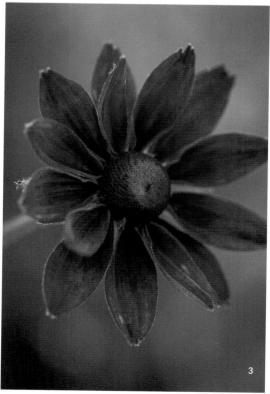

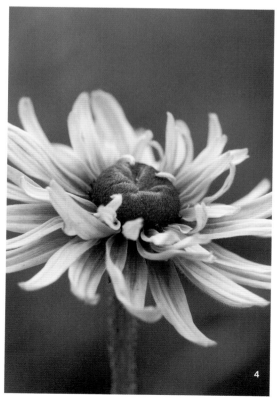

Mexican sunflower (*Tithonia rotundifolia*)

- Half-hardy annual
- Height: 0.8–2 m
- Sow: under cover in early spring
- Site: full sun, well-drained soil
- Flowers: midsummer to autumn

Relatively new to European gardens, this is a wonderful, vigorous, easy-to-grow annual, with velvety-orange flowers in late summer and autumn. Hailing from Mexico, it needs a good, hot summer to do its best, but if you're lucky with the weather it can form a huge, bushy plant up to 2 m tall. You would be extremely lucky for it to reach this lofty height, but at even half the size it should produce a good number of daisy-like flowers that are excellent for cutting.

The ideal weather scenario for Tithonia is a long, hot summer, so give it a position in the garden that can maximize these conditions – perhaps against a south-facing wall or within a sheltered walled or hedged garden.

Varieties

The species *Tithonia rotundifolia* is widely grown in the US, but a cultivar called 'Torch' is more popular in cooler climates. This is a shorter version of the species, able to produce flowers before the plant reaches the species' triffid-like proportions. 'Torch' has large, dark-orange flowers with golden centres. 'Yellow Torch' is also available, with pure-yellow flowers that are somehow not as special as the orange version. 'Arcadian Blend' is a seed mix with golden-yellow and orange flowers.

Sowing and growing

Sow seed under cover in early spring, into modular trays, two or three seeds to a module. Germinate in warm temperatures of 18–21°C and grow on in slightly cooler conditions, but preferably in a sheltered greenhouse or cold frame. Pot on into 7 cm pots when the seedlings get too big for the modules, and plant them out in late spring or early summer when all danger of frost has passed. Give them a sheltered spot in full sun, and ensure that the soil is well-drained. Don't over-fertilize, or the plant will produce too much foliage at the expense of flowers. In a very hot summer, the plant may get very tall and need some kind of support.

1 'Torch'

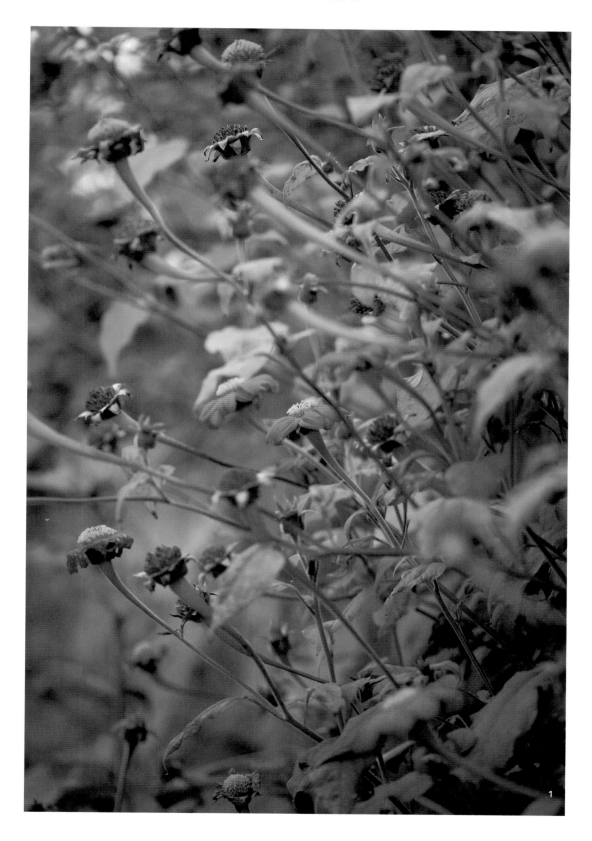

Zinnia (*Zinnia elegans*)

- Half-hardy annual
- Height: 50–80 cm
- Sow: under cover in mid spring or direct in early summer
- Site: full sun, fertile, moist but well-drained soil
- Flowers: midsummer to autumn

Zinnias bring exotic colour to our gardens, but are extremely easy to grow from seed. Native to South America, they were introduced relatively late to European gardens, in the eighteenth century, when they were known as 'poorhouse flowers' because they were so common and easy to grow. The original species were not that special, but as breeding began in the nineteenth century, many more colours became available and zinnias became the stars of colourful Victorian bedding schemes.

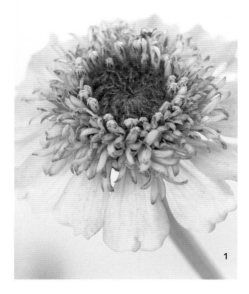

1

Varieties

There are dozens to choose from, in single, semi-double and double forms of varying size, and in almost every colour except blue. Here, we pick out a few that are particularly good for cutting. Growing up to 1 m, plants in the 'Benary's Giant' series are sturdy, with large double flowers in colours including lime, white and scarlet. Another recently developed group is the 'Zinderella' series, which have interesting raised double centres with a frill of larger single petals round the edge. 'Zinderella Peach' has lovely apricot-salmon flowers. 'Queen Red Lime' has the most unusual colour combination, with double flowers of pale red fading to lime at the edges of the petals. Finally, for a mixture of bright, cheerful colours, try 'Fabergé Mix', which has double flowers in shades of cream, salmon, rose-pink, magenta and scarlet.

1 'Fabergé Mix'
2 'Zinderella Lilac'
3 'Zinderella Peach'
4 'Queen Red Lime'
5 'Benary's Giant'

Sowing and growing

Don't sow too early under cover, or the seedlings will fill their modules before it is time to plant them out. Leave it until mid spring, then sow two or three seeds to a module, covering them only very lightly with vermiculite, since they need light to germinate. Start them off at 20–23°C and move them to a cooler place once the seedlings emerge. They can be prone to damping off, so don't overwater them, and keep the atmosphere dry. Plant out in early summer in a sunny spot with rich soil.

Zinnias are rather fussy about having their roots disturbed, so plant them out directly from their modules.

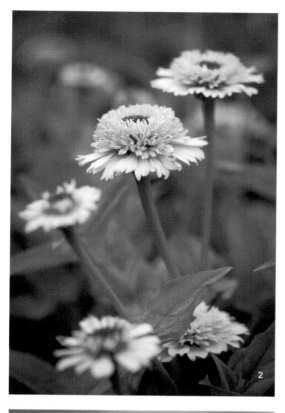

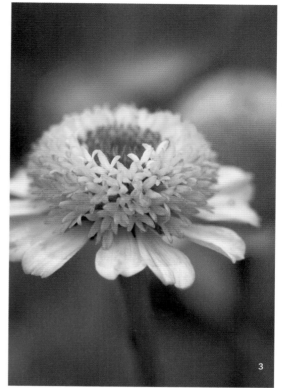

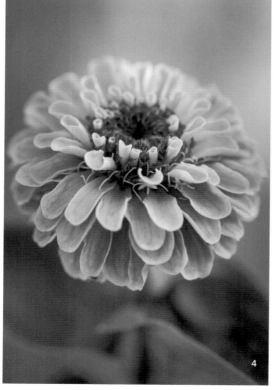

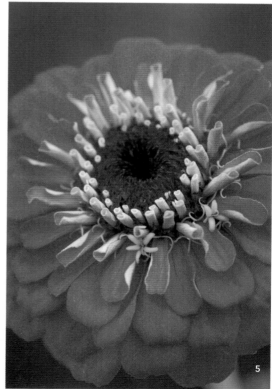

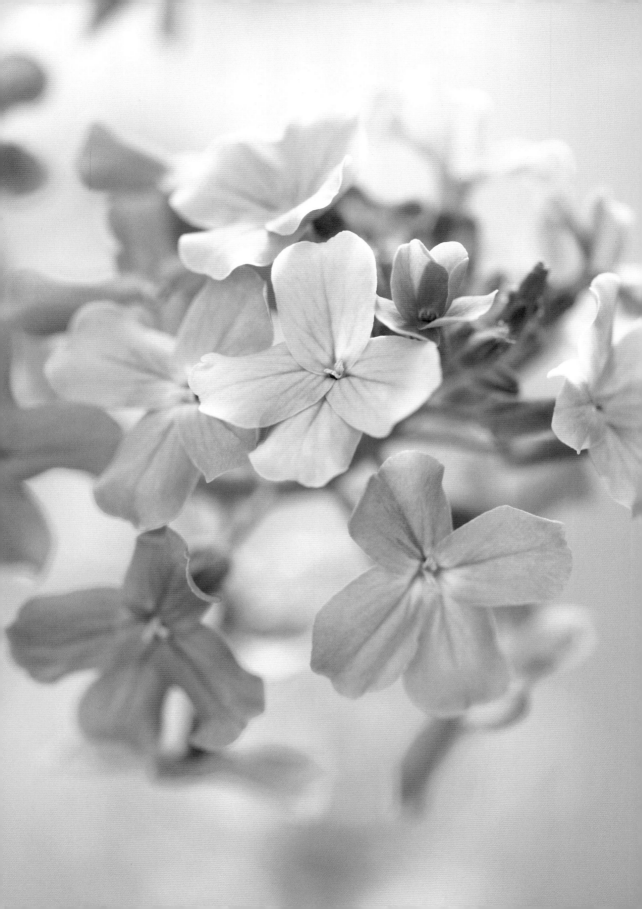

Sweetly Scented

Sweet rocket (*Hesperis matronalis*)

Sweet pea (*Lathyrus odoratus*)

Stocks (*Matthiola*)

Tobacco plant (*Nicotiana*)

Hesperis matronalis

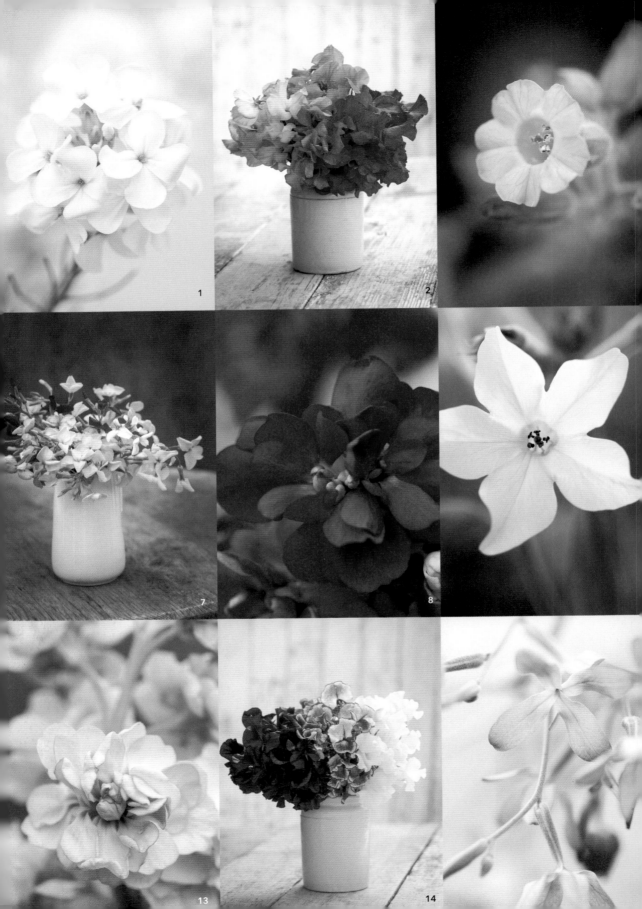

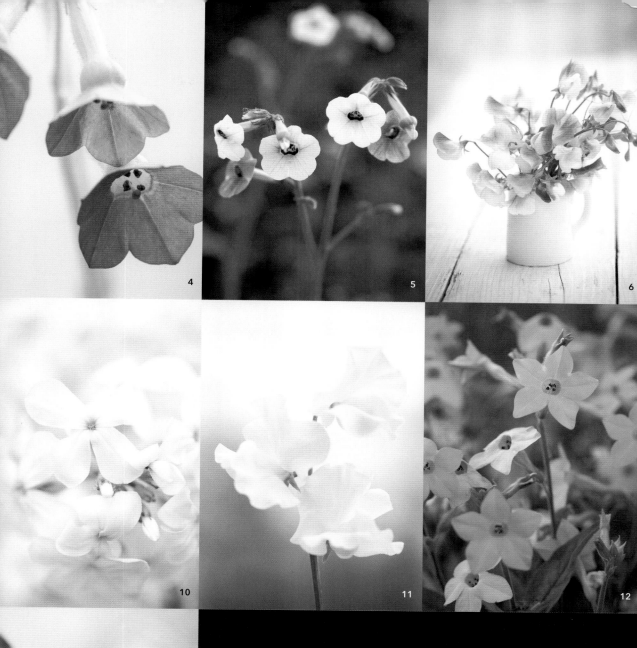

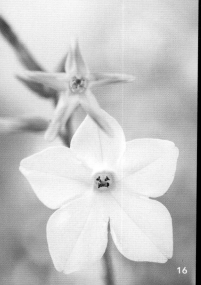

1	*Hesperis matronalis* 'Alba'	9	*Nicotiana sylvestris*
2	*Lathyrus odoratus* 'Gwendoline', 'Prince of Orange' and 'Henry Thomas' arrangement	10	*Hesperis matronalis* 'Alba'
		11	*Lathyrus odoratus* 'Jilly'
		12	*Nicotiana alata* 'Lime Green'
3	*Nicotiana rustica*	13	*Matthiola incana* 'Hot Cakes Mix'
4	*Nicotiana* 'Tinkerbell'		
5	*Nicotiana mutabilis*	14	*Lathyrus odoratus* 'Wiltshire Ripple' and 'Jilly' arrangement
6	*Lathyrus odoratus* 'Painted Lady' arrangement		
		15	*Matthiola bicornis* 'Starlight Scentsation'
7	*Matthiola* arrangement		
8	*Matthiola incana* 'Hot Cakes Mix'	16	*Nicotiana affinis*

Sweet rocket
(*Hesperis matronalis*)

- Biennial
- Height: 1.5–2.5 m
- Sow: under cover in spring or direct in late summer or early autumn
- Site: sun, well-drained soil
- Flowers: mid to late summer

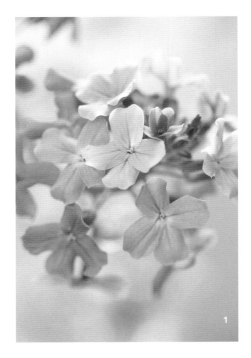

Like the wallflower, *Hesperis matronalis* is a member of the brassica family. Originally from central Europe, it has a long history of cultivation in Britain and has been grown in North America since at least the seventeenth century. The plants are a little like honesty, but taller and more willowy, with loose clusters of simple, sweet-smelling flowers in mauve or white, each with four rounded petals. As biennials, they produce rosettes of leaves in their first season, and flower the following year.

Varieties
Today it is just the single-flowered varieties that are grown, favoured for wild gardens or as a filler in naturalistic borders, where the plants can be left to seed around to form fragrant drifts. Only two forms are commonly grown: *H. matronalis* itself, which is pale mauve, and a white form, *H. matronalis* 'Alba'.

Sowing and growing
Sow *Hesperis* seed in modules or outside in seed beds in late spring or early summer, and plant out in early autumn. If they are happy in their home they will let you know by seeding generously around, meaning that after that initial sowing, the only attention you'll have to give them is to weed out unwanted seedlings.

1 *H. matronalis*
2 'Alba'

Relaxed and easy-going, the plants will do well in sun or dappled shade, and don't need rich soil. Their only foible is that they don't like to be waterlogged, so plant them in an area where the soil is well-drained.

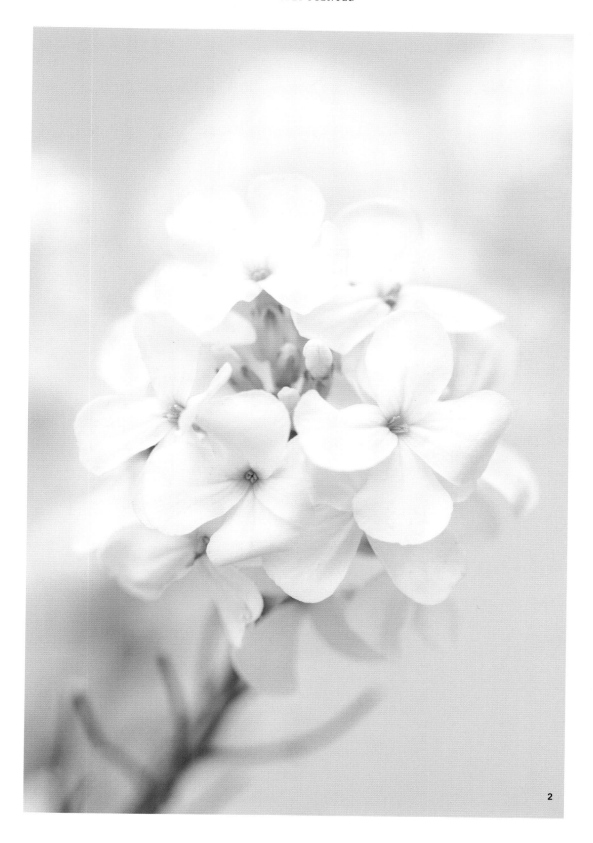

2

Sweet pea (*Lathyrus odoratus*)

- Hardy annual/climber
- Height: 1–2 m
- Sow: in pots or root trainers in autumn or early spring
- Site: full sun, fertile, moisture-retentive soil, with a support of some kind
- Flowers: early to late summer

How can you *not* love sweet peas? Other plants go in and out of fashion, but sweet peas are a consistent and universal favourite. Their sweetly scented flowers have enchanted generation after generation of garden-lovers, and they are brilliantly easy to grow, germinating willingly, growing swiftly and flowering lavishly, all within a few months.

Varieties

One of our top tips is to grow different varieties that will complement one another in the vase. This way you can mix the smaller-flowered, strongly scented varieties with the showier, larger-flowered varieties. For example, you could mix the highly perfumed 'Cupani' or 'Matucana', which have small maroon and purple blooms, with the larger-flowered 'Beaujolais' or the even more flamboyant Spencer sweet pea 'Windsor'. 'Lady Grisel Hamilton', one of the original *Grandiflora* sweet peas dating back to the nineteenth century, is a real old-fashioned beauty, with deeply scented, elegant lavender-blue flowers. One of the most recent and successful additions to the family is the cultivar 'Erewhon', which combines strong scent with pale pink and purple bi-coloured flowers. Often, it can be best simply to go for a sweet pea mix – if scent is most important to you, choose a highly scented mix, or if you want flower size and stem length, look for a Spencer mix.

Sweet peas are cool-climate plants, so don't give them too much heat once they have germinated, or the seedlings will grow weak and spindly.

1 'Cupani'
2 'Beaujolais' and 'Cupani' arrangement

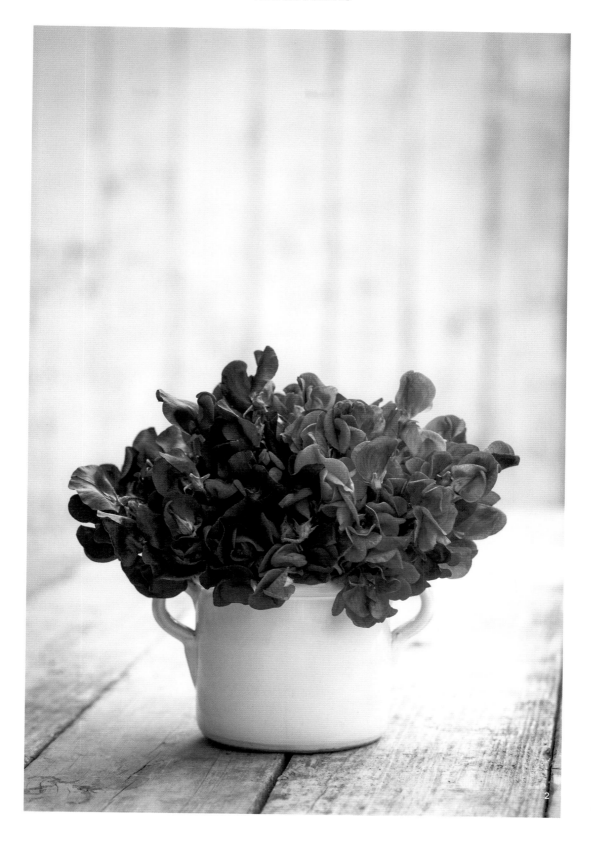

2

Sowing and growing

Sweet peas are easy to grow, but there are a number of ways to maximize your success. The first is to sow the seed into deep root trainers (see page 188), which allow the roots the space they need to develop, as well as making it easy to remove them. Sow the seed in autumn or in early spring; if you sow in autumn, you'll get earlier, stronger plants. Some people soak the seed overnight in warm water, which is said to improve germination, but I have never found this to be necessary. Simply push the seed into moist compost and leave to germinate in a warm place (18–21°C). As soon as the shoots appear, put the tray in a cooler place – ideally an unheated greenhouse or cold frame – so they don't become too leggy. Another way to produce stronger plants is to pinch out the growing tips when they reach about 10 cm tall; this will encourage more side shoots to appear, so that you end up with a branching plant. When the roots have filled the root trainer, it's time to plant the seedlings outside in well-prepared soil in full sun, giving them some kind of support to climb. As tendril-producing plants, sweet peas need something fine to cling to, so rig up some netting, twiggy pea sticks or chicken wire around the frame to get the plants started, and tie them in as they start to climb. Water them well until they are established, otherwise they can sulk and turn yellow. Mulching with compost can help to keep the moisture locked in. As the plants climb, keep tying them in, and then all that remains is to pick the flowers obsessively as they appear. The more you pick, the more they will flower, so pick fanatically and give away plenty of posies to share the joy.

3 'Lady Grisel Hamilton'
4 'Erewhon'
5 'Windsor'
6 'Gwendoline'
7 'Mrs Collier'
8 'Senator'

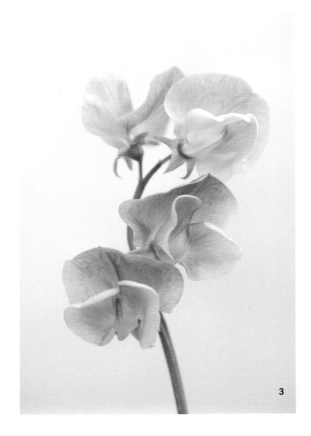

3

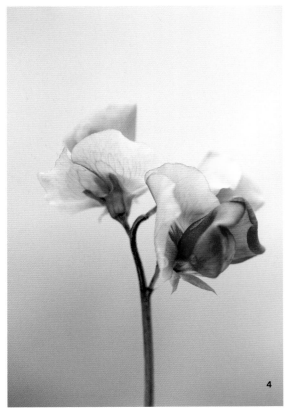

4

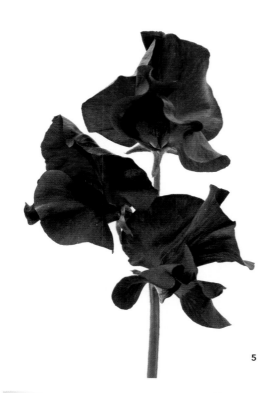

5

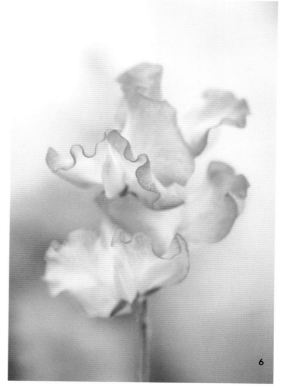

6

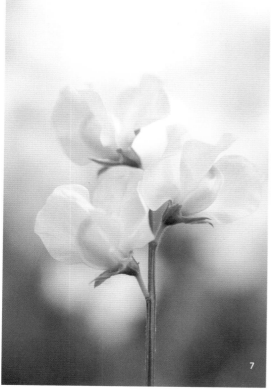

7

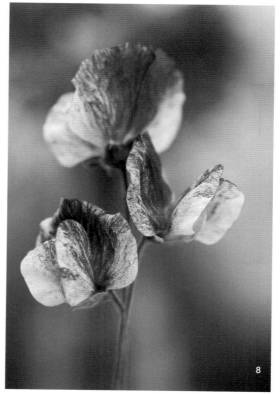

8

Stocks (*Matthiola*)

- Hardy annual/biennial
- Height: 30–50 cm
- Sow: direct (*M. longipetala* subsp. *bicornis*) or under cover (*M. incana*) in early spring. For biennials, sow in late spring or early summer
- Site: a sunny spot or container in well-drained soil
- Flowers: early to late summer

Stocks have had bad press in the past, not helped by the double varieties of *Matthiola incana*, with their chintzy colours and rather graceless, squat habit. But these easy annuals are worth growing for their phenomenal scent alone, and there are certain varieties that are much more pleasing to the eye. Pick a bunch for the kitchen and the sweet perfume will hang in the air for days – it is even better than the sweet peas!

Varieties

Of the double-flowered *M. incana* types, which flower throughout the summer, the variety 'Appleblossom' is our favourite. With antique-pink flowers clustered on a single stem, it is more subtle than many others, blending into a border and combining easily with other plants in a pot. There is also a single white form of *M. incana* called 'Pillow Talk', a biennial or short-lived perennial. Night-scented stocks (*M. longipetala* subsp. *bicornis*) are very different, flowering earlier in the season, from mid spring, with tiny flowers on longer, floppier stems. They are not the showiest of plants by day, but their starry flowers open in the evening to release their scent and attract night pollinators such as moths. Try the variety 'Starlight Scentsation', which has flowers in pastel shades of lilac, pink and white.

1 *M. bicornis* night-scented stocks
2 'Starlight Scentsation'
3 'Appleblossom'
4 'Pillow Talk'

Sowing and growing

If you're growing night-scented stocks, scatter the seed outdoors in early spring, where they are to flower. You can sow in a seed tray, but they grow so quickly that they can easily become leggy and floppy. For the double *M. incana* types, sow under cover in early spring at 18–20°C and plant out in late spring. For the biennial 'Pillow Talk', sow in modules in late spring or early summer and plant out in late summer or early autumn.

All stocks are unfussy when it comes to the ground they grow in, but will welcome a sheltered, sunny spot, ideally close to your house or seating area, where the scent can be appreciated.

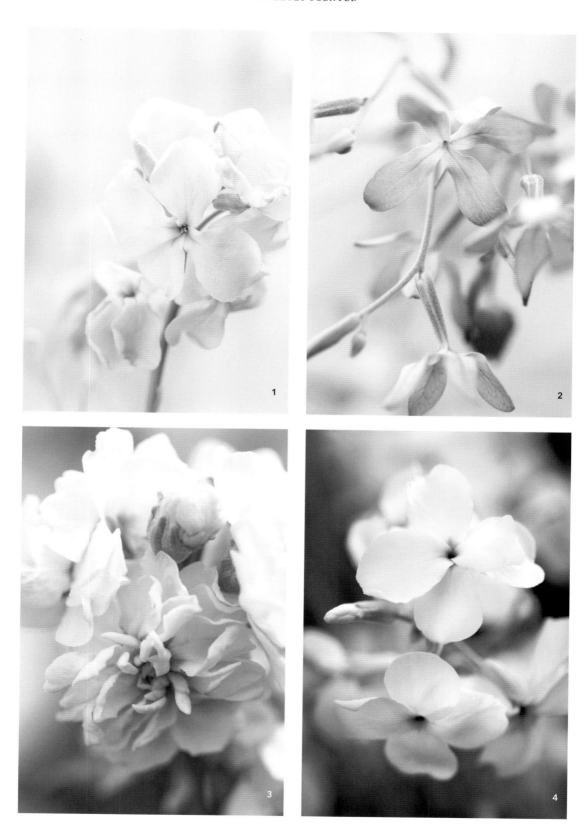

Tobacco plant (*Nicotiana*)

- Half-hardy annual
- Height: 30–150 cm
- Sow: under cover in mid spring
- Site: full sun or partial shade, most normal soils
- Flowers: early to late summer

The wild tobacco plant, *Nicotiana rustica*, was the original source of pipe tobacco brought back to Britain from South America by Sir Walter Raleigh in the sixteenth century. However, the species we grow in our gardens are important for their ornamental value and often for their scent, not for their nicotine. Growing swiftly from seed to become tall and statuesque, tobacco plants are perfect for summer bedding, and ideal for pots and containers, where they can be mixed with other annuals and grasses.

Varieties

N. sylvestris is the most common tobacco plant in our gardens. Growing up to 1.5 m tall, it produces tall, willowy stems with lime-green buds opening into clusters of long, scented, tubular white flowers like little lanterns. *N. alata* has more open flowers and possibly an even sweeter scent. 'Lime Green', with its curious green flowers, is popular, while the dwarf *N. alata* 'Roulette', in crimson, rose and white, is useful for containers. Other green-flowered tobacco plants include the lanky *N. langsdorffii* (1.2 m), with lime-green tubular flowers, and the even taller *N. knightiana*, with smaller, paler flowers, elegant and understated. One of the newest in cultivation is *N. mutabilis*, which was discovered in Brazil in 2002. Its multi-shaded – but unscented – flowers start off white, morphing through shades of pink to a striking magenta, and appear in various stages of colour on the same plant. For something different, try 'Tinkerbell', a small plant ideal for a container, with dark, rusty-red flowers held at the end of pale-green trumpets.

The best way to germinate these minute seeds is to scatter tiny pinches on top of moist seed compost – or mix them with a little sand before sowing.

1 *N. rustica*

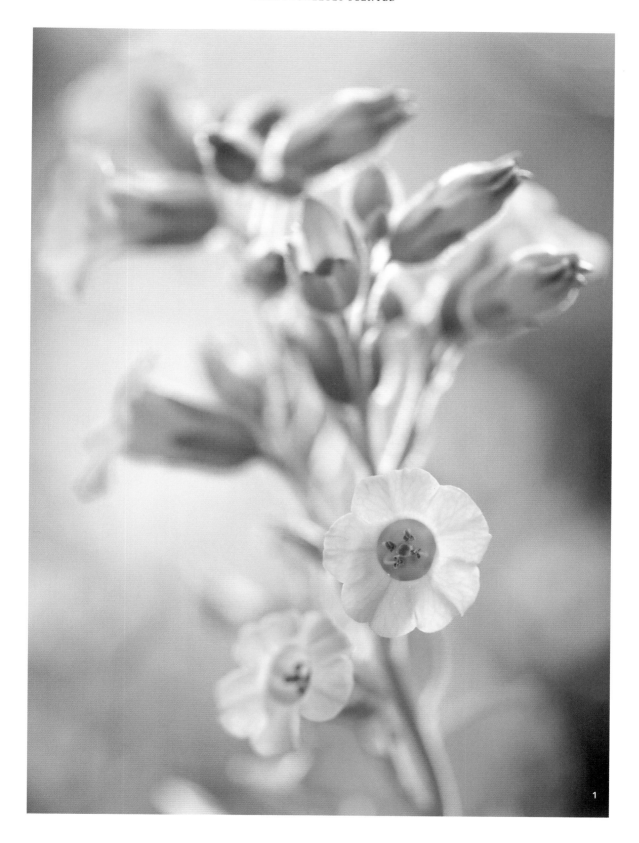

1

Sowing and growing

The seeds need warmth and light to germinate, so after sowing leave them at 20–22°C and keep the compost moist but not too wet. The seedlings must be pricked out when they are big enough to handle, but the leaves grow more swiftly than the roots, so you can leave it until the leaves are as big as the top of your forefinger. Sow in mid spring and grow on in a greenhouse or conservatory before hardening off in late spring and planting out once all danger of frost has passed. Tobacco plants grow best in full sun in moist but well-drained soil, and will tolerate light shade.

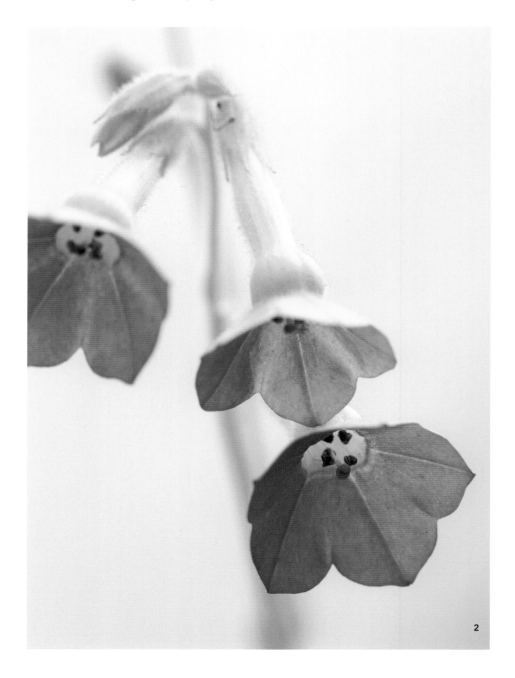

2

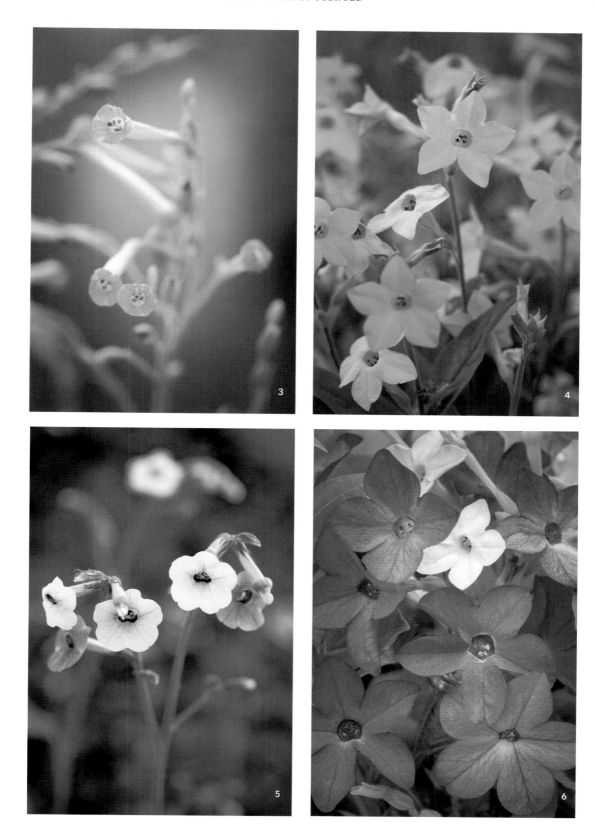

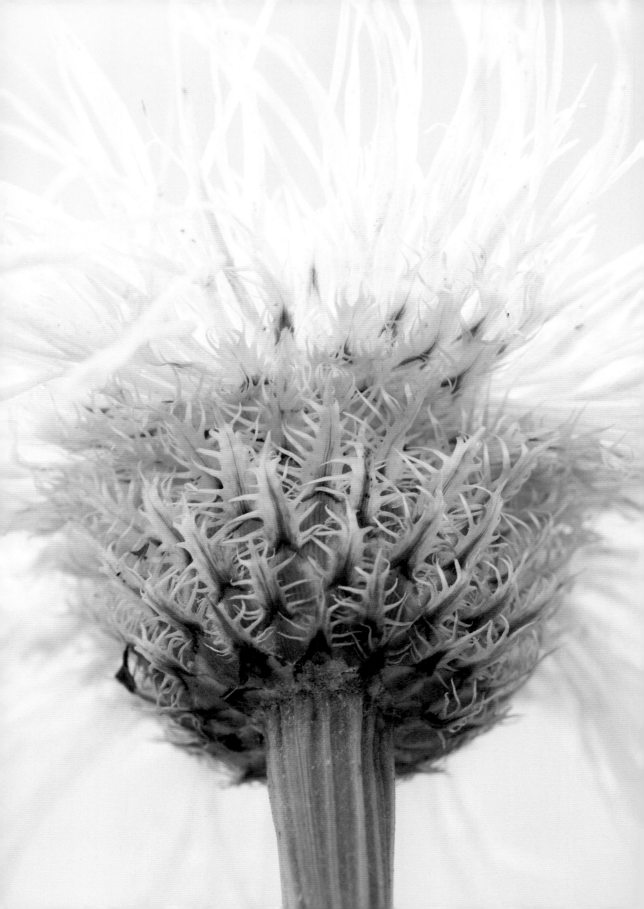

Exotic Beauties

Love-lies-bleeding (*Amaranthus caudatus*)

American basket flower (*Centaurea americana*)

Spider flower (*Cleome hassleriana*)

Cup-and-saucer plant (*Cobaea scandens*)

Dahlia (*Dahlia*)

Morning glory (*Ipomoea*)

Bells of Ireland (*Moluccella laevis*)

Centaurea americana
'Aloha Blanca'

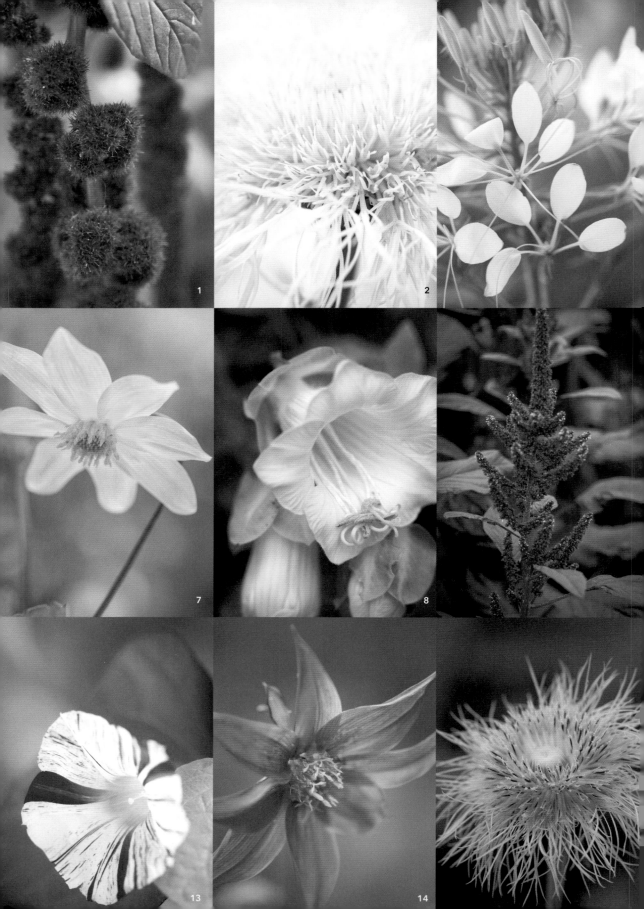

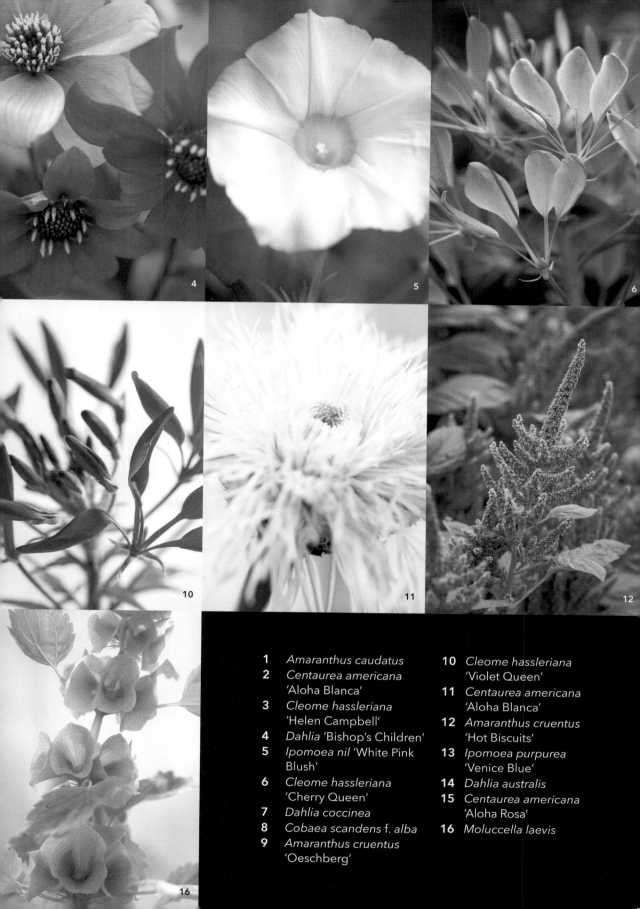

Love-lies-bleeding
(*Amaranthus caudatus*)

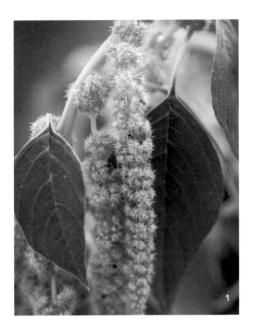

1

- Half-hardy annual
- Height: 1 m
- Sow: under cover in mid spring
- Site: sun, well-drained but moist soil
- Flowers: late summer to autumn

Amaranthus is a tropical plant with a wide geographical spread. The most common species grown in temperate climates is *A. caudatus*, a tall, upright plant with dramatic claret-red tassel flowers and large, tropical-looking leaves. In the UK it is used mainly as an ornamental or cut flower, but its leaves can also be eaten like spinach. In fact, almost every part of this plant is edible: in central and Latin America its seeds have been used as a grain since ancient times. Gluten-free as well as extremely rich in protein and minerals, and full of omega-3 oils, it could well be the next super-grain. The seeds can even be used like popcorn.

Varieties
The US has a wider selection of *Amaranthus* seed than the UK, with flowers in colours ranging from coral-pink to purple-black. In the UK, if you hunt around you can find seed of interesting cultivars, such as 'Viridis', which has slim green tassels (and is great as foliage for flower arrangements), or 'Autumn Palette', with intensely coloured bronze flowers. *A. caudatus* 'Pony Tails Mix' produces a mixture of red and green plants, while 'Red Army' has very dark maroon flowers and deep-red foliage – another good variety for cutting.

Sowing and growing
Sow *Amaranthus* in mid spring, for planting out in early summer. The small seeds can be sown on top of moist

compost in a seed tray, or in small pinches in modular trays, pulling out all but the strongest seedling in each module. Germinate the seeds at 20–25°C and cover them only lightly, since they need light to germinate. In the right conditions they will germinate easily. Remember that these are tender plants, so keep them under cover until summer has really started, potting them on if necessary and hardening them off.

Amaranthus is a warm-climate plant, and grows swiftly if it has plenty of warmth. Keep the seedlings under cover in a greenhouse or conservatory until you are ready to plant them out.

1 'Viridis'

American basket flower
(*Centaurea americana*)

- Hardy annual
- Height: 1.5 m
- Sow: direct or under cover in early autumn or early spring
- Site: full sun, poor soil
- Flowers: mid to late summer

This beauty is related to the humble English cornflower, but is altogether different, with large, thistle-like flowers in shades of pink or white – yet without the thorns associated with other thistles. In southern states of America, and in Mexico, the wild species forms large colonies along roadsides and in pastures, with huge pink, fringed flowers that exude a sweet honey scent. In the UK, it is rather a rarity, available only to grow from seed. Try it in a meadow setting, where it should do well among other sun-loving plants.

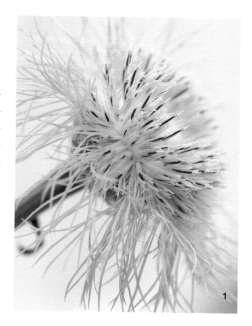

Varieties
In the UK, two varieties are available to grow from seed: 'Aloha Blanca', with fluffy, ivory-white flowers, and the very pale pink 'Aloha Rosa', whose inner petals are often tipped with black. Both can produce blooms up to 15 cm in diameter, and are even beautiful in bud, with a wonderful interlacing effect that lends it its common name.

Sowing and growing
C. americana is easy to grow as an annual sown in early autumn or early spring. It can be sown direct but, as always, you will have more control if you sow under cover. Sow two or three seeds to a module, cover with a fine sprinkling of compost and germinate at 18–20°C. Plant out the seedlings in early summer, giving them a spot in full sun and well-drained soil.

1 'Aloha Rosa'

Despite its exotic looks, Centaurea americana is a humble meadow flower, and does best in poor soil. Too much richness will mean more foliage at the expense of flowers, so treat it mean and it will be happy.

Spider flower
(*Cleome hassleriana*)

- Half-hardy annual
- Height: 1–1.2 m
- Sow: under cover in mid to late spring
- Site: full sun, fertile, well-drained soil
- Flowers: late summer to autumn

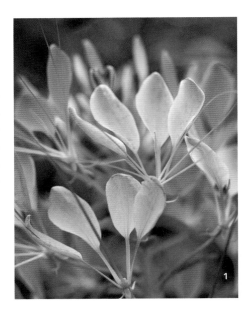

The wonderful-looking *Cleome hassleriana (syn. C. spinosa)* comes from the pampas lowlands of South America, where it grows widely on the open, fertile plains. Its large, faintly scented flower clusters add an exotic touch to a late summer border, with long, spidery stamens and narrow seed pods developing lower down on the flower. The palmate leaves are exotic-looking, too, but do be careful of the spines that develop at the base of each leaf; they can be a hindrance if you're using it as a cut flower. *Cleome* grows tall, so it can pack a real punch in a border, especially if planted en masse, or with other half-hardies such as *Amaranthus* and *Tithonia* to create a colourful throng of plants that will go on flowering until the first frosts.

Sowing and growing
Despite its striking appearance, *Cleome* is easy to grow from seed, although – as with all half-hardy annuals – it is helpful to have a greenhouse or conservatory to house the seedlings in the first few weeks. In mid spring, germinate at 21–25°C and barely cover the seeds, since they need light to germinate. Once the seedlings appear, move the trays to a cooler place and grow on, hardening them off gradually and finally planting them out in early summer. Give them an open, sunny spot in rich, well-drained soil and keep them well watered until they are established.

Varieties
One of the loveliest is 'Helen Campbell', which produces tall, sturdy stems topped with airy white flowers. 'Violet Queen' is another widely grown variety, dramatic and architectural, with deep violet flowers, while 'Mauve Queen' has paler, more subtle blooms. If you want a mixture of all three colours, choose 'Odyssee Mix'.

Cleome doesn't like having its roots disturbed, so is best planted out direct from the modules rather than being potted on.

1 'Cherry Queen'
2 'Helen Campbell'

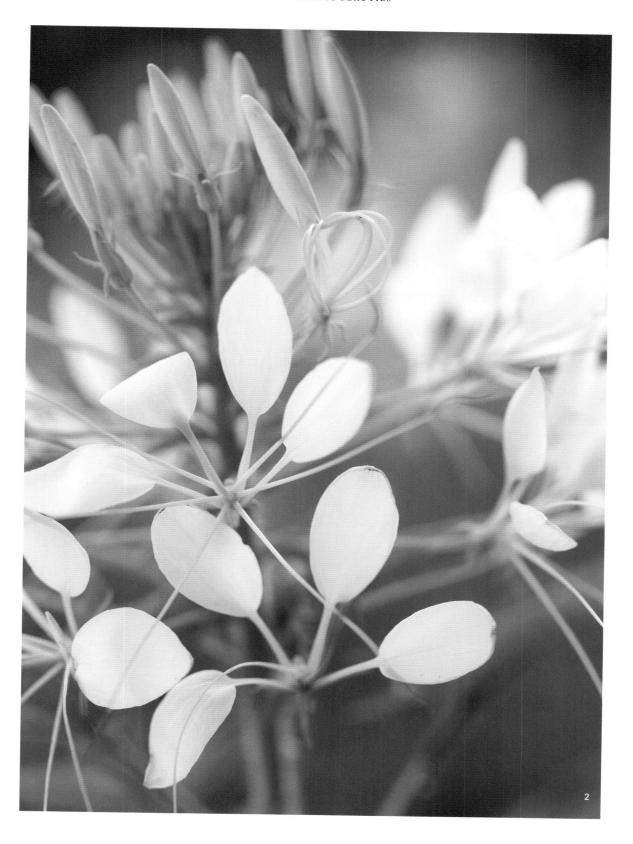

2

Cup-and-saucer plant
(*Cobaea scandens*)

- Short-lived perennial grown as a half-hardy annual in cool climates
- Height: up to 4 m
- Sow: under cover in late winter or early spring
- Site: sheltered, south-facing wall or tall fence
- Flowers: late summer to autumn

This vigorous climber from Mexico will grow prodigiously in a single season, flowering on and on from midsummer until the first frost. It is reasonably easy to grow and widely available, yet not often seen, and its large, bell-shaped flowers held on longish stalks away from the foliage are guaranteed to attract attention. In its natural home in tropical South America it is pollinated by bats, and at dusk the flowers give off a scent to attract them. *Cobaea* needs a sunny, sheltered spot to thrive, and will clamber over any kind of support, often putting on several metres of growth in a season.

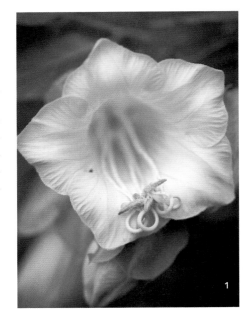

Cobaea is a tender plant that must be sown early in the year and kept under cover until the last frosts have passed. Because it sometimes takes a few weeks to germinate, it should ideally be sown in late winter in order to get it flowering by late summer.

1 *C. scandens* f. *alba*
2 *C. scandens*

Varieties
There are two forms, the purple *C. scandens* and the less commonly seen white *C. scandens* f. *alba*. The flowers of the purple form are perhaps the most spectacular, starting off greenish white and maturing to inky purple as the season goes on. They look like silk-covered lampshades, with petals that flare elegantly at the ends, and a ruff of green bracts at the top.

Sowing and growing
Cobaea seeds are large and can be sown individually in modular trays in late winter or early spring. Soak them for a couple of hours before sowing, then push the seeds into the compost on their sides, just covering them with a layer of compost. These South American beauties need heat, so keep them at 20–23°C until they have germinated. Grow them on inside on a windowsill, or in a conservatory or greenhouse, potting them on until they are substantial enough to be planted outside, in late spring or early summer. As you increase the pot size, harden the plants off before planting them out to continue growing up a wall, trellis or fence, tying the shoots in as necessary.

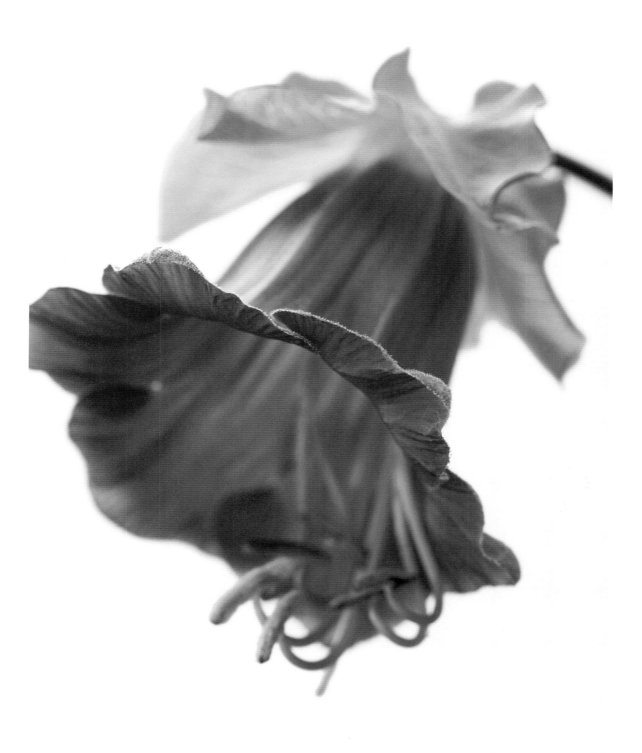

Dahlia (*Dahlia*)

- Short-lived perennial grown as a half-hardy annual in cool climates
- Height: 40–150 cm
- Sow: under cover in late winter or early spring
- Site: full sun, well-drained soil
- Flowers: midsummer to autumn

Dahlias were introduced to Europe and North America from Mexico in the late eighteenth century. Their tendency to mutate led horticulturists to hybridize them obsessively to create increasingly outlandish varieties in an infinite variety of colours and shapes. Named strains are usually grown from tubers, but dahlias can also be raised from seed to flower the same year. Bear in mind, however, that you will not be able to grow named varieties from seed. Most seed-raised dahlias will be from seed mixes with flowers in a range of colours and shapes, or the species themselves, which come true from seed.

Varieties
Many seed mixes are available, some of them fairly gaudy. One of the most attractive is 'Bishop's Children', which produces single, daisy-like flowers in rich shades of red, magenta and burnt orange. *D. variabilis* 'Sunny Reggae' has single and semi-double flowers in shades of apricot and orange, and is great for pots. The seeds germinate readily and grow quickly to produce flowers in a matter of months, and the plants form tubers that can be lifted and replanted the following year to flower again. Species you can grow from seed include crimson-orange *D. coccinea* and pink *D. australis* and *D. merckii*. These tall, airy dahlias produce small, delicate flowers; they aren't as showy as some of the others, but they are excellent border fillers for late summer, and will flower until the first frosts.

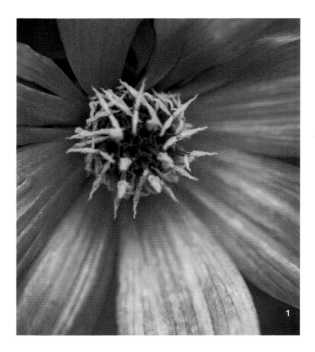

1

Deadhead or pick dahlias regularly to keep them blooming until the first frosts.

1 *D. coccinea*
2 'Sunny Reggae'

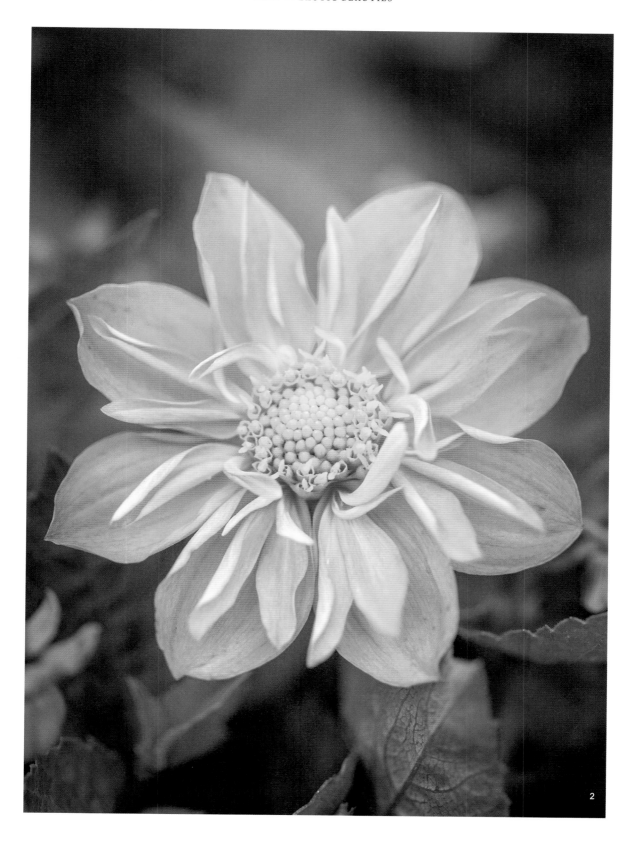

2

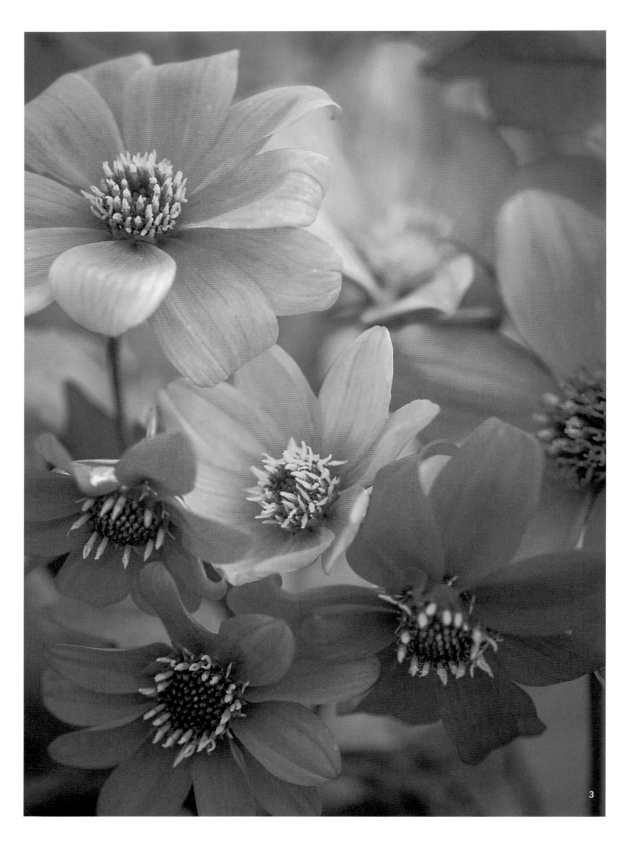

3

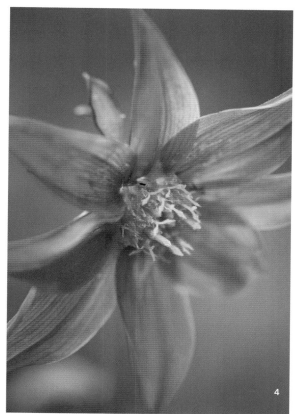

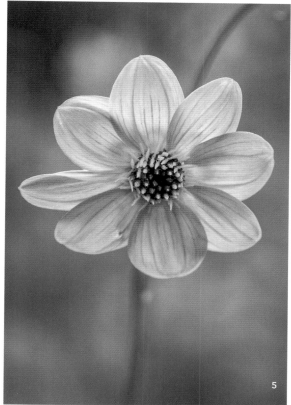

Sowing and growing

Dahlia seed should be treated as that of any other half-hardy annual: sown indoors in late winter or early spring, and planted out in late spring or early summer when all danger of frost has passed. The elongated seeds can be sown in individual modules, germinating readily at 18–21°C. Move the seedlings to an unheated greenhouse to grow on, but bring them in again if there is a prolonged frost. If the modules become congested, pot the seedlings on into 9 cm pots, and plant them out eventually in a sunny, sheltered position with fertile, well-drained soil.

3 'Bishop's Children'
4 *D. australis*
5 *D. merckii*

Morning glory (*Ipomoea*)

- Half-hardy annual/climber
- Height: 3–4 m
- Sow: under cover in early spring
- Site: a sheltered wall or fence in full sun
- Flowers: late summer to autumn

Ipomoea is a huge genus found in tropical and subtropical regions around the world, containing over 500 different species. In temperate climates, we have adopted a handful of these attractive climbing species to grow as annuals, particularly forms of *I. purpurea* and *I. tricolor*, which originated in Mexico and Central America. Both have heart-shaped leaves and wide, saucer-shaped flowers, and grow quickly through the growing season if they have enough warmth, twining around canes or over an arch as they grow. The reason for the common name becomes apparent when you watch the plant flower: its large blooms unfurl slowly in the morning sun and fold up as the day draws to a close.

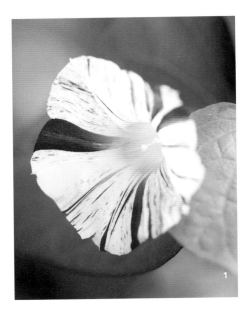

Varieties

I. tricolor 'Heavenly Blue' is one of the most widely available morning glories, but we think there are other more unusual varieties to get excited about. Two derived from *I. purpurea* spring to mind: 'Venice Blue' has huge white flowers splashed and striped with purple-blue, while 'Dacapo Light Blue' has powder-blue flowers with a distinctive purple-blue line down the centre of each petal. Another unusual one is *I. nil* 'Chocolate', which has huge flowers in dusky chocolate-pink.

Sowing and growing

Growing *Ipomoea* from seed is easy. Sow in early spring in individual small pots, at 20–25°C, and grow on in a sheltered greenhouse. Pot them on as the seedlings grow, taking care not to disturb their roots too much, since they are pernickety about being moved. Beware of leaving the greenhouse door open at night – single-digit temperatures will leave the seedlings looking sick and wilted, and they may not recover. Plant them out when temperatures have risen and the forecast is consistently warm. Don't give them an over-rich soil or they will produce too much foliage at the expense of flowers.

In a warm, sunny summer, these twining climbers will put on masses of growth and flower profusely, draping themselves over any climbing frame you provide: trellis or wires on a fence, a metal or wooden arch, or you could even try growing them up a tree.

1 'Venice Blue'
2 'Dacapo Light Blue'

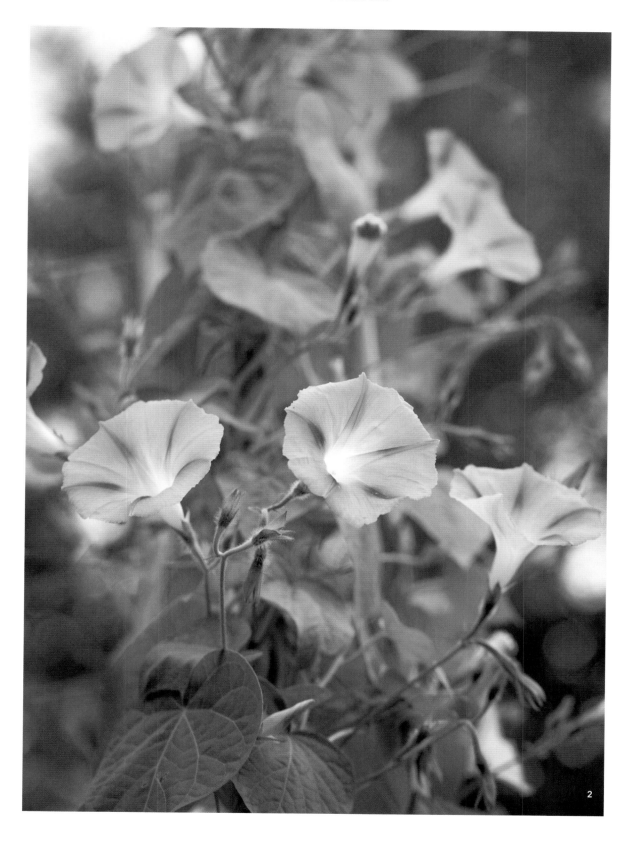

2

Bells of Ireland (*Moluccella laevis*)

· Half-hardy annual
· Height: 60–90 cm
· Sow: under cover in mid spring
· Site: full sun in moist but well-drained soil
· Flowers: mid to late summer

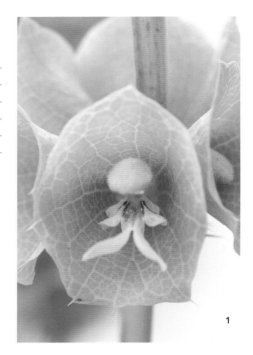

1

This one-off plant is a member of the mint family native to Turkey, Syria and the Caucasus – the common name arose because of its fresh green colour, not because of its origin. Beloved by flower-arrangers, who use it both fresh and dried, it is a swift-growing half-hardy annual that produces tall spikes of apple-green flowers. Strictly these flowers are calyces, the outer casing of the bud and flower; the real flower is tiny and white, visible if you peer into the centre of each bell-shaped calyx. An excellent addition to the cutting garden, it can also look good in a border to break up blocks of brighter colour with its green spires.

Moluccella is classified as half-hardy, but its seeds benefit from a spell in the fridge before sowing.

1 and **2** *M. laevis*

Sowing and growing

Once the seeds have been stratified, sow them under cover in mid spring, in modules or coir pots that can be planted straight out into the ground, at 18–21°C. Wait until early summer to plant them out, and be very careful when you do so: *Moluccella* produces tap roots that don't like too much disturbance. Give them a position in full sun, and water them well as they grow. You may need to stake them as they grow taller, since their willowy form makes them susceptible to wind damage.

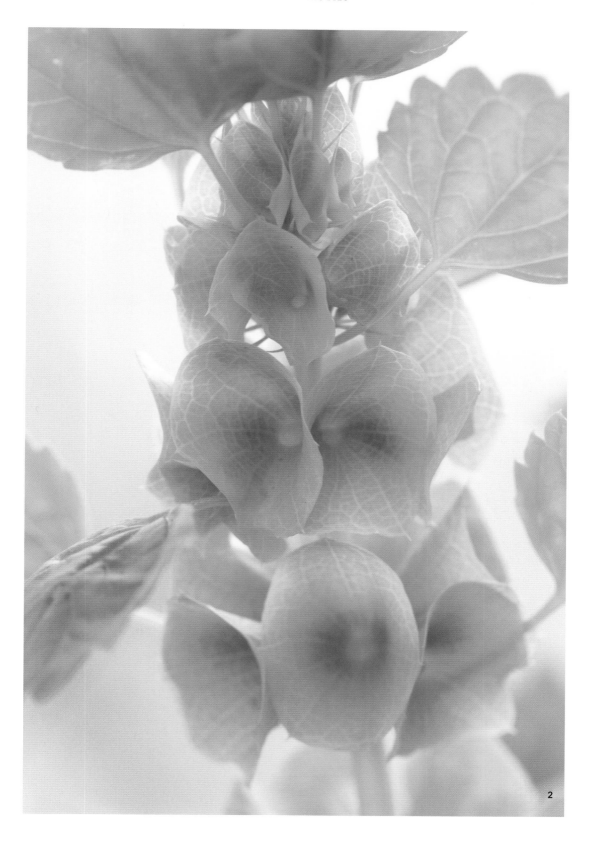

2

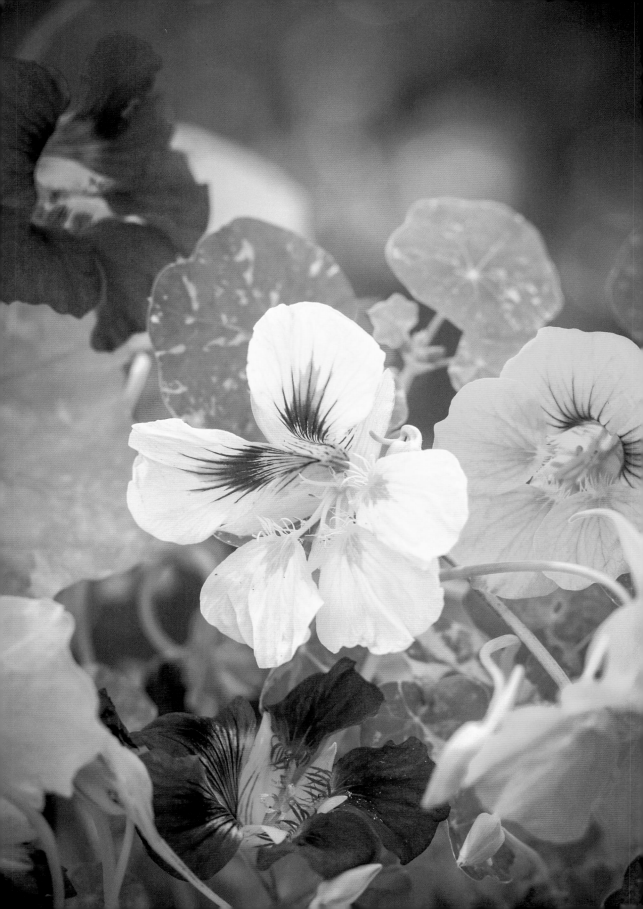

Edible Flowers and Herbs

Chives (*Allium schoenoprasum*)

Dill (*Anethum graveolens*)

Borage (*Borago officinalis*)

Coriander (*Coriandrum sativum*)

Basil (*Ocimum basilicum*)

Pot marjoram (*Origanum onites*)

Parsley (*Petroselinum crispum*)

Nasturtium (*Tropaeolum majus*)

Heartsease (*Viola tricolor*)

Tropaeolum majus
'Jewel of Africa'

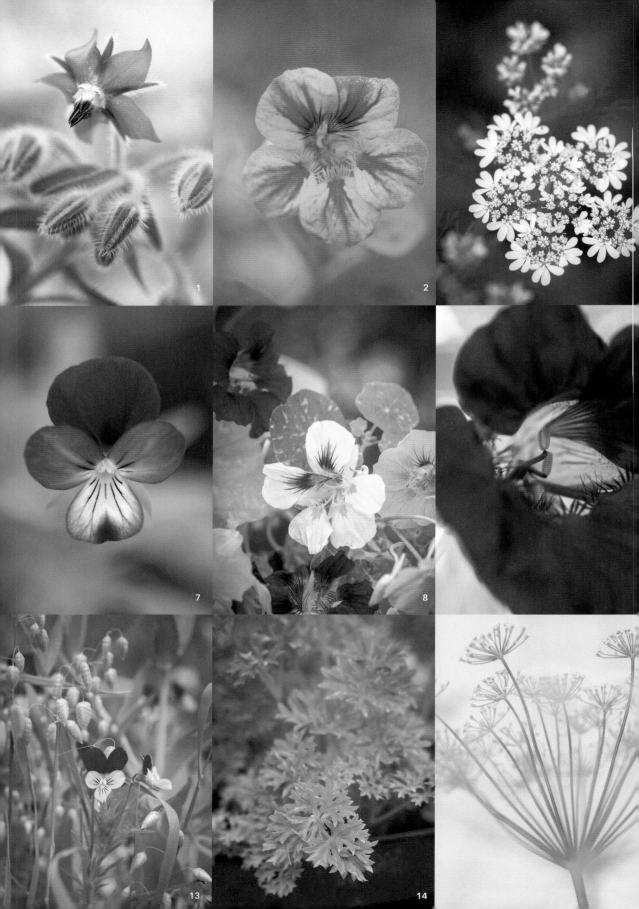

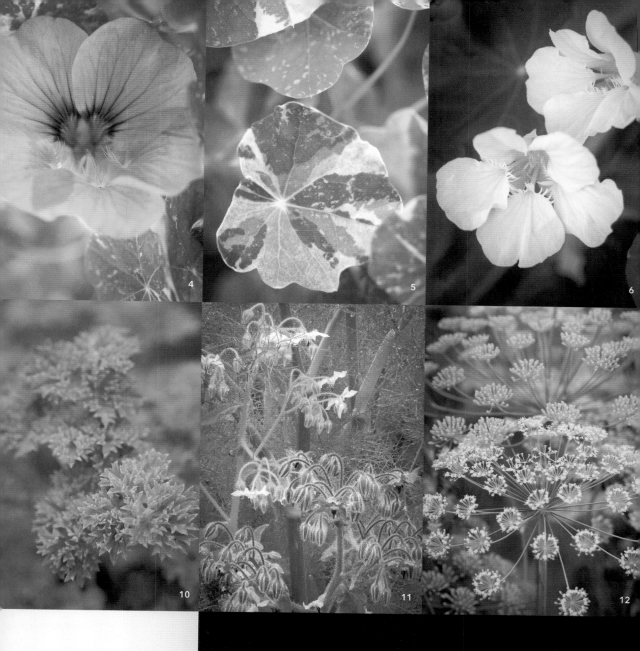

1 *Borago officinalis*
2 *Tropaeolum majus*
3 *Coriandrum sativum*
4 *Tropaeolum majus* 'Alaska Mix'
5 *Tropaeolum majus* 'Alaska Mix' leaves
6 *Tropaeolum majus* 'Milkmaid'
7 *Viola tricolor*
8 *Tropaeolum majus* 'Jewel of Africa'
9 *Tropaeolum majus* 'Black Velvet'
10 *Petroselinum crispum*
11 *Borago officinalis*
12 *Anethum graveolens*
13 *Viola tricolor* and *Briza maxima*
14 *Petroselinum crispum*
15 *Anethum graveolens*
16 *Borago officinalis* 'Alba'

Chives (*Allium schoenoprasum*)

- Perennial
- Height: 30 cm
- Sow: under cover or direct in spring
- Site: sun, in fertile, moist soil
- Flowers: mid to late summer

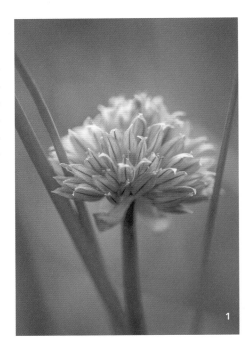

1

A member of the *Allium* family, including leeks and garlic, chives are a staple of the herb garden and very easy to grow from seed. Grown for their pungent, onion-flavoured leaves, they are used to flavour various dishes, salads and cheeses. They also produce attractive, edible purple flowers that can be used as a garnish. Although not grown commercially, they have been cultivated on a domestic scale since at least medieval times, and were referred to in writing as early as AD 80, when the Roman poet Martial amusingly recorded: 'He who bears chives on his breath/ Is safe from being kissed to death.'

Sowing and growing

Chives are hardy perennials, so once you have sown them they will reappear year after year. If you are sowing chives direct, sow thinly in spring into a well-prepared seed bed, in rows 30 cm apart. Thin the seedlings to about 20 cm and keep well watered. If you choose to start them off under cover, sow onto the surface of the compost in seed trays, covering them with a sprinkling of finely sieved compost or vermiculite, and germinate them at a temperature of 18-21°C. Prick them out into 7 cm pots when they are large enough to handle, with four seedlings to a pot, and plant out into larger pots or into the ground in late spring or early summer. Chives like a moisture-retentive soil, so make sure you have prepared their final resting place by digging in plenty of compost or manure before you plant.

Chives have insect-repelling qualities so are often used as a companion plant in vegetable gardens to ward off aphids and other pests.

1 *A. schoenoprasum* in flower

Dill (*Anethum graveolens*)

- Biennial
- Height: 45–120 cm
- Sow: direct in mid spring
- Site: sun, moisture-rich soil
- Flowers: mid to late summer

This useful kitchen herb originated in Eastern Europe, and its ferny leaves are used most often to flavour fish dishes. It is also an attractive addition to a border, producing striking acid-yellow umbels in midsummer that are also useful for cutting.

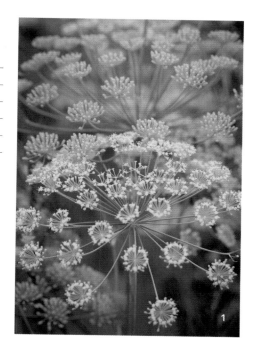

1

Varieties
Common dill (*Anethum graveolens*) grows to about 90 cm and produces numerous flowers and seeds, so this is the perfect variety for anyone using it ornamentally. If you are growing it for culinary purposes, however, you don't necessarily want it to flower too quickly. In that case, choose the cultivar 'Dukat', which many people say has leaves with a superior taste and is slow to bolt (produce flowers and seed). If you are growing in a small space, 'Fernleaf' and 'Bouquet' are dwarf varieties (45 cm) that are ideal for containers.

Sowing and growing
Sow the seed thinly outdoors after the soil has warmed up in mid spring, and thin the seedlings to 30–40 cm apart. If the thinning seems wasteful, you can always use the seedlings in your next meal to make the most of them! Keep them well-watered and weeded as they grow, and you should be harvesting the delicious leaves 8–10 weeks after sowing.

1 *A. graveolens* in flower

Dill is easy to grow from seed, but is best sown direct, since it resents disturbance to its roots.

Borage (*Borago officinalis*)

- Hardy annual
- Height: 50–90 cm
- Sow: direct in late spring
- Site: sun, poor soil
- Flowers: early to midsummer

Borage (also known as starflower) is one of the easiest plants to grow from seed, maturing very quickly into a tall, robust plant. The stems and leaves are rather coarse and prickly, but the starry, sapphire-blue flowers make up for this ungainliness, catching the eye with spots of intense colour. The oil from the seeds is used widely in herbal medicine to reduce inflammation and balance hormones. The flowers and young leaves are edible, with a fresh, cucumber-like flavour. The flowers can be scattered on salads, infused in drinks or candied to decorate cakes or biscuits.

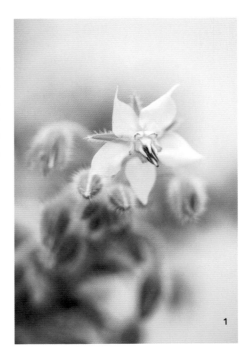

1

Varieties
The flowers of common borage, *B. officinalis*, can vary in colour, and often open pink before changing to blue. A white form, *B. officinalis* 'Alba', is also available.

Sowing and growing
Borage likes full sun and a poor soil, and it will self-seed freely if it is happy; in fact, it seeds around so readily that you will almost certainly find yourself having to pull out unwanted plants. Grow it as a filler for gaps in a border, or let it self-seed around the edges of your vegetable patch to provide insect-friendly flowers as companion plants.

1 *B. officinalis* 'Alba'
2 *B. officinalis*

Sow borage seed direct into the soil as soon as it has warmed up in late spring, scattering it thinly wherever you want it to flower.

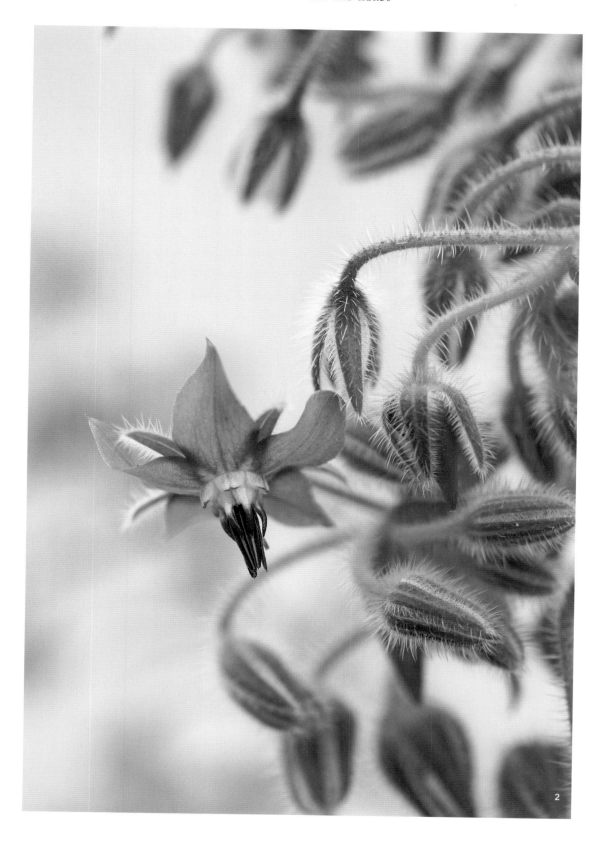

2

Coriander (*Coriandrum sativum*)

- Half-hardy annual
- Height: 40–50 cm
- Sow: direct or under cover in late spring
- Site: moist soil and partial shade
- Flowers: midsummer

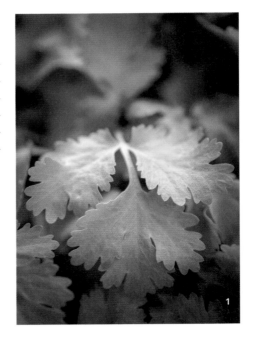

Coriander is a staple leafy herb for Indian, Thai and other Asian food, and it's worth making successive sowings so that you can pick it regularly during summer. Native to southern Europe, it was brought to the UK by the Romans, who used it to preserve meat, and both its leaves and its seeds have been used in British cuisine ever since. The flowers have a milder taste than the leaves and are used to decorate salads.

Varieties

If you're growing coriander for its leaves, there are several varieties to look out for. 'Calypso' is a recently bred variety that is said to be slow to bolt, so you can harvest it up to four times as a cut-and-come-again plant. 'Slobolt' and the large-leafed 'Leisure' are similar, but the advantage of 'Calypso' is that the leaves emerge lower down the stem than in other varieties, so you can start cutting it earlier, and then return to cut more a week later.

Sowing and growing

Coriander has carrot-like tap roots that don't like being disturbed or transplanted (that can make them bolt or run to seed too early), so it's best to sow either direct in the ground in late spring, or in pots large enough for the seedlings to grow for their whole life cycle – at least 25 cm in diameter, and deep enough to contain the long root. If sowing direct, sow finely in drills in well-prepared soil; in a pot, sow the seeds thinly on the surface of moist compost and cover with a fine layer of compost or vermiculite. Germinate at 16–21°C.

Coriander needs a reasonably moist soil and doesn't like to be baked dry, so it's best to give it a spot that gets a little light shade at some point during the day.

1 *C. sativum* leaves
2 *C. sativum* flowers

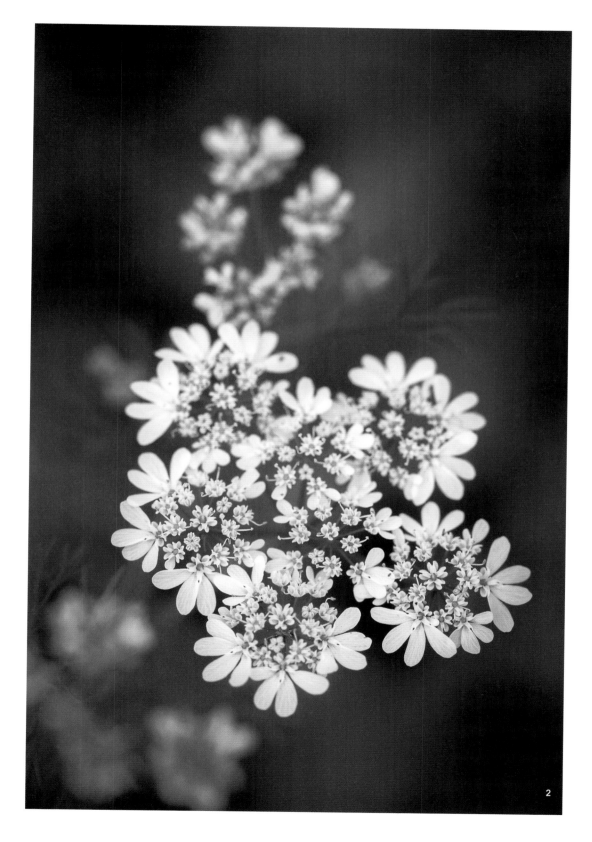

2

Basil (*Ocimum basilicum*)

- Short-lived perennial grown as a half-hardy annual in cool climates
- Height: 40–50 cm
- Sow: under cover in late spring or direct in early summer
- Site: full sun, well-drained soil
- Flowers: grown for its leaves

If, like me, you're someone who buys endless pots of basil from the supermarket and doesn't look after them properly, you should think about sowing your own for a limitless summer supply. A staple of Italian cookery, it is used to flavour a huge spectrum of dishes, including pesto, so having a source from which to pick generous handfuls is a bonus. A native of Asia, basil is grown as an annual widely throughout America and Europe.

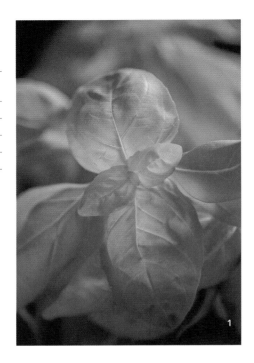

1 *O. basilicum*

Varieties

It makes perfect sense that this herb should have varieties with Italian names, and you can't go wrong with 'Napoletano', which has big, fat, rounded leaves, sweet and fragrant. Forming dense mounds of bright green, Greek basil, *O. minimum*, is an ornamental addition to the herb garden as well as a source of tasty leaves, smaller than the classic basil and delicious in soups and stews. Another ornamental basil is *O. basilicum* var. *purpurascens* 'Purple Ruffles', whose dark, glossy leaves have fringed edges; it also produces very attractive purple flowers if left to its own devices in the summer. The taste, as you might expect, is different from that of green basil, with a spicier flavour underpinned with liquorice, and it makes an excellent garnish for green salads.

Sowing and growing

In warmer climates, basil can be perennial, but in temperate climates it is grown as a half-hardy annual, since it will be damaged and killed by even the lightest frost. Because of this, it's best to sow it under cover in late spring, on a warm windowsill or in a greenhouse or conservatory, at 20–25°C. Sow in small pots and pot the seedlings on as they grow bigger. If you are growing basil outside, don't sow until early summer, and choose a warm, sheltered spot in full sun. Once the plant is established, pick the leaves regularly to stop it from flowering and going to seed.

Pot marjoram (*Origanum onites*)

· Perennial
· Height: 40–45 cm
· Sow: under cover in early spring
· Site: sun, well-drained or poor soil
· Flowers: mid to late summer

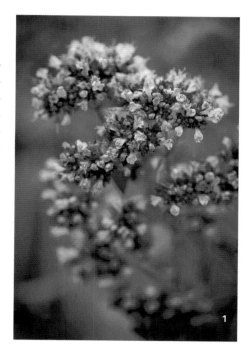

This tasty herb is a relative of the oregano plant (wild marjoram) that grows in scrubland in the UK and further south in the Mediterranean. While oregano can be used as a dried herb, pot marjoram is more versatile, with excellent flavour in both fresh and dried forms. The flowers can also be used to impart a more subtle taste in salads or other dishes, and both leaves and flowers can be used to flavour oils and vinegars. With small, soft green leaves, it forms a neat mound of foliage, with attractive, pale pink flowers in summer. Use it as an edging plant or grow it in a large tub with other herbs.

Varieties

Origanum onites is widely available as seed. A golden-leaved variety called *O. onites* 'Aureum' is also in cultivation, but less often grown from seed.

Sowing and growing

Pot marjoram is easy to grow from seed and is best sown under cover in early spring. The seed is very small so should be sprinkled sparingly on the surface of the compost in a small seed tray, and germinated at a temperature of 18–21°C. Don't cover the seed, watering the tray from below. Carefully prick out the seedlings when large enough to handle, transplanting them to small 7 cm pots before planting out after all danger of frost has passed. As a Mediterranean-climate plant, it thrives in full sun and well-drained soil, and once established will tolerate very dry conditions with little maintenance required. As a perennial, it should survive the winter; it will die right back and may need some protection if the weather is especially cold and wet. To harvest the leaves, keep cutting the herb in spring and summer as the flavour is best before the flowers appear.

As its name suggests, pot marjoram is an excellent candidate for a container, where it can be placed near the kitchen for easy harvesting.

1 *O. onites* in flower

Parsley (*Petroselinum crispum*)

- · Biennial
- · Height: 25–50 cm
- · Sow: direct or under cover in mid spring or early autumn
- · Site: full sun or semi-shade, moist but well-drained soil
- · Flowers: grown for its leaves

Parsley is the foodie's stalwart, and it can be grown to edge beds in the kitchen garden, or in small quantities in pots on a windowsill. Native to the Mediterranean, it has been cultivated for thousands of years; wreaths of it were worn on the head by the Romans to ward off intoxication, and it was fed to war horses to give them magical strength. Today parsley oil is used in commercial shampoos, soaps and skin lotions, and the leaves – which are high in vitamin C and iron – are used widely to flavour food.

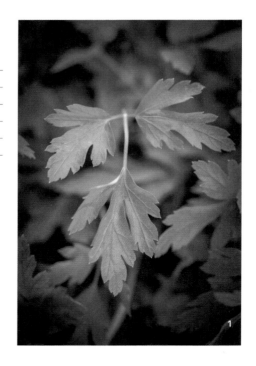

Varieties

There are two types of parsley: curly-leaved and flat-leaved. The former, also known as moss parsley, is traditionally used as a garnish. Its compact shape and emerald-green colour make it an excellent edging plant in the kitchen garden or border. Flat-leaved parsley is more tasty, and its flavour defines Middle Eastern dishes such as tabbouleh. Of the cultivars we have come across, 'Moss Curled' is the most widely available curly parsley, while 'Gigante d'Italia' and 'Gigante di Napoli' are good, flavoursome flat-leaf varieties.

Sowing and growing

Parsley has a reputation for tardiness, being slow to germinate. The biological reason for this is that the seeds are coated with chemicals that inhibit nearby weed seeds. Washing the seeds in warm water and drying them overnight before sowing can help. Sow in mid spring or early autumn, either direct or in modular trays, with several seeds to a module in case of sporadic germination, and germinate at 20–23°C. Remove all but the strongest seedling, and grow them on until you are ready to plant them out, giving them plenty of space in a sunny spot.

Parsley is a great companion plant for asparagus as it provides good ground cover to help suppress weeds, and is said to improve the crop's flavour.

1 'Gigante di Napoli'
2 'Moss Curled'

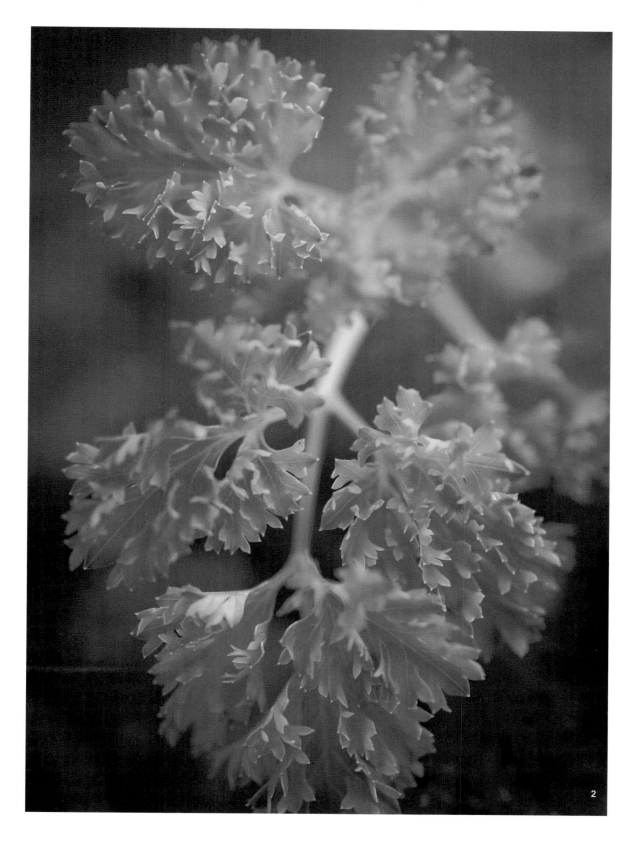

2

Nasturtium (*Tropaeolum majus*)

- Hardy annual
- Height: various
- Sow: direct in mid spring
- Site: full sun, poor soil
- Flowers: mid to late summer

Nasturtiums are one of the easiest annuals to grow, with cheerful flowers and a happy-go-lucky scrambling habit. They are also deliciously edible. All parts can be eaten – leaves, buds, flowers and seed pods – and their almost sweet, peppery flavour jazzes up salads in both taste and looks. The common name is derived from the Latin *nasus tortus*, meaning 'twisted nose', a reference to the effect the wasabi-like flavour has on one's nasal passages. All nasturtiums have large, attractive flowers with long spurs, and circular leaves like little parasols, each supported by a central stalk.

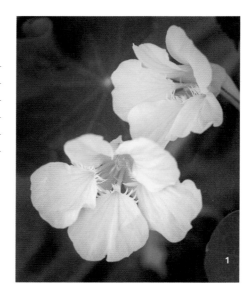

Varieties

Tropaeolum majus is the species from which nasturtium cultivars are derived, a swift-growing South American annual that scrambles over the ground or up a support. Many cultivated varieties are available, with flowers in a huge range of colours from deepest crimson-purple to creamy white. The trailing 'Milkmaid' is one of our favourites, with flowers in a subtle pale yellow. It makes an eye-catching contrast when mixed with the dark-mahogany nasturtium 'Black Velvet'. Some of the most striking new varieties have marbled or variegated foliage, and 'Alaska Mix' is one of these, with white-splashed and speckled leaves set against tangerine-orange, crimson and yellow flowers. 'Just Peachy' is a good choice for those seduced by pale apricot colours.

Sowing and growing

Scrambling varieties can be grown in and around vegetable plots, climbing varieties planted to hide ugly fences or walls, and dwarf or mounding varieties in pots and containers. As the saying goes, 'be nasty to nasturtiums' and you will succeed. Too many nutrients in the soil will cause them to produce far too much leaf and not enough flower, so a poor soil is preferable. Sow the large seeds direct in mid spring, and they should germinate within days. Keep them watered and watch daily as they grow.

The best thing about nasturtiums is that they thrive on neglect. You can pop a seed in and it will grow.

1 'Milkmaid'
2 'Alaska Mix'
3 'Alaska Mix' leaves
4 'Black Velvet'
5 'Just Peachy'

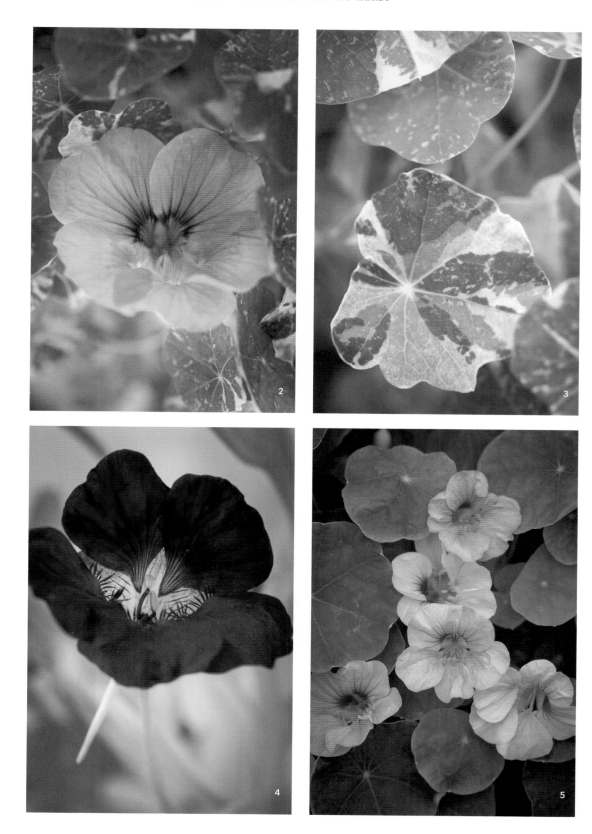

Heartsease (*Viola tricolor*)

- Short-lived perennial
- Height: 15–20 cm
- Sow: under cover in early autumn or early spring
- Site: partial shade, moist but well-drained soil
- Flowers: throughout the year

The wild pansy is the progenitor of the cultivated pansy, and with its pretty little flowers is a perfectly charming addition to pots or the front of borders. It has been used for hundreds of years as an edible flower, and its small, jewel-coloured blooms in a combination of violet, lavender, yellow and white can be used to garnish dishes, add to salads or float in drinks. Native to a large part of Europe, including the UK, it grows in short meadow grass and wasteland, usually in partial shade. This makes it ideal for shady corners of the garden, perhaps edging a path, or as part of a herb garden in pots and containers.

1 and **2** *V. tricolor*

Varieties
As an edible flower, *Viola tricolor* is the best species to choose, with its fresh, almost pea-like flavour. The leaves can also be added to salads. The wild violet, *V. odorata*, can also be eaten, and it has a sweeter flavour that makes it more suitable for garnishing desserts. It is also used for making violet syrup and teas.

Sowing and growing
Sow under cover in early autumn or early spring, but be aware that germination might be erratic, since the seed needs a period of cold to mimic the natural seasons. If you are sowing in autumn, sow in modular trays, covering the seed with a fine layer of sieved compost, and leave in a cold frame or cold greenhouse over winter. Some of the seed may germinate immediately, some the following spring, but it's a slow process, so be patient. If you are sowing in the spring, chill the seeds first in the fridge for a week or two to imitate winter conditions, then sow in the same way, keeping them at 10–15°C. Transplant the seedlings when they are big enough to handle, and plant them out in a cool spot, ideally in a moist but well-drained soil.

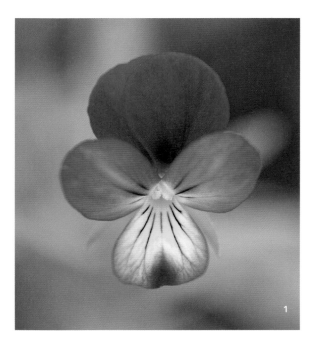

1

Pretty and easy going, heartsease will flower for months on end.

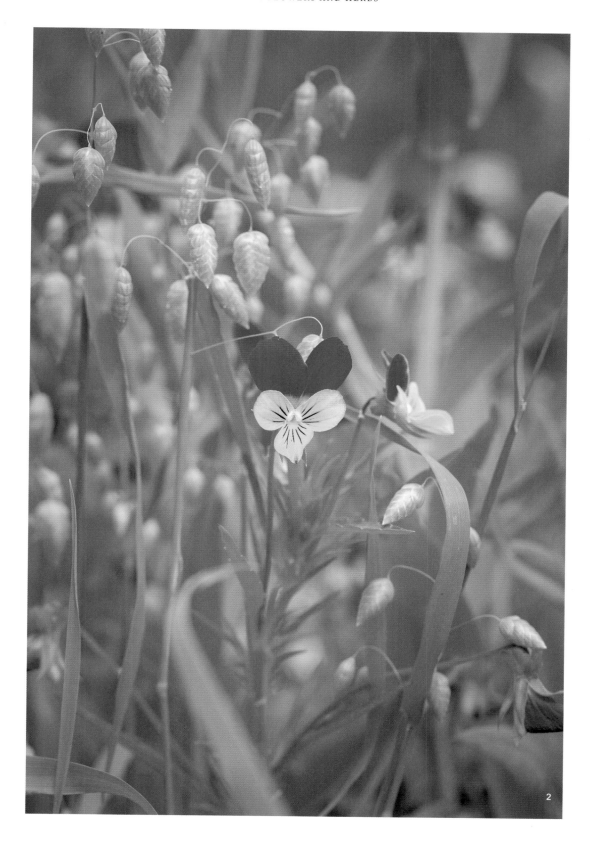

2

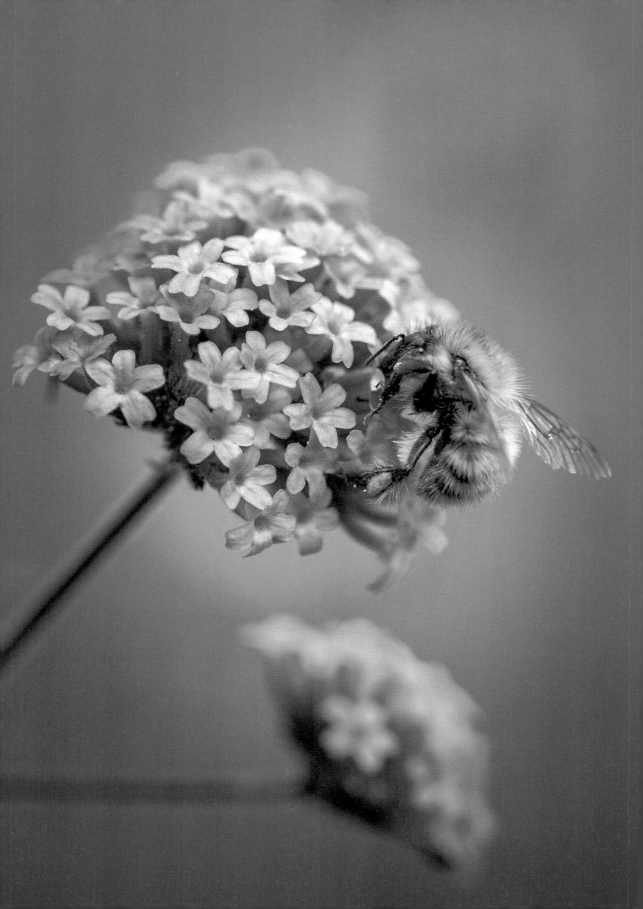

Bee-Friendly Flowers

Korean mint or hyssop (*Agastache*)

Corncockle (*Agrostemma githago*)

Cupid's dart (*Catananche caerulea*)

Cornflower (*Centaurea cyanus*)

Honeywort (*Cerinthe major*)

Fiddleneck (*Phacelia tanacetifolia*)

Sage (*Salvia*)

Clustertop vervain (*Verbena*)

Verbena

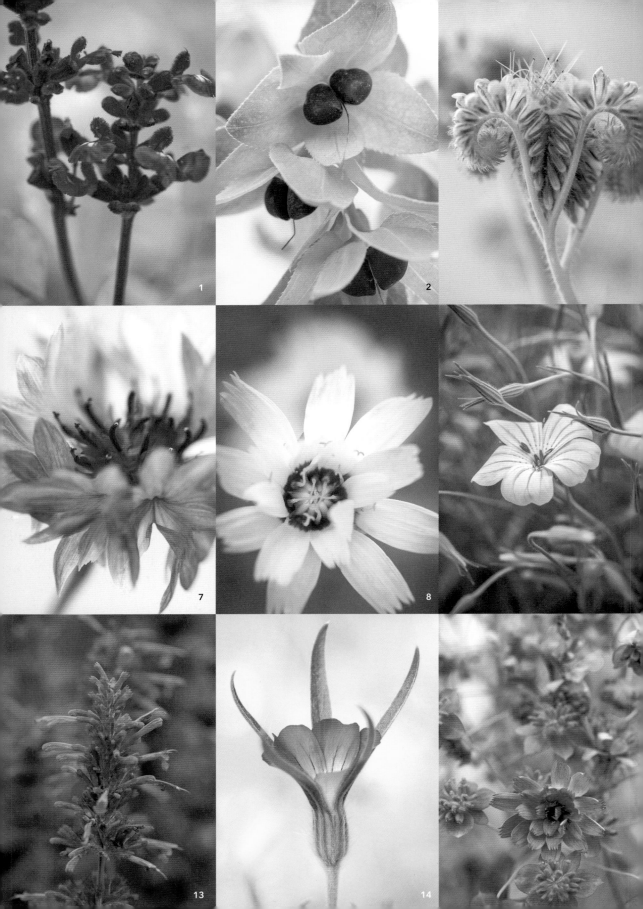

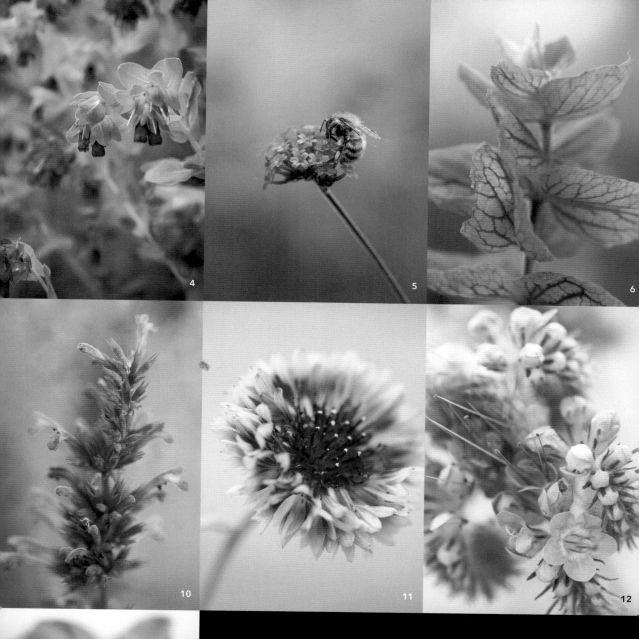

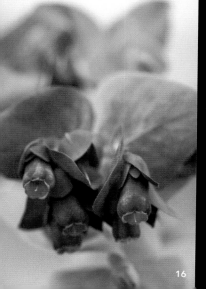

1	Salvia farinacea 'Blue Bedder'	9	Agrostemma githago 'Pink Queen'
2	Cerinthe seeds	10	Agastache 'Pink Pop'
3	Phacelia tanacetifolia	11	Centaurea cyanus 'Frosted Queen'
4	Cerinthe major 'Purpurascens'	12	Phacelia tanacetifolia
5	Verbena bonariensis	13	Agastache 'Heather Queen'
6	Salvia viridis 'Pink'	14	Agrostemma githago
7	Centaurea cyanus 'Classic Fantastic'	15	Catananche caerulea
8	Catananche caerulea 'Alba'	16	Cerinthe major 'Purpurascens'

Korean mint or hyssop (*Agastache*)

- Perennial
- Height: 30–90 cm
- Sow: under cover in early spring or direct in autumn
- Site: sun, well-drained, fertile soil
- Flowers: mid to late summer

Agastache **is an easy-going aromatic plant, excellent for attracting bees and other pollinating insects. There are a number of species that are easy to grow from seed, flowering two or three months from sowing and giving a good summer's worth of blooms before dying back. Although they are perennials, these species hail from Japan and Korea and may be borderline hardy, especially if your soil is heavy and prone to waterlogging. If that is the case, treat them as annuals, since they flower easily in the first year.**

Agastache is an easy-going plant that will do well in moist soil as long as it is well drained. It prefers a sunny site, but will tolerate a little dappled shade.

1 *A. anisata*
2 'Bolero'
3 'Navajo Sunset'
4 'Apache Sunset'

Varieties

Many of the *Agastaches* are blue, such as *A. foeniculum* (also known as *A. anisata*, the anise hyssop), which forms a branching plant with dense bottlebrush flowers in dusky lavender-blue set against dark-green leaves with a strong liquorice scent. But there are other colours, too, and they are less often grown. 'Bolero' has striking pink flowers, while *A. aurantiaca* and its cultivar 'Navajo Sunset' have orange flowers. Easy to grow and quick to flower, this species has unusual grey-green, peppermint-scented leaves and small, tubular coral-orange flowers set off by dusky purple calyces, giving a pretty two-tone effect. A smaller form, *A. aurantiaca* 'Apricot Sprite' is good for containers. For brick-red flowers, try the striking *A. rupestris* 'Apache Sunset'.

Sowing and growing

Seeds vary in size among the species, but if they are big enough to handle they can be sown in a modular seed tray in early spring, covered with a sprinkling of compost or vermiculite; otherwise, sow thinly in a small seed tray and prick out the seedlings in due course. Germinate at 18–21°C and once the seedlings have emerged, keep them in a cooler place to grow on. Harden them off as they grow bigger, and plant them out in early summer. The seeds can also be sown direct in the autumn for earlier flowering the following year.

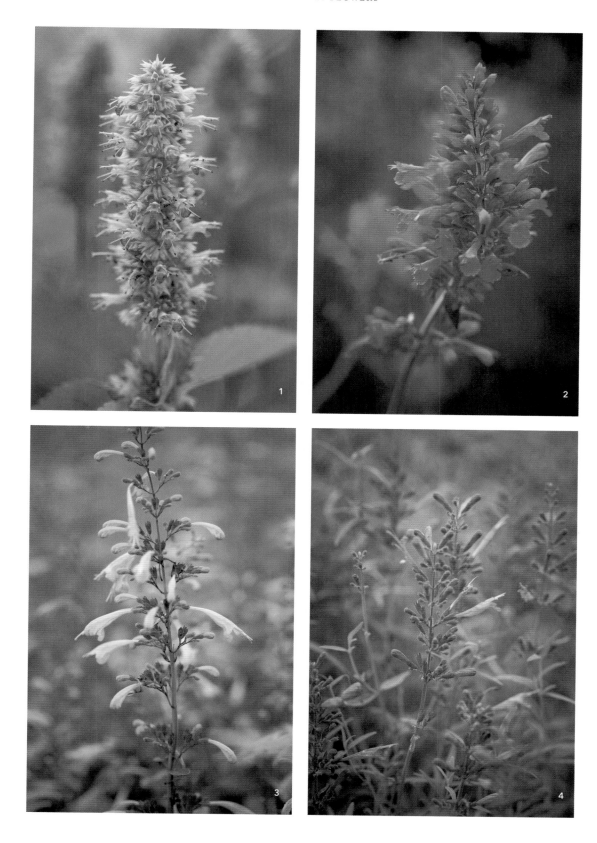

Corncockle
(*Agrostemma githago*)

- Hardy annual
- Height: 30–50 cm
- Sow: direct in late spring or late summer
- Site: sun, poor soil
- Flowers: early to late summer

The corncockle is a pretty, delicate annual, once common in British meadows, but now sadly rare in the wild. It is also known, slightly less poetically, as bastard nigella. Often included in wild-flower seed mixes, it is also easy to grow from seed on its own, in a meadow setting or in a cottage garden. It is excellent as a filler plant, but more importantly a magnet for bees, butterflies and other insects. Like some other wild flowers, including the foxglove, this flower is poisonous if ingested.

Corncockle is a meadow flower that is best sown direct where it is to bloom. Like many meadow plants, it does best in full sun on poor, stony soil.

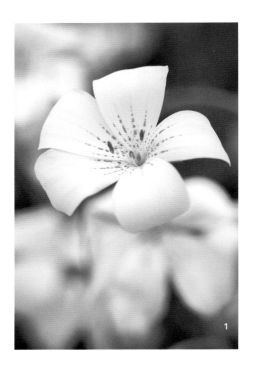

Varieties

These delightful flowers have five rounded petals in shades of magenta, pink or white, each with a white eye and radiating dark lines that look as though they have been painted on with the finest paintbrush. The whole is set off by five narrow, pointed green calyces. This really is something you have to look closely at to appreciate how nature creates these works of art. En masse, the effect is soft and airy, the flowers hovering in a cloud on wiry stems. The species itself, *Agrostemma githago*, is the most widely available, but a cultivar called 'Milas' is worth looking out for, with larger flowers, as well as 'Milas Purple Queen', nearer purple than pink, and 'Milas Snow Queen', with silvery-white petals. 'Ocean Pearl' is another white form, with slightly larger flowers.

Sowing and growing

Sow corncockle in late summer, or in spring when the soil has warmed up, broadcasting the seed in a border or wild-flower meadow.

1 'Milas Snow Queen'
2 'Milas Purple Queen'

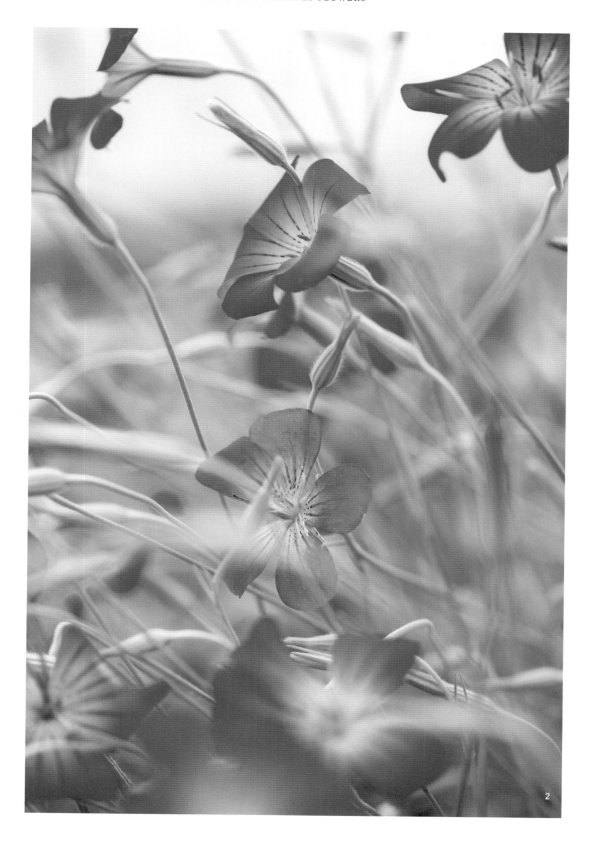

2

Cupid's dart
(*Catananche caerulea*)

- Short-lived perennial
- Height: 60–75 cm
- Sow: under cover in late winter or early spring, or direct in late spring
- Site: sun, well-drained soil
- Flowers: early to late summer

Hailing from the Mediterranean, *Catananche* was used by the ancient Greeks as an aphrodisiac, hence its common name. Robust and easy to grow, it is a pretty plant, unassuming and delicate-looking, with papery, fringed lavender-blue or white flowers on top of wiry stems. Although strictly perennial, it flowers in its first year from seed, so it can be treated as an annual. Grown as a meadow flower among grasses, or with other prairie-style perennials such as *Achillea*, *Echinacea* and *Rudbeckia*, it looks best grown in clusters or ribbons that weave through the other plants. It also makes a useful cut flower, both fresh and dried.

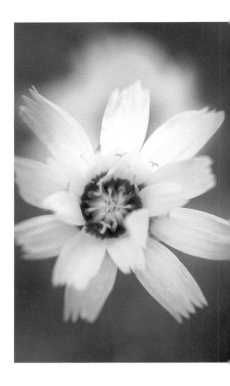

Varieties
There are two forms: the mauve *C. caerulea* and a white form, 'Alba'. Both have attractive grey-green foliage and stems; the flowers of the white form have dark purple centres with golden stamens.

Sowing and growing
Catananche seeds are large enough to grow in individual modules, and will germinate easily within a week or two at 18–21°C. Grow the seedlings on before hardening them off and planting them out in late spring. Alternatively, sow direct in late spring to produce plants that may flower by late summer, or the following year. These plants need lots of sun, so put them in an open spot, with well-drained soil.

To ensure that the plants flower in their first year, it's best to sow Catananche seed indoors in late winter or early spring.

1 *C. caerulea* 'Alba'
2 *C. caerulea*

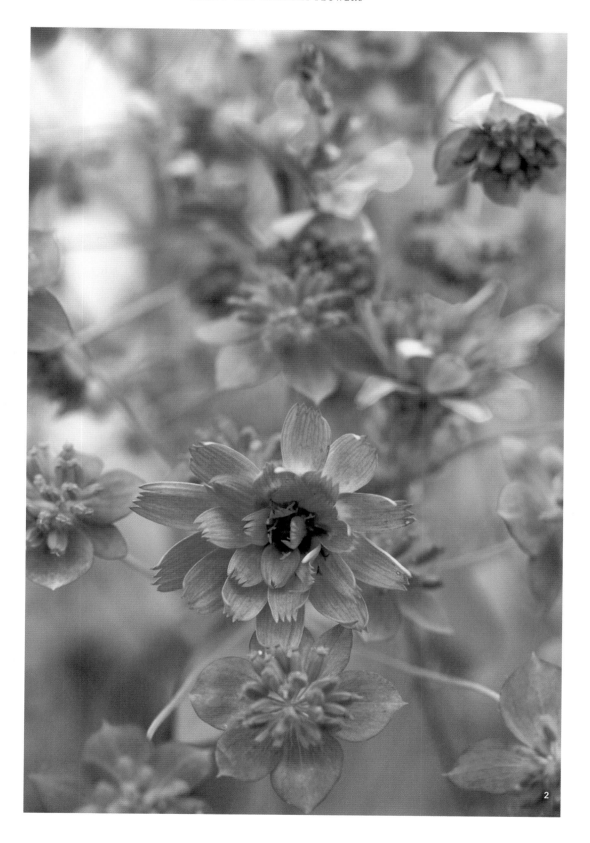

2

Cornflower (*Centaurea cyanus*)

- Hardy annual
- Height: 70–120 cm
- Sow: direct in early autumn or mid spring
- Site: sun, well-drained, poor soil
- Flowers: early to late summer

This European native was once a common sight in arable fields, but it has declined dramatically in the wild in the past half-century owing to the increased use of chemical fertilizers and pesticides in modern agriculture. Thankfully, the revival of meadow gardens and the fashion for natural planting mean that this beautiful flower is now widely grown again, especially as a cut flower – and it is fantastically easy to grow from seed.

Varieties

The wild form has handsome cobalt-blue, buttony flowers on tough, straight stems. There are also cultivars with bigger, showier flowers, as well as a host of other varieties in different colours, from deep purple-black to pale pink. Nothing beats that electric sky blue of the true cornflower, but the double-flowered 'Blue Boy' is worth seeking out as it has larger blooms than the species and is particularly free-flowering, going on and on from early summer until autumn if you keep picking it religiously. 'Black Ball' has dark berry-purple flowers that can look sophisticated both in the border and in arrangements, while 'Snowman' is, as its name suggests, a snowy-white cornflower. If you're not a purist, choose a seed mix such as 'Frosty Mix', with bi-coloured flowers in shades of blue, red, pink, white and lavender.

Sowing and growing

Cornflowers are one of the easiest annuals to sow direct, so, to avoid the fuss of raising seedlings for later transplanting, sow them outdoors in early autumn or in mid spring, as soon as the soil has warmed up. If you sow in autumn, your plants will be taller and stronger. Sow in drills, and take care to thin the seedlings as they grow, to an eventual spacing of about 30 cm. Although their stems are strong, these tall, willowy plants will need some sort of support (pea netting or canes and twine) or the wind will topple them.

Cornflowers are undemanding creatures, growing swiftly and easily in most soils as long as they don't become waterlogged. They thrive in poor soil.

1 *C. cyanus*
2 'Black Ball'
3 'Snowman'
4 'Frosty Mix'

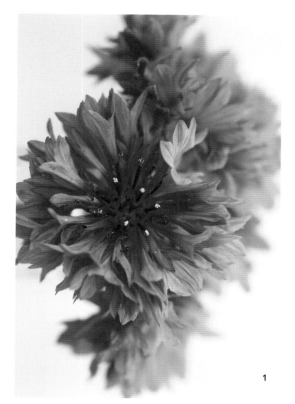

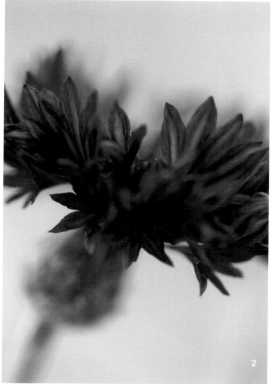

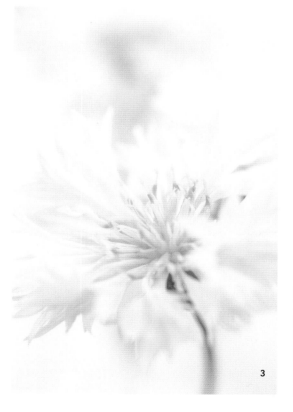

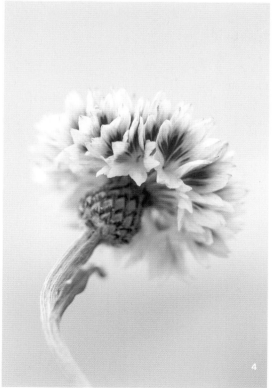

Honeywort (*Cerinthe major*) ☀

- Hardy annual
- Height: 45–60 cm
- Sow: under cover in early spring, or direct or under cover in late summer
- Site: full sun, sheltered spot
- Flowers: late spring to midsummer

Cerinthe is a prima donna – beautiful, unusual and opulent – yet pleasingly easy to grow from seed. It originated in southern Europe and, although it is often classified as a hardy annual, in its natural form it can be perennial. It will revel in a warm, sunny spot, where it will seed around, and in particularly mild areas its glaucous evergreen foliage will survive over winter, as long as the temperature doesn't drop below about -5°C. Its common name refers to the fact that it is a rich source of nectar, and in summer you'll see bees buzzing happily from plant to plant.

Sow the large seeds in modules, soaking them overnight in warm water to help germination.

1 *C. major* 'Purpurascens'

Varieties

By far and away the most commonly grown form in cultivation is *C. major* 'Purpurascens'. Known in the US as the blue shrimp plant, it has wonderful, arching swathes of damson-purple flowers offset by handsome blue-green leaves. Look more closely and you'll see that the flowers themselves are violet purple, with layers of darker blue bracts above them, hanging down like a set of plush curtain tassels. The leaves, too, can be speckled with silver, so the overall colour effect is incredibly rich, like an illuminated manuscript. It looks wonderful with silvery-leaved plants such as *Stachys* or *Perovskia*, or with other late-flowering blue flowers, such as *Agapanthus*, which will pick up the *Cerinthe*'s metallic blue tones.

Sowing and growing

Like many hardy annuals, *Cerinthe* can be sown in late summer or in spring. Sow in late summer direct or in modular trays, to be planted out before the first frosts, and you will have flowers in late spring. Alternatively, sow the seed under cover in early spring for slightly later-flowering plants. Germinate the seeds in a warm place at 18–20°C, then move the seedlings to a cooler spot to grow on. They can be planted out when all danger of frost has passed. Choose a sheltered, sunny spot in well-drained soil.

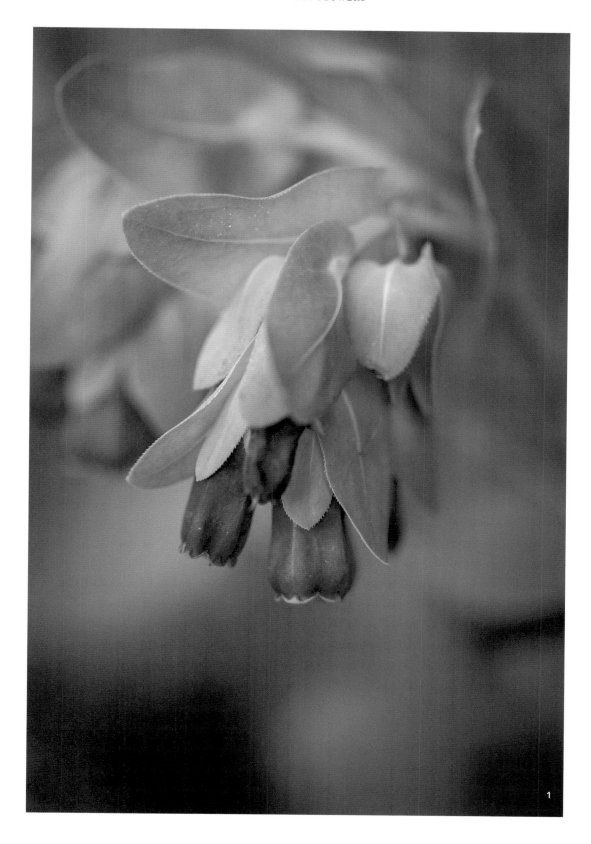

Fiddleneck (*Phacelia tanacetifolia*)

- Hardy annual
- Height: 80–100 cm
- Sow: direct in early autumn or spring
- Site: full sun, well-drained soil
- Flowers: early to late summer

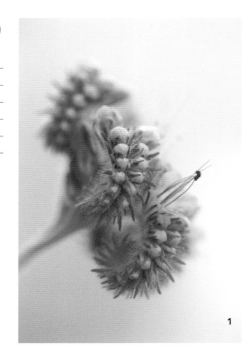

1

Phacelia is often grown as a green manure or cover crop (a nitrogen-rich plant that is grown for a short period and then dug back into the soil to improve nutrient levels), but it is also an excellent plant for the wildlife garden, as its nectar-rich flowers attract bees in droves. It is used increasingly as a cut flower. Its pretty, pale-lavender blooms unfurl from coiled spikes as the buds open, with long, spidery stamens that give a hazy effect from a distance.

Sowing and growing

Native to California, Arizona and Mexico, this plant colonizes dry, stony hillsides and needs very little care. It is useful for a patch of ground that has been cleared, or for scattering among other summer annuals; it is also a good cut flower. Grow it in an open, sunny spot in well-drained soil and prepare the ground by digging it over lightly. Sow the seed direct in rows, or by broadcasting it over the soil, and raking it in gently. As the flowers grow, use them for cutting, and then as the crop goes over, chop the stems at ground level and dig all parts of the plants back into the soil as a nutritious green manure.

1 and **2** *P. tanacetifolia*

Phacelia will set seed readily, so if you don't want a rash of new plants, cut the flowers before they go to seed to use in your summer arrangements.

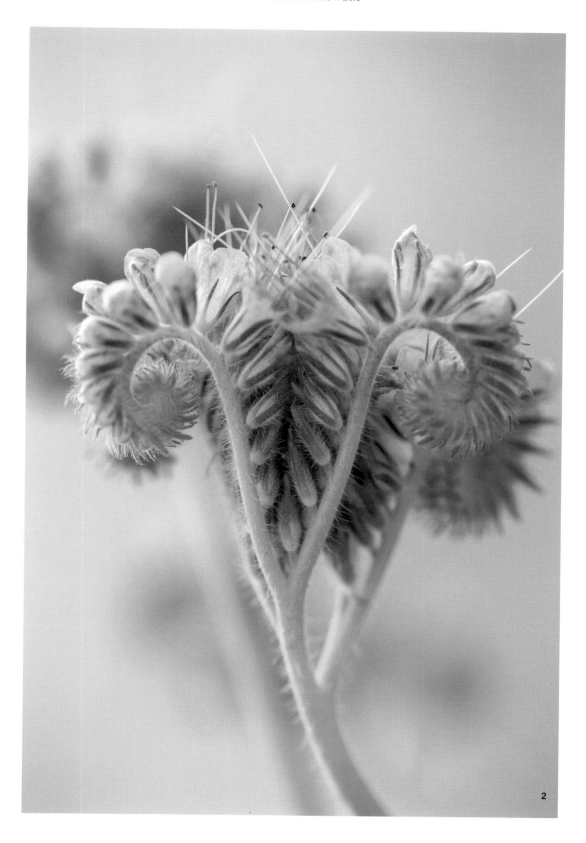

2

Sage (*Salvia*)

- Annual/biennial/tender perennial
- Height: 40–100 cm
- Sow: direct or under cover in early autumn or mid spring (annuals); under cover in early summer (biennials); under cover in late winter (tender perennials)
- Site: full sun, will tolerate poor soil
- Flowers: early to midsummer

Salvia **is a huge genus, containing species from both Mediterranean Europe and South America, but only a handful of species are available to grow from seed, since few set seed readily. For those that do, the seed is easy to germinate and grow, forming sturdy seedlings and flowering within a few months of sowing. The common sage,** *S. officinalis,* **is used widely as a culinary herb.**

Varieties

Among the easiest salvias to grow from seed is the annual *S. viridis* (previously *S. horminum*), which produces multiple stems of coloured bracts with darker veining. *S. viridis* 'Oxford Blue' is a vivid shade of blue, while *S. viridis* 'White Swan' is a beautiful greenish-white. Growing to about 60 cm tall, these cut-and-come-again flowers will bloom for weeks on end and last well in the vase. The biennial *S. sclarea* var. *turkestanica* is one of the larger salvias, growing up to 1 m tall, with architectural sprays of small blue flowers with pale-pink bracts. There is also a white form, 'Alba'. One of the few New World salvias available from seed is *S. farinacea*, a tender perennial from Mexico that in temperate climates can be grown as an annual, since it flowers the same year from an early sowing. The cultivar 'Fairy Queen' is our top pick, with its gorgeous spires of bi-coloured blue-and-white flowers on dark stems.

1 *S. sclarea* var. *turkestanica*
2 'Oxford Blue'
3 'White Swan'
4 'Alba'

Sowing and growing

Sow the annual salvias in early autumn or mid spring, either under cover or direct. If sowing under cover, sow in modules or small pots and germinate at 16–18°C. Plant the seedlings out in late spring after hardening them off. Sow the biennial salvias in early summer, planting them out in autumn to flower the following year. Finally, sow the tender perennials in late winter in the warmth, and plant the seedlings out once all threat of frost has passed.

All Salvias are sun-loving plants, so give them a spot where they can bask in it. They are also fairly drought-tolerant, so good candidates for the low-maintenance garden.

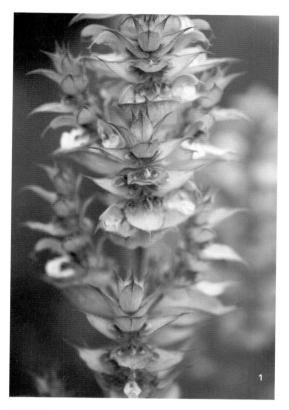

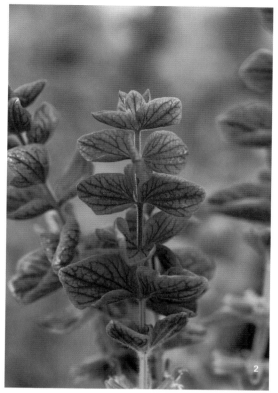

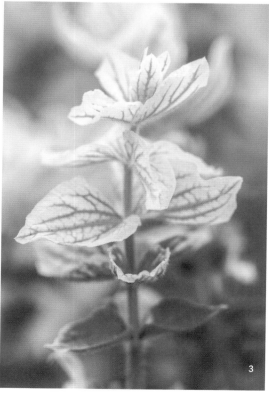

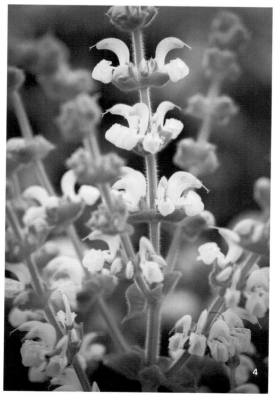

Clustertop vervain (*Verbena*)

- Short-lived perennial
- Height: 1–1.8 m
- Sow: under cover in early spring or direct in autumn or mid spring
- Site: dry, well-drained soil or gravel
- Flowers: midsummer to autumn

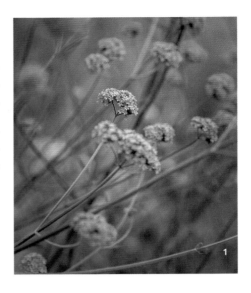

Verbena rose meteorically in popularity at the beginning of this century. A tall, airy perennial with small lavender-coloured flowers that appear in midsummer, it looks best planted en masse, perhaps with other dry-loving plants such as *Dianthus carthusianorum*, *Verbascums* and *Cosmos*, and is perfect for a gravel garden. This South American native can be short-lived in cool, wet climates, but it self-seeds readily, so you should always have a ready supply of new plants once it is established. It is found as an expensive pot plant in garden centres, and many people don't realize how easy it is to grow from seed, flowering in its first year.

Verbena doesn't always tolerate extreme cold, and it can be short-lived, but it will self-seed and is an excellent candidate for a gravel garden.

Varieties

V. bonariensis is a species that people have not found the need to breed from, so there is very little deviation from it. In recent years a dwarf form, 'Lollipop', has become available, more suitable for pots and small spaces at only 60 cm high. *V. hastata* is also excellent, with branching flower spikes that frill out and then taper at the top like little witch's hats. It comes in a different range of colours: 'White Spires', 'Blue Spires' and f. *rosea* 'Pink Spires'.

Sowing and growing

Sow both *V. bonariensis* and *V. hastata* under cover in early spring in a small seed tray, sowing on the surface of the compost and just covering the seeds with a fine layer of sieved compost. Germinate at 18–20°C, but if germination is slow, try giving the seeds a period of cold to kickstart it, returning them to the warmth if nothing happens. Prick out the seedlings and grow them on until they are big enough to plant out in the garden, where they need an open, sunny spot in well-drained soil. You can also sow the seed direct in autumn or mid spring. Once established, the plants will be reasonably drought-tolerant, but they will need watering for a few weeks after planting out to encourage a good root system to form.

1 *V. bonariensis*
2 'Pink Spires'

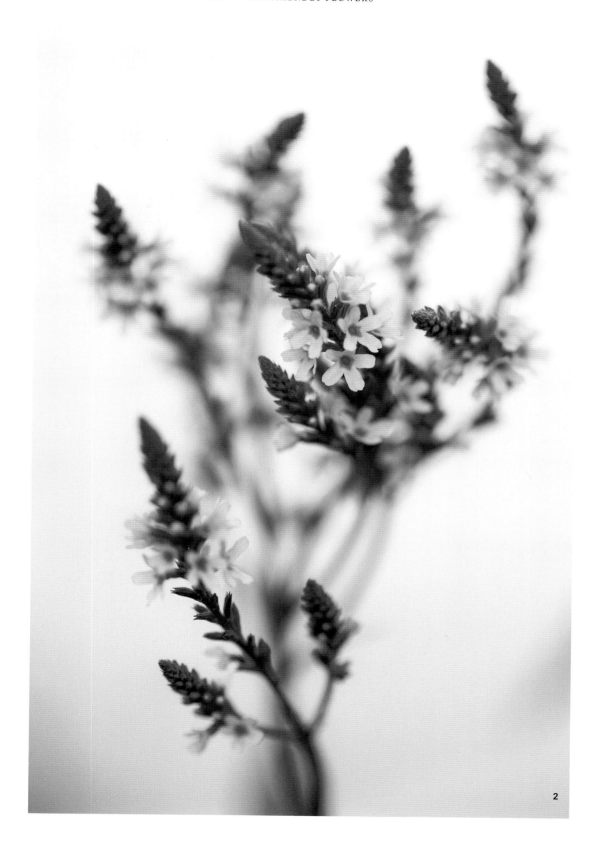

2

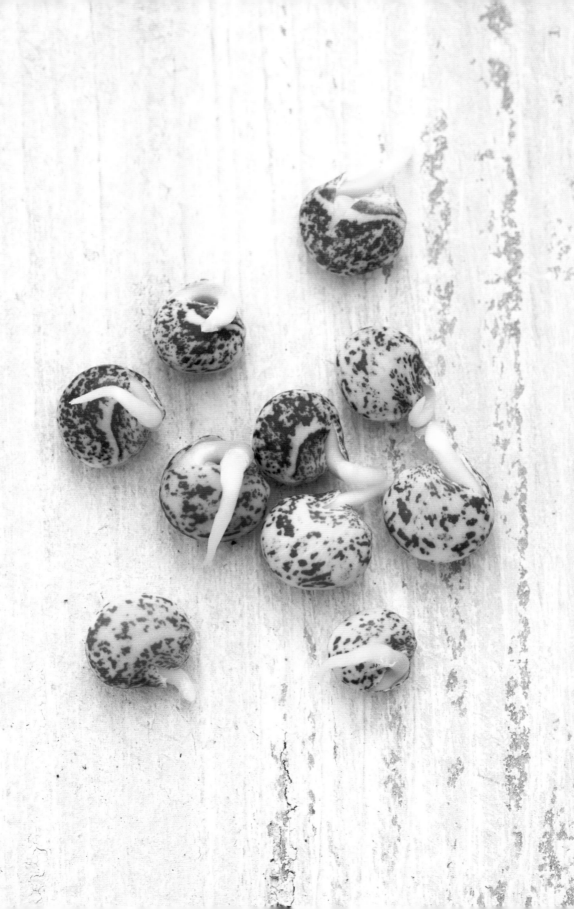

Part II

Sowing and growing

Introduction, Sowing under cover, Sowing direct,
Pests and diseases

Introduction

This section is designed to guide you through the process of sowing and germinating your seeds successfully, and eventually growing them on and watching them flower. The first thing to remember is that plants inherently want to grow, so if you give them the right conditions, nine times out of ten they will do what you want them to do. The second is that gardening is not an exact science. One person's failsafe method for germinating one particular plant might not work for another, while unpredictable weather can mean huge variations in success, particularly with direct-sown plants. We have found that a process of trial and error is an essential part of growing from seed, so don't be afraid to use your initiative and be prepared to experiment and develop your own methods.

There are two basic methods of sowing seed: sowing direct outside in the ground and sowing under cover in pots or seed trays, inside on a windowsill or in a greenhouse or conservatory. The method you choose depends on what you are sowing and when, but before you start it helps to have an understanding of the broader plant groups: annuals, biennials and perennials. It is also worth noting here that, somewhat confusingly, there can sometimes be more than one plant type within a genus. So for example, there can be both annual and perennial *Rudbeckias*, or biennial and perennial foxgloves. In this book we focus on those that are easiest to grow from seed.

Hardy annuals, summer-flowering plants that bloom and die within a year's cycle, and can be sown direct in the ground or in seed trays. They are tough enough to survive frost, so many of them can be planted out in the autumn to overwinter in the garden. This is the best group of plants to focus on if you are starting out

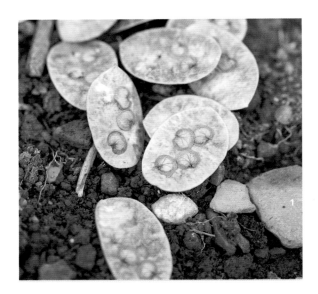

and don't have a greenhouse or any other form of winter protection.

When to sow: Annuals can be sown in late summer or early spring. Those sown in late summer can be overwintered in pots kept in a cold frame, or sown direct in the ground. If you're sowing direct at this time of year, it's best to sow before the equinox so there are enough hours of light for the plant to make sufficient growth before winter. They may not appear to be doing much as the weather gets colder, but underground the root systems will be bulking up, so that when the warmer weather arrives they are ready to spring into growth. These plants will be taller and sturdier and will flower earlier than spring-sown plants.

Making two sowings of the same plant, in late summer and early spring, will lengthen their flowering season considerably. If sowing direct in spring, wait until the ground has warmed up a little – you can tell when this happens as the soil starts greening up with annual weeds. Hardy annuals often self-seed, producing seed that falls around the plant and germinates the following year of its own accord. When this happens all you have to do is remove the seedlings you don't want.

1 Honesty seeds
2 Annuals

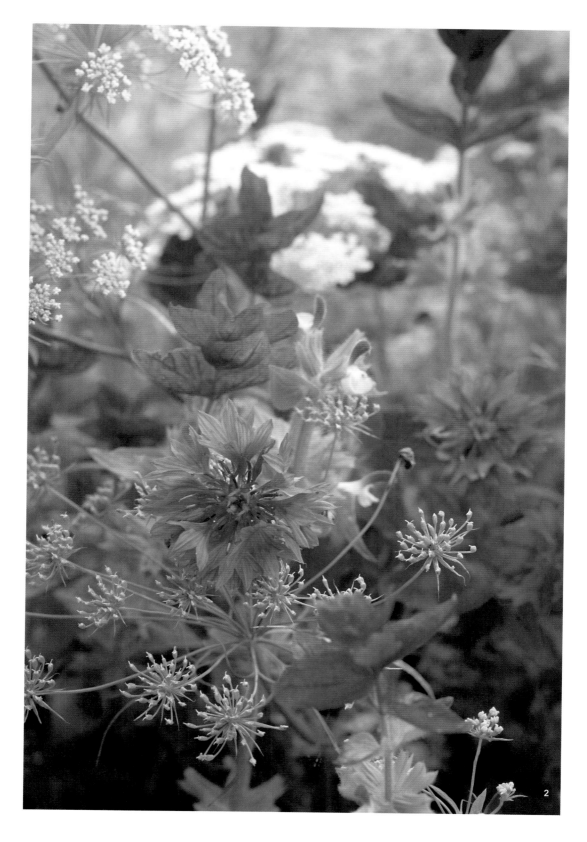

2

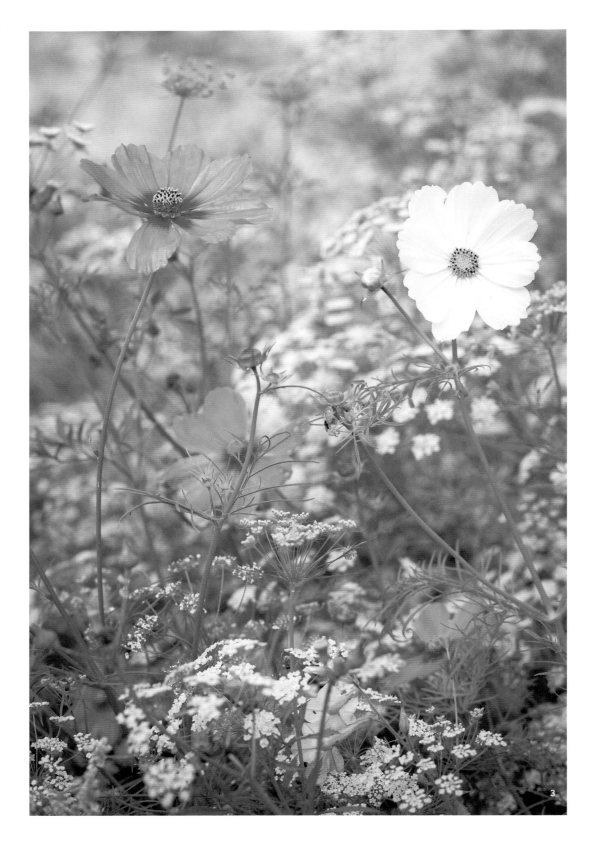

Biennials germinate and form foliage one year, then flower the following year. They are hardy plants that can tolerate a cold winter.

When to sow: Biennials are usually sown in late spring or early summer, to be planted out or kept in a cold frame over the winter, to flower the following year. They can be sown in modules or pots, or direct, but we think the best method is to sow under cover, since there will be so many other plants flowering in the garden that you may not have space in beds or borders. Grow the seedlings on in pots over the summer, and plant them out in their final growing places in autumn. Their leaves will continue to grow, and in late spring they will produce flowers.

Half-hardy annuals or tender perennials aren't hardy enough to survive when the temperature drops below freezing, so they are usually raised under cover, to be planted out after the last frosts, in late spring or early summer. Flowering in mid to late summer, this useful group will bloom on and on until the first frosts, often producing more flowers the more they are cut.

When to sow: Half-hardies should be sown indoors in early to mid spring, and need heat to germinate (20–25°C). The source of this heat can be an electric propagator or, more simply, a room with central heating. After germination, the seedlings should be moved to a slightly cooler place but still kept under cover, so for this group of plants it really helps if you have a greenhouse, cold frame or conservatory where you can keep them until they are ready to be planted out in the ground. While you could sow these plants direct in early summer, they are unlikely to have long enough to develop and flower before the first frosts of winter arrive, so we recommend sowing most under cover. They will probably need potting on once or even twice before they are planted out (see p.176).

Hardy perennials are plants that return year after year, and while many species can be raised from seed, they form the smallest group in this book. That is because many garden perennials are hybrids or cultivars, which either fail to produce seed (they are sterile) or produce seed that does not come true (it won't look the same as the parent plant, so flower colour and so on is a lottery). Some perennials take longer to mature and won't flower in the first year, while others are trickier to germinate, sometimes needing a period of cold (stratification) to trigger them into growth. Those that are included in this book are largely species that are easy to germinate, swift-growing and known to flower in the first year of growth.

When to sow: Hardy perennials can either be sown in late summer or autumn and then overwintered in a cold frame, or in early spring. At either time it is best to sow perennial seed in seed trays, pots or modules, which can be potted on as the seedlings get larger. Plant them out as soon as the soil has warmed up in spring. As a general rule, perennial seed germinates more readily when it is fresh, so be aware of this when buying seed. Collecting seed from your own plants and sowing it immediately is one of the best solutions.

Sowing times
Precise sowing and planting out times can vary depending on where you live. If you are sowing under cover, you can start in late winter; if you are sowing hardy seeds outdoors, wait until the soil warms up in mid-spring (indicated by a flush of green, annual weeds in the soil). Planting tender seedlings out shouldn't be done until after the last frosts, and this will vary from year to year; just keep an eye on the weather forecast.

3 *Cosmos* (a half-hardy) and *Ammi*

Sowing under cover

'Under cover' is the term generally used for sowing in a greenhouse or conservatory, or on a windowsill inside the house. These are seeds that need a little protection or nurturing before they are planted out, either because they are tender or because planting them out as seedlings is a way to give them the best possible start in life. It allows them to germinate and grow to a decent size without being affected by the lottery of weather, soil, slugs or any other hazards that nature might to throw at them. It's safer, for example, to sow unusual or difficult-to-get-hold-of seeds (where there may be only a precious few in the packet) under cover to increase your chances of raising more plants.

This is not the best method for every single plant – some don't like their roots to be disturbed, for example, and are best sown direct so they don't have to be moved – but it does work for a large percentage of plants that grow quickly and easily in seed trays or modules before being planted out into the garden.

Greenhouses and cold frames
You don't need to have a greenhouse to raise seeds in this way, but if you're growing more than just a couple of trays of seedlings, it does help to have at least a cold frame or mini-greenhouse outside (both are relatively cheap to buy and take up little space). Many a gardener will germinate their seeds on a windowsill in the warmth of the house, and move them to a cooler conservatory or cold frame once they have sprouted.

Compost
Choosing compost can be bewildering as there are many different types available. The safest bet is to go for one that is specifically labelled as a seed compost, which is designed to give germinating seeds the nutrients they need for the first few weeks after they

have emerged. Avoid using compost formulated for potting plants, which contains too much fertilizer and may scorch the seedlings. Generally, the bigger the seeds are, the less the grade of the compost matters, so if you're sowing large seeds such as sweet peas, it is fine to use a multipurpose compost (these are also cheaper than the finer-grade seed composts).

Choose a coir-based, peat-free compost if you are concerned about the environment, but be aware that these composts dry out very quickly, so keep a watchful eye on your seedlings. You can make your own seed compost by mixing sieved multipurpose compost in equal proportions with sharp sand or vermiculite (a lightweight mineral medium that is very water-retentive).

Seed size
Seeds come in all shapes and sizes, and this will dictate how you sow them. Seeds such as sweet peas, morning glory and sunflowers are large and easy to handle, and can be sown directly in small (7 cm) pots. Medium-sized seeds, such as cosmos, scabious and *Dianthus*, can be sown in modular trays. Tiny seeds, such as tobacco plant and foxglove, are best sown in a traditional open seed tray. The size of the seed generally dictates the depth at which it is sown. Large pea-like seeds can be pushed down into the compost to about half a knuckle's depth; medium seeds should be covered with a light sprinkling of compost or vermiculite; and tiny seeds should be sown on the surface.

Modular seed trays
Modular seed trays with 12 or 24 cells are widely available in different sizes, and are incredibly useful for sowing medium or large seeds because they remove the need to prick out the seedlings at a later stage, thereby

1 Young plants in a cold frame
2 Seeds ready to be sown
3 Cloches
4 Seeds of varying sizes

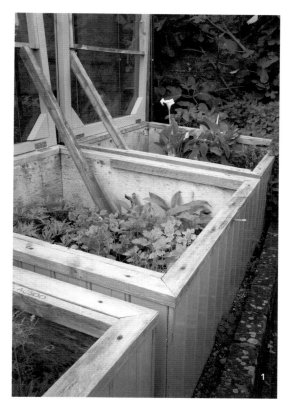

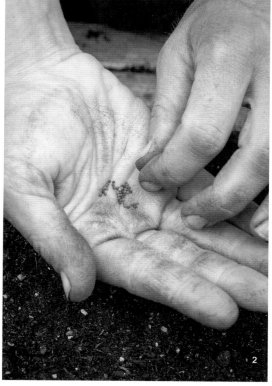

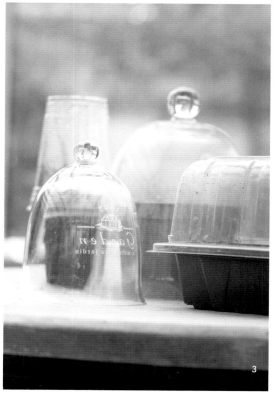

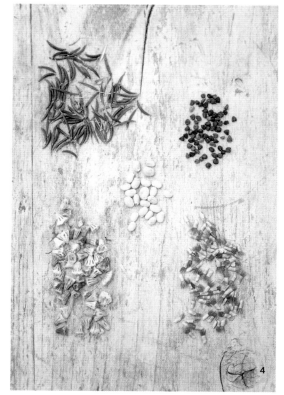

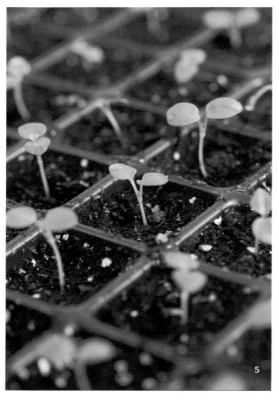

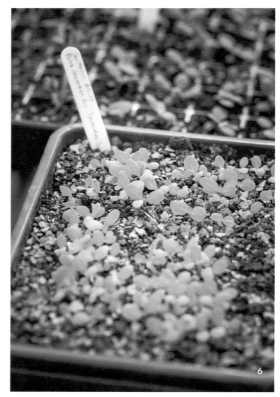

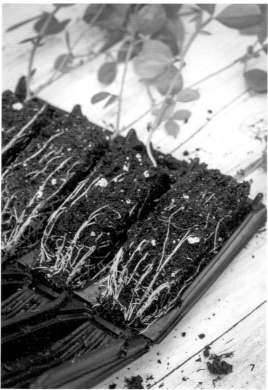

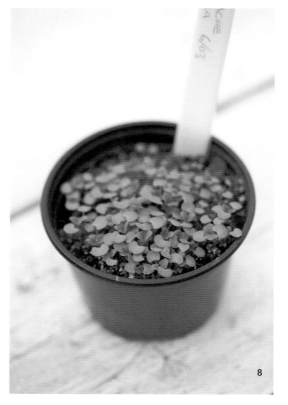

minimizing root disturbance. Most of our seedlings are raised this way. Fill the modules with compost, gently flattening it with a pot tamper. (Beware of packing the compost too tightly, or air will be pushed out and the seedlings will dwindle.) Place the tray in a 'gravel tray' (despite its name, this tray does not contain gravel but is simply a seed tray without holes) half-filled with water, so that the water soaks into the compost from below. Sow two seeds to a module, either by pushing them gently into the compost, or by sowing on the surface and then covering with a fine layer of sieved compost. Once they have germinated, take out the weaker seedling, allowing the other to grow on without competition. It can be planted out in the garden once its roots have filled the module.

Open seed trays

Traditional oblong seed trays can be used for smaller seeds, such as *Digitalis*, which should be scattered on the surface of the compost. Water the compost first so that you are sowing on a moist surface, or place the seed tray in a water-filled gravel tray to water from beneath. A word of warning: it is very easy to produce far too many seedlings from tiny seeds, so consider using half-size seed trays (approximately 23 x 17 cm) instead.

Root trainers

Root trainers are special deep, narrow modules that split open so that the plants can be extracted easily. These are excellent for sweet peas, which have long roots that need plenty of depth to grow. Simply fill the root trainers with multipurpose or seed compost and push the seeds in using your forefinger or the end of an old pencil. When the seedlings have grown and the roots have filled their spaces (you will see them starting to appear through the hole at the bottom), it is time to plant them out. Simply open the root trainers as you would a book and tip out the seedlings.

Biodegradable pots and pellets

You can buy small coir or other biodegradable pots that can be planted straight into the ground when the seedling is big enough. These are great for tap-rooted plants such as *Ammi* and *Orlaya* that sulk when their roots are disturbed. Alternatively, sow seeds direct into coir pellets, which expand when you water them. Jiffy-7 propagation pellets are surrounded with light netting, which can be cut away when the roots have filled them and they are ready to be planted out.

Sowing seed in pots

Fill the pots with compost and firm it down very gently with a pot tamper or the bottom of another pot. Take care not to over-firm, or air and water channels will be excluded, making it much more difficult for the plants to thrive as they grow. Sow the seeds according to their size: the tiniest on the surface of the compost, or covered with a very fine sprinkling of vermiculite; medium-sized seeds with a sprinkling of fine compost over them (ideally shaken through a garden sieve); and larger seeds pushed into the compost at twice the depth of the seed size. Always sow as thinly as possible – with smaller seeds this will just be a pinch between thumb and forefinger. You can buy special seed dispensers to control the number of seeds you sow, but they aren't strictly necessary. If you sow too many seeds they can rot, or not have enough space to develop properly, so be as mean as you like when you sow.

Tiny seeds, such as tobacco plant and foxglove, are best sown in a traditional open seed tray.

5 Modular seed trays
6 Seedlings in an open seed tray, covered with vermiculite
7 Sweet pea seedlings in a root trainer, shown split open
8 Seedlings in a plastic pot

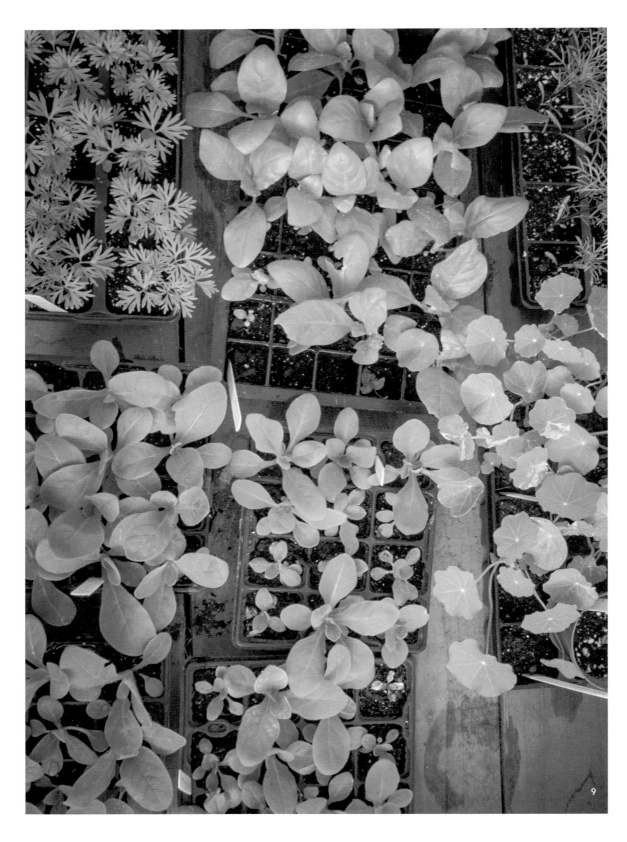

9

Germination requirements

Once you have sown your seeds, whether in modules, seed trays, root trainers or pots, they need to be given the right conditions if they are to germinate. Moisture, temperature, air and light levels need to be correct, and each plant has different requirements that will trigger them into growth.

The first element, water, is essential for all germination, so make sure the compost is moistened before you sow. The moisture must be kept in by putting a plastic lid on the tray, or plastic bag or piece of plastic wrap over the pot. Plastic propagator lids are widely available to fit most standard seed trays, and often this is all you need. The seeds also need oxygen, and if the compost is over-saturated or compacted, air is excluded and germination can be inhibited.

The next consideration is temperature. It would be easy to get bogged down with technical detail here, but let's keep it simple: most seeds need a little warmth to germinate. Some, particularly the half-hardy annuals and tender perennials, need more than others. Some perennials need a period of cold before the temperature is brought up to trigger the seed into growth, but most of the flowers that we include in this book don't need this more specialized treatment.

As a general rule, germinate hardy annuals at 16–20°C and warmer-climate half-hardies and tender perennials at 20–23°C. Let's face it, though, not many of us will be looking at thermometers and checking precise temperatures; it's usually a case of juggling seed trays around the house from warm room to slightly cooler room – trial and error again. To produce a more even heat for the seedlings, you can buy electric propagators and heat mats from a wide range of sources, but it's easy to do without.

The final consideration is light. Not all seeds have the same light requirements. Most don't need light to germinate, and it is therefore fine to cover them with a layer of compost (while still leaving the seed tray somewhere light). Some seeds are actually inhibited by light, and may need to be covered with a layer of newspaper or black bin liner to encourage them to germinate. Others are the opposite and need light to germinate, and should therefore be sown on the surface of the compost without covering at all. Finally, don't confuse germinating seeds with the seedlings themselves. Once they have emerged, all seedlings need sunlight otherwise they will become spindly and etiolated. If that all sounds a bit confusing, don't worry. As a rule, most seeds will germinate without specialist treatment, and if there are specific requirements they will be mentioned in the instructions on the seed packet.

Chitting

Some larger seeds can be chitted (sprouted) before sowing. This is a very simple process of placing the seeds on several layers of damp kitchen paper, and putting them in a plastic container or plastic bag in a warm, dark place. Once chitted, the seeds can be carefully planted in compost to continue growing. Try this with sweet peas, sunflowers, morning glory and even marigolds. This process is especially useful for seeds that may have been hanging around for some time and may or may not still be viable: if you don't want to waste compost, test them this way first.

After germination

As soon as the seedlings emerge, take off the lid of the seed tray or the plastic bag, and move the tray to a cooler place. If they have too much heat at this stage, they will grow too quickly and become weak and leggy. If you're lucky enough to have a greenhouse or cold frame, you can move hardy annuals outside; for more tender seedlings, move them to a cooler windowsill. The cooler conditions will decelerate growth in the top half of the plant and encourage a strong root system to develop instead. If the lid or

9 Trays of seedlings

plastic is kept over the seedlings for too long, they may suffer from 'damping off', a fungal infection that kills tiny seedlings. Newly emerged seedlings need air, light and moisture, so keep them lightly watered at all times to ensure the compost doesn't dry out.

Pricking out

You will only need to prick out seedlings that have been sown in traditional seed trays. When seeds germinate, they first form a pair of seed leaves (cotyledons), small, rounded leaves that bear no resemblance to the final shape of the foliage. The received wisdom is to wait until the second set of leaves has formed before pricking out, so that the seedling is strong enough to put up with the disturbance, but if you are careful you can prick them out before then, as long as the seedling is big enough to handle. The main thing is not to wait too long, or the root systems will become too tangled.

First of all, fill a modular seed tray or several 6 or 7 cm pots with multipurpose compost, as above. Using a pencil or a plastic plant marker, gently loosen the soil around the seedling and, holding the tiny plant by its leaves rather than its stem or roots, ease it out of the compost. Plant it in its new module or pot, making a hole large enough to accommodate the roots, dropping it in and firming the compost very gently around the roots and stem. As when sowing, take care not to firm the compost too much, or you will exclude air and water channels. Keep the new seedling watered from below, or by using a small watering can with a fine rose.

Caring for your seedlings

The most important requirement of any seedling is, of course, water, so be prepared to be around for a month or two at this stage, as modules and small pots can dry out very quickly. However, as always, it's a fine balance, and overwatering can cause damping off. It is always best to use mains water for seedlings, since saved water may be contaminated with leaf or soil debris, which also increases the risk of damping off and other disease. Being watchful is essential, but you'll soon discover that germinating your own seedlings and watching them mature is addictive. Like babies, they need to be nurtured and cosseted, and if you give them the time they need, you will be rewarded with strong, healthy plants for your garden. The nutrients in the compost may start to run out as the plants grow, and after about six weeks you may notice that the plant is looking increasingly unhealthy, perhaps even yellowing. If it's not warm enough to plant them outside at this stage, you may need to give them a liquid feed. General tomato fertilizers, which are high in potash, are the best to use, as high-nitrogen feeds will encourage too much leggy growth.

Potting on

If your seedlings grow too big for their modules or pots before they are due to be planted outside, you will need to pot them on: in other words, move the seedlings to larger pots to give the roots more space to spread out. Root-bound plants may droop or display yellowing leaves, and if you turn the pot or module upside down and can see roots appearing through the drainage holes at the bottom, it's time to pot on. Choose a pot in the next size up – not too much bigger – and remove the seedling by turning its pot over and loosening the root ball gently so that it falls out whole. Place it in the new pot, on a layer of fresh compost if necessary, and fill in around the sides with more fresh compost.

Hardening off

If your seedlings have been raised in warm conditions, they will need to be hardened off – acclimatized to cooler temperatures outside – before they are finally planted out. Much of this process is common sense, and sometimes it is dictated by space. If your plants have been languishing in a warmish greenhouse, you can start the process by opening the door overnight when the weather is warm enough, and then perhaps moving them to an open cold frame, and finally to a table outside. Obviously if there is a frost forecast and you have half-hardies or tender perennials outside, they must be whipped back inside or given some protection using fleece. This can involve some juggling, particularly in the UK, where the season often tricks us into thinking it is summer in mid spring, and then throws another frost or storm at us before the weather finally becomes reliably warm. Looking at the weather forecast can become something of an obsession when you have trays of precious seedlings to think about.

Planting out

Hardy annuals such as marigold, honeywort and *Ammi* can be planted out in mid spring, as they will tolerate a light frost, while half-hardies shouldn't be planted out until late spring or early summer, after all danger of frost has passed. If you've sown hardy annuals in modules, you shouldn't have to pot them on; they can go straight out into the garden from the modules. If you've planted half-hardies in modules, you may need to pot them on before they go out, since they'll grow too big too quickly.

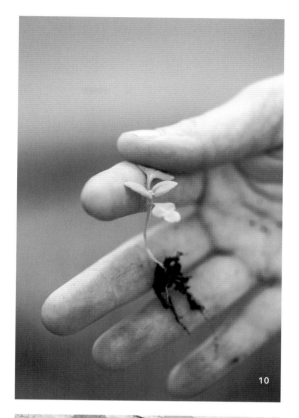

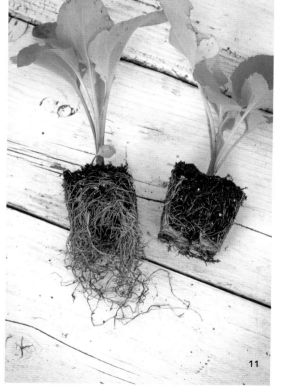

10 A seedling pricked out and ready to transplant
11 Young plants grown on in small pots. Roots on the left have been gently teased out, ready for planting outside

Sowing direct

Sowing direct – sowing directly into the soil outside – is the best method to use for some hardy annuals, especially those (such as poppies or love-in-a-mist) that dislike root disturbance, and also for meadow seed mixes covering large areas. It is, of course, much less time-consuming than sowing under cover, but the downside is that germination can be sporadic, varying from year to year depending on the weather and other conditions.

Preparing the soil

The single most important factor in successful germination outside is the condition of the soil. If it's heavy and wet, the seeds will rot. If it's compacted and dry, it will form large clods that the seeds won't be able to break through. Even sometimes if the soil is fine, a hard crust or pan can form on the surface or just underneath if the weather is dry, again preventing the germinating seed from pushing through. The best you can do is to prepare your soil early by incorporating plenty of organic matter (humus) in the form of well-rotted compost or manure, which will improve the structure of the soil and make it more workable and moisture-retentive, as well as adding nutrients.

If the soil is particularly heavy or full of clay, sharp sand or grit can also be dug in to improve the texture. Try to do all this weeks or even months in advance; preparing beds in the autumn, for example, makes sense for a spring sowing. When you are ready to sow, dig over the soil and rake it to break the particles down, removing large stones and weeds as you go. Keep working away, breaking down large clods with the back of the rake, until the surface of the soil has a fine, crumbly consistency or 'tilth'. Now the soil is ready to receive your seeds.

Seed beds

If you have room, it can be a good idea to create a small bed specifically for raising seedlings, where they can be sown in drills (rows) and later transplanted to their final flowering position. However, many annuals are unhappy to be moved, and in the case of poppies and love-in-a-mist, seed should be scattered (broadcast) on the soil where you want them to flower. The only drawback with this is that the seedlings can be difficult to distinguish from annual weeds, so it helps to mark the spot by sprinkling the soil with sand.

With all seeds, sowing thinly is the key. Too many seeds competing for the same light, nutrients and water will produce weaker plants that run to seed too quickly, so be sparing when you sow, using finger and thumb to take a delicate pinch of smaller seeds rather than broadcasting whole handfuls. You can also mix tiny seeds with a handful of sand before broadcasting, which will dilute them and lessen the chance of seedlings being clumped together.

It goes without saying that you must keep the seeds well-watered – but not overwatered – when they are germinating, so if the weather is dry, water the ground using a watering can with a fine rose. Seeds of hardy annuals should germinate in a week or ten days, so watch them closely.

As the seedlings grow, they must be thinned out. Remove the smaller seedlings and leave the larger ones to grow at an eventual spacing of 20–30 cm apart, so that the plants can spread out and thrive. Plants that are too close together go into panic mode, and will run to seed too quickly. Generally, give them more space rather than less, and your plants will be bigger and flower more generously for you.

Pests and diseases

Pests

Aphids include blackfly and greenfly, and are very common. These sap-sucking insects feed on foliage, stems and flowers. Aphid infestation is easy to spot, as they colonize shoot tips, flower buds and the underside of leaves. They cause stunted growth with curled leaves, and can quickly weaken the plant. Aphids have many natural predators, including ladybirds, lacewings and hoverfly larvae, and if you garden organically you should have good quantities of these, at least by midsummer. However, an early spell of warm weather can allow aphids to multiply rapidly. Keep an eagle eye out for them, and if you see any signs, pinch out the growing tips or rub the insects off by hand. If they've managed to start taking over, spray them with an organic pest-control spray or washing-up liquid and water.

Mice can be a problem in greenhouses and cold frames, and they have a penchant for sweet pea seeds and young, succulent seedlings of almost any kind. Some people soak sweet pea seeds in paraffin or methylated spirits before planting, to make them unpalatable to mice. Protecting seedlings is more difficult, and you may have to resort to good old-fashioned traps.

Slugs and snails are a real nuisance, wreaking havoc in beds of young seedlings and doing their best to destroy even quite large plants. Generally, though, the larger the plant the safer it will be, and a lot of heartache can be avoided just by starting seeds off in pots. There are various methods of control, from copper rings or tape to wool matting. Chemically based slug pellets containing metaldehyde will harm other wildlife, so should not be used, but other pellets contain ferric phosphate, which is less harmful. If you can manage without, so much the better.

Diseases

Damping off is the most common problem with seedlings, occurring in moist, humid conditions. Caused by various fungi in the compost, it will swiftly kill an emerging seedling, making it wilt and collapse. You can take measures to avoid this fungal disease by keeping your seedlings in a dry, well-ventilated place, and not overwatering them. Use fresh tap water rather than water from a water butt, which may introduce infection.

Powdery mildew can affect some annuals, including marigolds and zinnias. While it isn't usually fatal, it can be unsightly, causing whiteish patches to spread on the leaf and stem, particularly in warm weather. Fungicides can be used to control it, but easy preventative measures can be taken: water the plant well and mulch around the base to make sure the moisture stays in the soil, and give it a liquid feed. A healthy plant is always less likely to succumb to disease.

Red spider mite can affect plants in warmer, drier climates, and particularly in greenhouses. The leaves appear mottled at first, damaged by the sap-sucking mites, and then the fine silk webs of the spiders may appear. To counteract the mites you can use a biological control such as *Phytoseiulus persimilis*, another mite that will prey on it.

Rust is a disease that affects only a small handful of plants, including hollyhocks and *Antirrhinums*. It causes deep-brown or rusty-red spots to appear on the underside of the leaves, which start to shrivel and may die. Hollyhocks can usually survive, although the rust is unsightly, but *Antirrhinums* can be wiped out completely. The rust is caused by a fungus that is spread by airborne spores, and can be controlled using fungicides.

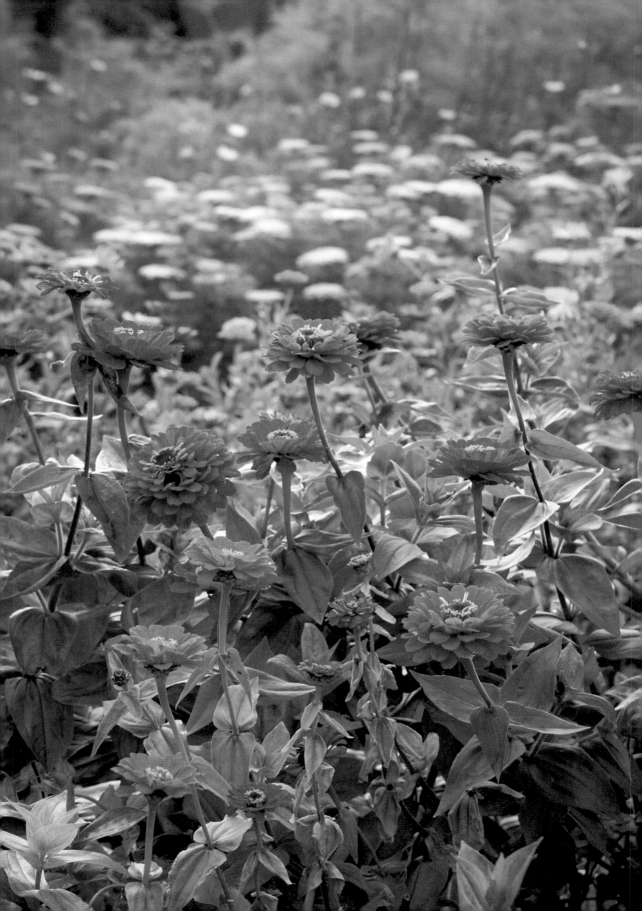

Part III

How to use your flowers

Using annuals and biennials in borders, Planting a mini meadow,
Making a sweet pea arch, Making a cutting garden,
Container planting, Arranging your flowers

Using annuals and biennials in borders

Annuals are great for padding out a summer border, while half-hardies can bring a zap of colour to the late summer garden. If there are gaps in the border in early summer, having a supply of seed-raised plants will allow you to create rivers of colour in the garden using colour-burst flowers such as marigolds or California poppies, or, if the garden is already colourful, tone it down with airy white or neutral fillers such as *Ammi*, *Orlaya*, *Gypsophila* or *Phlox drummondii* 'Crème Brûlée'.

Biennials are useful fillers for late spring borders, because they flower earlier than many perennials and annuals, at a rather green time in the garden. Honesty and wallflowers are the first to bloom, and are excellent as a companion for tulips, while Icelandic poppies, foxgloves and *Aquilegias* flower in May, bridging the gap between spring and summer.

1 A sea of poppies in a naturalistic border
2 *Nicotiana* can fill gaps in a summer border
3 A purple-leaved form of honesty combines with *Euphorbia* in a spring border

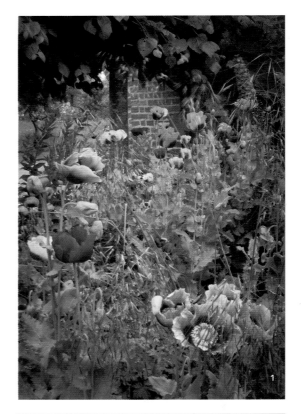

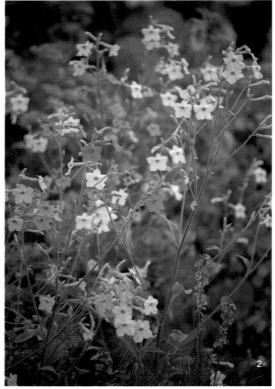

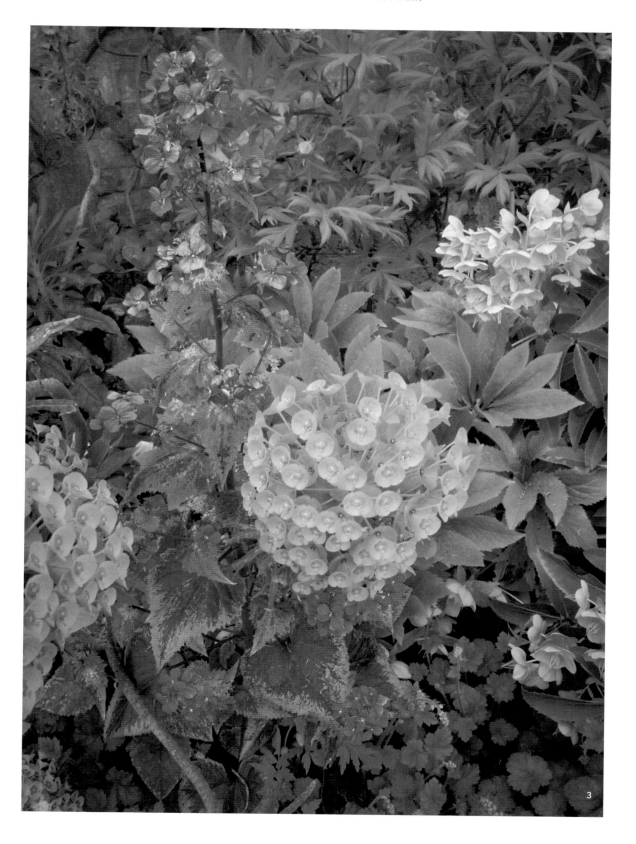

3

Planting a mini meadow

By direct-sowing annuals such as cornflowers, *Ammi* and ox-eye daisies, you can create your own patch of summer meadow, even if you have only a small space. This is easy to do in a border, but less so in existing turf, since the grass species will always be stronger than the flowers. If you're using annuals, some will self-seed, but the grass will always start to win over again, so you may need to repeat the process every year. If you want a sustainable meadow that develops naturally from year to year, consider planting yellow rattle only in the first year. This is a small, insignificant meadow annual whose size belies its ability to muscle the strongest grass species out of the way. Once you have a good crop of yellow rattle, you can start introducing other wild-flower seeds; they will have more space to thrive once the grasses' monopoly loosens.

Start in spring by preparing the area you are planning for your meadow. If it's turfed, strip back the turf and weeds completely, then leave the area for a couple of weeks and continue to pull out the weeds as they return (or use a weedkiller if you don't garden organically). Leave the ground again for a couple of weeks before digging it over, removing any big stones and raking the soil. Don't add organic matter; meadow annuals flower best on poor soil, and if the soil is too rich the grass and weeds will be too strong for your flowers to compete with.

Then, in mid to late spring, you can sow your meadow seeds. The easiest way to do this is by mixing them with sand to dilute them and broadcasting the mixture evenly over the area. However, there is a flaw in this method for those (and that includes most of us) who don't recognize the weed seedlings that will inevitably germinate at the same time. To get round this, you can sow the mixture in rows or in a grid 30 cm square, marked out with a cane to make shallow drills. Sowing the seeds in lines may sound counter-intuitive for a naturalistic meadow, but as the plants grow the lines soon merge, and this way you will be able to see where the right seedlings are, and pull out the wrong ones that come up in between. Cover the lines of seeds with a layer of sand and gently firm them in, then water using a watering can with a fine rose so as not to dislodge the seeds. If the weather is dry, keep the area watered as you watch your seedlings appear.

Many different meadow seed mixes are available in varying quantities, and you can choose from native and non-native ones. In Britain, the mixes that include non-native annuals and perennials give the most colourful result.

Some suitable meadow flowers
Agrostemma githago (corncockle)
Ammi majus (bishop's flower)
Asclepias syriaca (common milkweed)
Centaurea americana (American basket flower)
Centaurea cyanus (cornflower)
Centaurea nigra (knapweed)
Chrysanthemum segetum (corn marigold)
Coreopsis tinctoria (coreopsis)
Echinacea purpurea (purple coneflower)
Geranium pratense (meadow cranesbill)
Knautia arvensis (meadow scabious)
Leucanthemum vulgare (ox-eye daisy)
Papaver rhoeas (poppy)
Rhinanthus minor (yellow rattle)
Rudbeckia hirta (black-eyed susan)

1 Field poppies, mallow and ox-eye daisies mingle with meadow grasses
2 *Centaurea nigra* (knapweed)
3 *Geranium pratense* (meadow cranesbill)
4 *Rhinanthus minor* (yellow rattle)

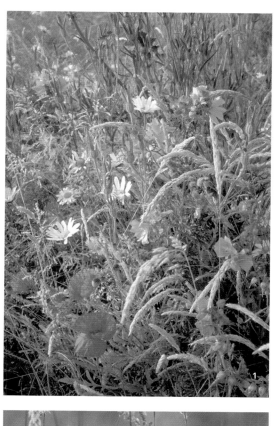

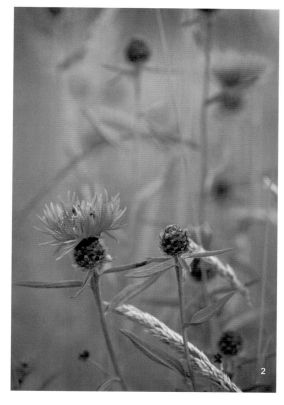

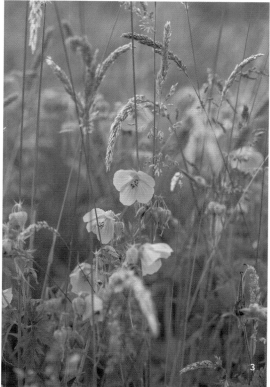

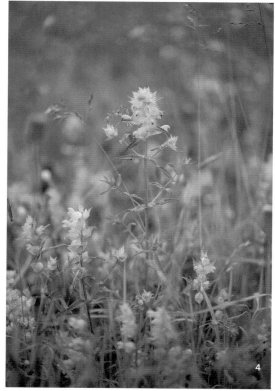

Making a sweet pea arch

There is nothing nicer than a rustic arch smothered with sweet peas in the summer, and if you make your own arch out of hazel coppicing, it won't cost you more than the hazel and a packet of seeds. Start in the autumn or early spring by planting sweet peas in root trainers (see p.172). You'll need a dozen or more plants, depending on how wide you want your arch to be. In mid spring, buy hazel from your local garden centre or find a thicket and cut your own long, straight stems – the ones that are growing from the base of the plant. For an arch 0.9 m long by 1 m wide, you will need 12 canes roughly 2 m long, plus smaller, twiggy branches to weave in for the lower layer. The canes must be flexible, so use them as soon as possible after cutting.

1 A sweet pea arch made of coppiced hazel
2 Sweet peas supported by netting

Push six long canes into the soil as deep as you can, in a line, leaving 15 cm between them. Do the same to make the other side of the arch, so you have two lines. Then bend each pair over to meet at the top to make the arch, weaving the canes around each other and securing them with a couple of plant ties. Do the same along the length of the arch. Weave in the shorter branches down below, to make the structure more sturdy as well as provide the initial twiggy surface for the sweet peas to cling to.

The arch is now ready, and it can wait until the sweet peas are big enough to be planted out, in mid to late spring. When the time comes, plant one or two seedlings to a cane. They may need tying in initially, but once they get going they will clamber over one another and the canes, covering the arch in no time. Give them plenty of water and pick the blooms regularly when they are in flower to ensure a lasting floriferous display.

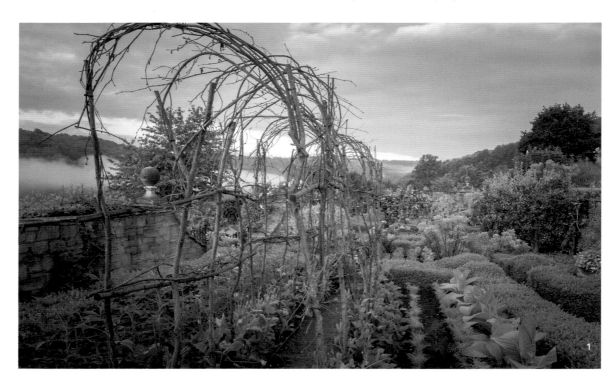

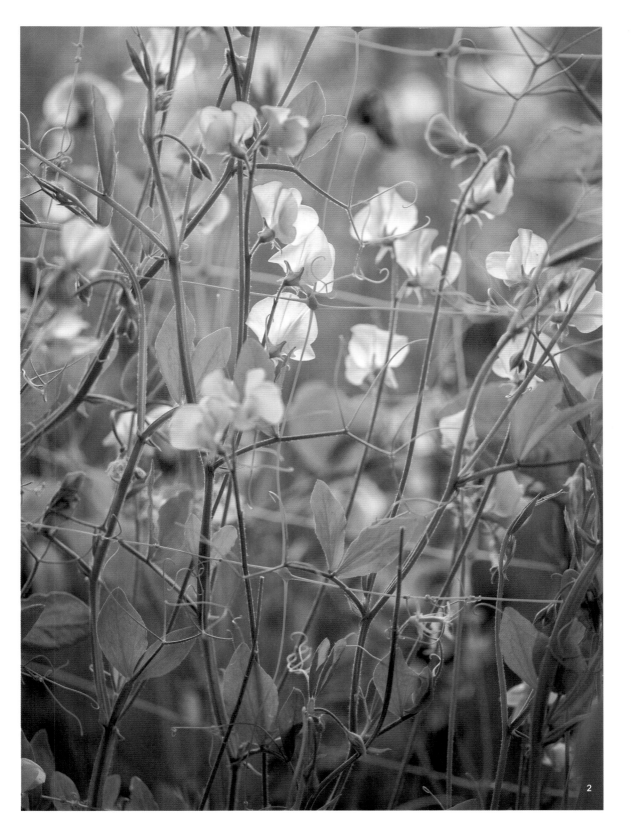

2

Making a cutting garden

Using your seed-grown plants to make your own cutting patch is hugely rewarding, and you don't need vast tracts of land to achieve it. You can create a very productive cutting garden with four raised beds, each 4 x 1.5 m, planted with a mixture of annuals and biennials, supplemented if you wish with spring and summer bulbs.

Plant the beds in a quadrangle and have a sweet pea arch connecting them at the centre. The following year, rotate the beds, planting one up entirely with *Phacelia tanacetifolia*, which will rest and nourish the ground as well as providing cut flowers.

Planting suggestions for a four-bed cutting garden

Bed One:
Biennials planted out in autumn
- *Dianthus barbatus* 'Auricula Eye Mix' (sweet william)
- *Digitalis purpurea* 'Sutton's Apricot' (foxglove)
- *Erysimum cheiri* 'Fire King' (wallflower)
- *Lunaria annua* 'Dark Form' (honesty)
- *Papaver nudicaule* 'Meadow Pastels' (poppy)

Bed Two:
Hardy annuals grown in modules
- *Ammi majus* (bishop's flower)

- *Calendula officinalis* 'Indian Prince' (pot marigold)
- *Calendula officinalis* 'Sherbet Fizz' (pot marigold)
- *Centaurea cyanus* 'Blue Boy' (cornflower)
- *Orlaya grandiflora* (white lace flower)
- *Scabiosa atropurpurea* 'Black Knight' (scabious)

Bed Three:
Hardy annuals, sown direct in rows
- *Consolida regalis* 'Blue Cloud' and 'Snow Cloud' (larkspur)
- *Gypsophila elegans* 'Snow Queen' (baby's breath)
- *Nigella damascena* 'Miss Jekyll' (love-in-a-mist)
- *Nigella papillosa* 'African Bride' (love-in-a-mist)
- *Papaver somniferum* 'Black Peony' and 'Flemish Antique' (poppy)

Bed Four:
Half-hardy annuals, planted out in early summer
- *Cosmos bipinnatus* 'Purity' and 'Rubenza' (cosmos)
- *Helianthus debilis* 'Vanilla Ice' (sunflower)
- *Moluccella laevis* (bells of Ireland)
- *Nicotiana langsdorffii* (tobacco plant)
- *Panicum* 'Frosted Explosion' (switch grass)
- *Zinnia elegans* 'Zinderella Peach' (zinnia)

1 Cut flowers planted in rows, surrounded by box hedges
2 Late summer cutting flowers, including dahlias and marigolds

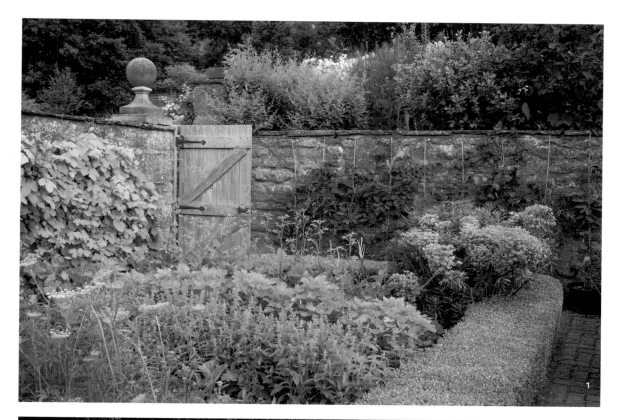

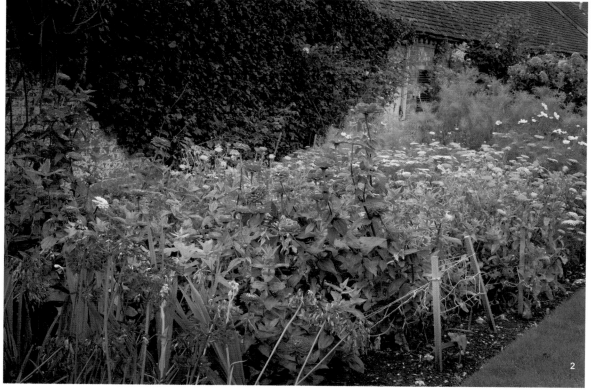

Container planting

If you have limited outdoor space, plant your seed-sown flowers in containers. Window boxes, tubs, pots and hanging baskets can all be used to create beautiful, floriferous summer displays. And even if you have a large garden, there are always areas that can benefit from groups of pots that can be moved around according to the season.

The variety of pots and tubs available to buy is limitless, so choose materials that suit the style of your garden: square-cut zinc for a modern, urban plot, for example, or traditional terracotta for a country kitchen garden. If you have a lot of space, go for the largest containers you can afford. A single large container in the middle of a courtyard will create a focal point, while three elegant long toms in a row make a design statement. In an informal garden, a collection of pots in different sizes and materials can soften a corner.

Be imaginative about what you plant, using perennials, grasses and small shrubs to anchor your pots and planting around them with your seed-sown annuals to give them that full, abundant look you are after. If your sole purpose is to grow plants for pots, make sure from the outset that the plants are suitable for the size of container you have. For example, *Cosmos bipinnatus* 'Xanthos' is more suitable than its taller cousin 'Purity', being shorter, bushier and easier to manage. Traditional annual bedding plants tend to be short-growing, so

these are ideal. For large or medium-sized containers, choose a combination of several plants with different shapes and forms; a bold focal point, a filler and a trailing plant, for example. Other pots look effective with a mass of just one plant.

Seed-grown plants for containers
Antirrhinum majus (snapdragon)
Briza maxima (quaking grass)
Calendula officinalis (pot marigold)
Cerinthe major (honeywort)
Cosmos bipinnatus 'Xanthos' (dwarf cosmos)
Dahlia variabilis 'Sunny Reggae' and 'Dwarf Amore Mix' (dahlia)
Dianthus species (sweet williams and carnations)
Erysimum cheiri (wallflower)
Ipomoea species (morning glory)
Lagurus ovatus (rabbit's tail grass)
Lathyrus odoratus (sweet pea)
Nicotiana species (tobacco plant)
Orlaya grandiflora (white lace flower)
Panicum 'Frosted Explosion' (switch grass)
Phlox drummondii (annual phlox)
Rudbeckia hirta (black-eyed susan)
Salvia viridis (ornamental sage)
Scabiosa 'Butterfly Blue' (scabious)
Stipa tenuissima (Mexican feather grass)
Tropaeolum majus (nasturtium)
Viola tricolor (heartsease)
Zinnia elegans (zinnia)

Herbs for pots
Anethum graveolens (dill)
Coriandrum sativum (coriander)
Ocimum basilicum (basil)
Petroselinum crispum (parsley)

1 Stone planter with annuals including sweet peas
2 Terracotta and aluminium pots filled with annuals, including cosmos, *Nicotiana* and *Phlox drummondii* 'Crème Brûlée'
3 Terracotta pot filled with a mass of annuals and perennials, including sweet peas
4 An urn forms a focal point in the centre of a garden room

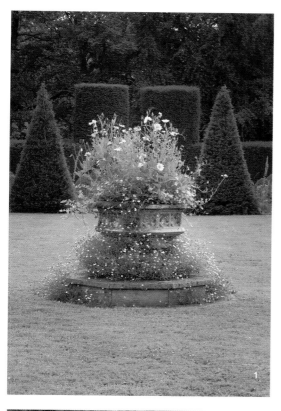

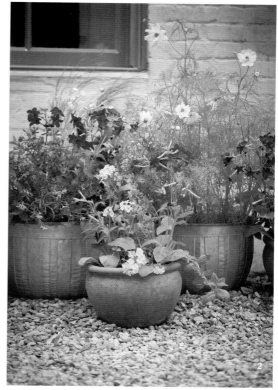

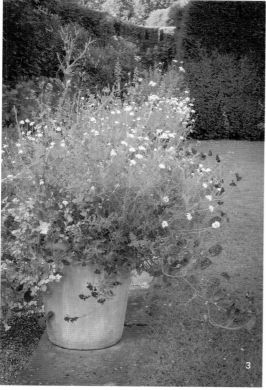

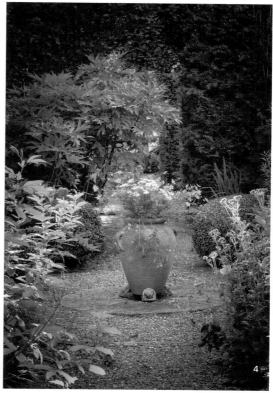

Arranging your flowers

One of the joys of growing your own plants from seed is that you can grow lots of flowers very cheaply, so that you always have a ready supply to cut and arrange for the house, or for giving to friends or family. From huge, blowsy bouquets to single blooms in tiny vases, the only limit to your creations is your own creativity!

Picking and conditioning

Cut your flowers with scissors or sharp secateurs. For best results, make sure your plants are well-watered beforehand and pick in the morning when the stems are full of water. Put the cut flowers in a bucket of water as soon as you have picked them, and ideally wait a couple of hours before arranging them.

When arranging, strip off the leaves from the bottom half of the stem and re-cut each stem at an angle, which increases the surface area to draw in water. Some flowers such as poppies and *Euphorbia* are prone to drooping, and benefit from being sealed. Simply boil a kettle, pour the water into a mug or bowl and dip the stems in for 20 to 30 seconds. It seems counter-intuitive, but it works.

Choosing your vase

You can never have too many vases, so scour antique markets, auctions and second-hand shops for bargains. Choose a large, plain ceramic or glass vase for an elaborate arrangement with many colours and textures or a more decorative one for a simple arrangement with one to three flower varieties. Use wide bowls with wire or oasis for large, statement arrangements, and tall, slim vases for willowy stems of larkspur or foxgloves. Recycle small glass bottles for single stems of any flower that might be in season. Old medicine bottles are ideal; I dug up three when making my new garden and have found others in a local antique market. And finally, keep all your jam jars and fill them with informal posies that can be made in five minutes.

Putting flowers together

Arranging flowers is like putting a planting plan together in the garden. For a well-balanced bouquet, choose a range of different textures and forms with plenty of visual contrast. Use filler plants such as *Ammi* or *Orlaya* (pp.58, 66) to contrast with strong shapes such as cosmos and sunflowers (pp.76, 82).

Try experimenting with colour themes and remember that tasteful is not always the way forward. The clashing pinks, oranges and purples of cosmos, zinnias and dahlias with acid-green fennel can look spectacular in late summer, but if you're in a quieter mood, select harmonious colours such as creams, lilacs and pinks.

A blocky arrangement can be broken up with lacy *Ammi* or the delicate filaments of *Panicum* 'Frosted Explosion', while a bunch of pale, icy cosmos and white *Nicotiana* can be lifted by a shot of colour from *Nicotiana alata* 'Lime Green'.

And if you're feeling under-confident about putting flowers together, start out by making small, jam jar posies for the centre of the table, or even single stems of large flowers. Arrange three or more of these along a long table, or cluster them together in the middle of a round table, and you have an instant stylish table decoration.

1 Scabious, *ammi* and *antirrhinums*
2 Cosmos and *nicotiana* with *senecio*
3 Cosmos, zinnias, dill and California poppies
4 Scabious and sweet peas
5 Sweet peas, clary sage and dill
6 *Rudbeckia*, sunflowers and nasturtiums
7 Borage, sunflowers and nasturtiums
8 Phlox and dill
9 *Cobaea* with hydrangea

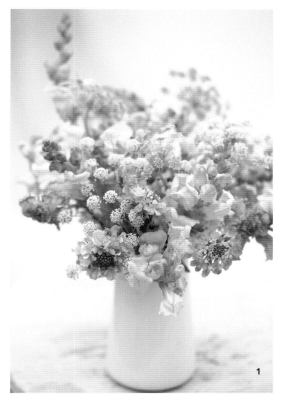

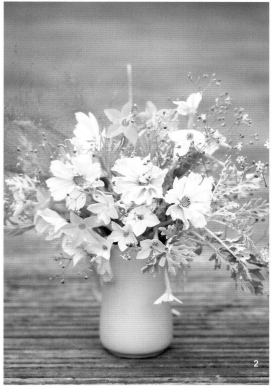

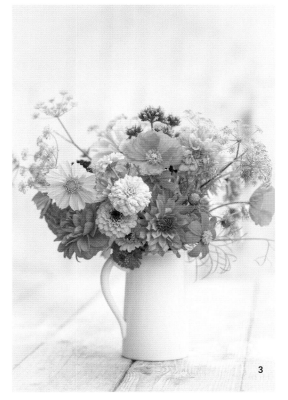

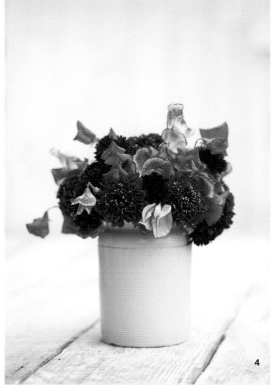

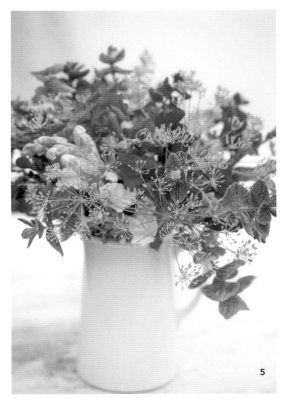

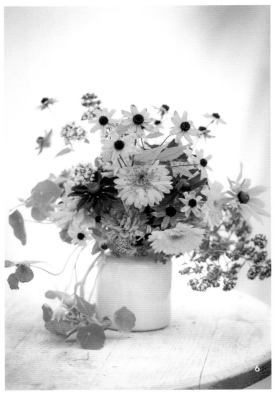

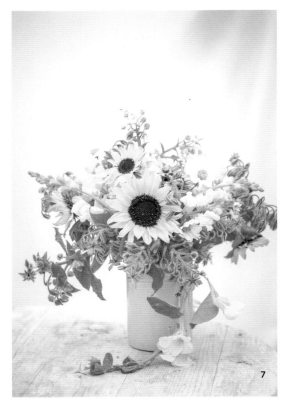

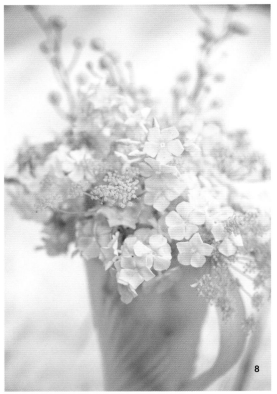

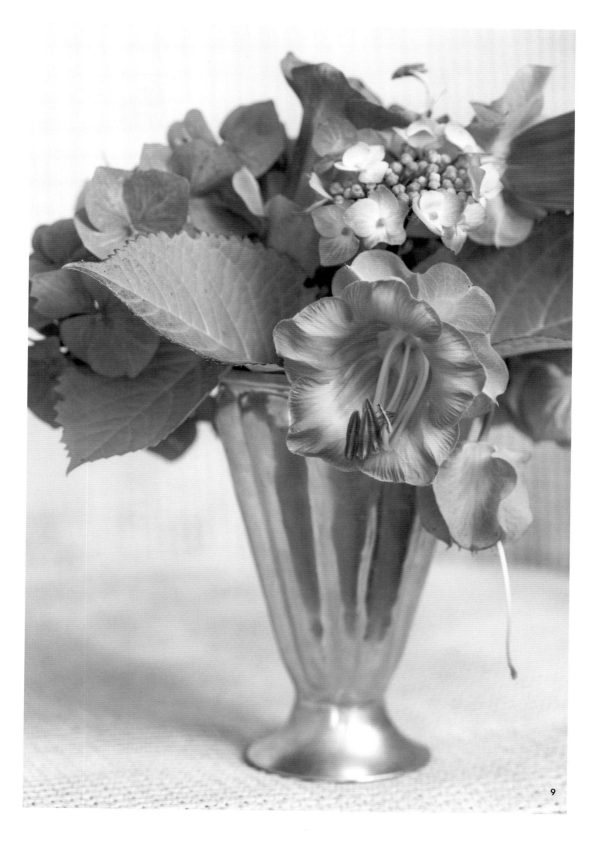

9

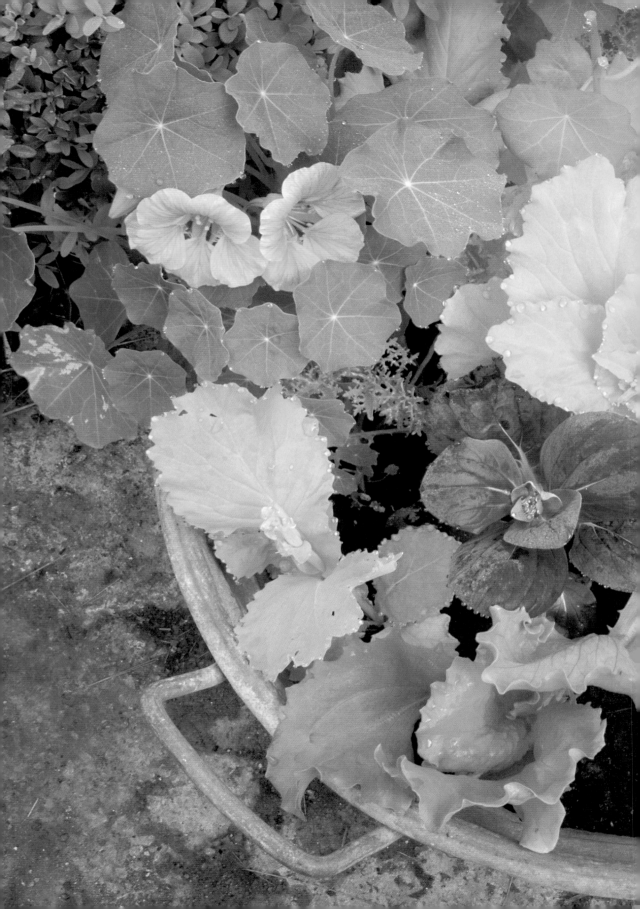

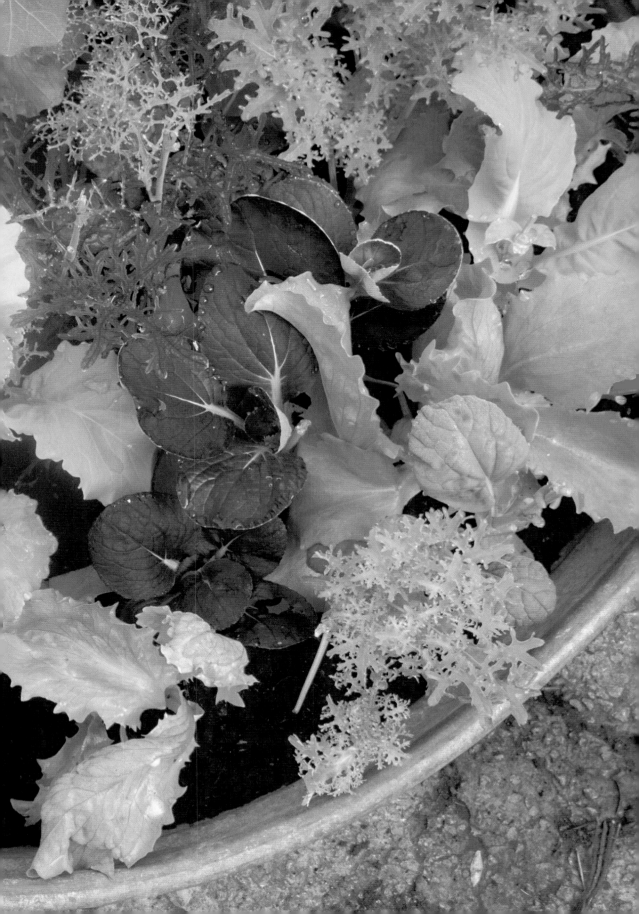

Glossary

Annual: a plant with a life cycle that lasts only one year, growing from seed, flowering, producing seed and dying within one growing season.

Biennial: a plant that takes two years to complete its biological cycle. In the first year the plant grows leaves and stem, while in the second it flowers, produces seed and then dies.

Bolting: a term applied to flowering or vegetable crops when they prematurely run to seed.

Broadcasting: to scatter seed by hand over an area of soil, as opposed to sowing in rows.

Calyx (calyces): comprised of separate sepals, this is the usually green outer whorl of a flower, forming a protective layer when in bud.

Cultivar: a plant variety that has been produced in cultivation by selective breeding.

Damping-off: a fungal disease that causes emerging seedlings to collapse, particularly those sown under cover.

Deadheading: the process of snipping off spent flower heads to encourage the plant to keep producing flowers.

Double flower: any flower with more than one layer of petals, resulting in a fuller appearance.

Drill: a row of seeds or seedlings produced when sowing direct into the ground.

Floret: a tiny flower that is one of masses making up a composite flower head.

Genus: a taxonomic category in plant nomenclature that is above the species and below the family, always in Latin, ie *Taxus baccata* (genus and species).

Germination: the growth and development of a plant from a seed after a period of dormancy.

Grow on: a term used to describe the progressive stages of growing plants under cover, re-potting them as they get bigger.

Half-hardy annual: a tender annual that can be grown outside but that will not survive a frost.

Hardening off: gradually acclimatizing plants that have been grown under cover to outside conditions, usually by using a cold frame or other protection.

Hardy: the term used for plants that are able to tolerate lower temperatures including frost and snow.

Humus: organic matter such as compost or any other rotted vegetable matter that gives soil nutrients and moisture-retaining properties.

Hybrid: a cross between two different, genetically dissimilar, species of plant.

Legume: a plant in the pea family.

Loam: a fertile, easy-to-work soil, with roughly equal proportions of sand, clay and silt, and with good humus content.

Palmate: having palm-like leaves with five or more lobes whose midribs all radiate from one point.

Perennial: a plant with a continuing life cycle that means that it grows back year after year. Typically, the top parts of the plant die back and become dormant in winter, with new growth appearing in spring.

Potting on: transferring seedlings sown under cover into larger pots as they outgrow their existing pots.

Pricking out: the careful removal of individual seedlings from a seed tray into individual cells or pots to give their root systems space to develop.

Root-bound: a plant that has outgrown its pot which may begin to show signs of stunted growth or yellowing.

Self-seed: the process of a plant propagating itself from seed.

Sepal: the green components of the calyx of the flower, which forms a protective layer around the bud and bloom.

Side shoot: a shoot growing from the side of a plant's stem.

Single flower: the simplest flower form, with a single set of petals around the central disc.

Species: in taxonomy, a botanical term used to classify a particular plant member of a genus, always in Latin.

Stamen: the male fertilizing organ of a flower, typically consisting of a pollen-containing anther and a filament.

Stem rot: a disease caused by fungal disease in the stem, causing the stem of a plant to wilt and rot.

Stigma: the section of the female part of a flower where pollen germinates.

Stratification: the process of treating seeds by simulating natural conditions, often with a period of cold.

Successive sowing: the process of sowing in batches over several weeks so that the flowering or harvesting period is prolonged.

Tap root: a straight, tapering root growing vertically downwards.

Thinning out: the process of removing excess seedlings in direct-sown rows, to give stronger seedlings the room to grow.

Tilth: the condition of tilled or raked soil after large particles have been broken down.

Umbel: a flower form typical of the carrot family (e.g. cow parsley) in which flower stalks radiate outwards with smaller florets to create an umbrella-like flower head.

Vermiculite: a lightweight mineral used as a moisture-retentive medium for growing plants, typically as a top-dressing when sowing seeds.

Resources

We live in the UK, so have listed below the mail order seed companies, kit suppliers and gardening courses local to us. If you live elsewhere, the internet is the first port of call for reviews of the best local suppliers.

Buying Seed
Flower seed is available in garden centres up and down the country, and there you'll find a good range of basic seeds to get you started, especially hardy annual seeds that are easy to grow. However, as you get more ambitious, you'll find that a much wider range of different annuals, as well as perennials, is available from mail order specialists. Here we list a few of the best mail order seed sources in the UK:

- Chiltern Seeds
A very comprehensive range of seeds including annuals, biennials and perennials. Their website is user-friendly with plants divided into various useful categories including 'first-year flowering perennials', 'scented', 'wild flowers' and 'pollinators'. Their catalogue includes some unusual species and varieties that you won't find elsewhere. Chilternseeds.co.uk.

- Higgledy Garden
A delightful small company run by Benjamin Ranyard who grows his own flowers in Cornwall and sells seed in hand-printed brown seed packets. He also offers an eccentric blog with his notes and tips on growing flowers from seed. Higgledygarden.com.

- Kings Seeds
Based in Suffolk, Kings Seeds offers a wide selection of flower seeds, and is an especially good source for sweet peas, with over 100 varieties listed. They are also known for their wide range of herb seeds. Kingsseeds.com.

- Seedaholic
Seedaholic has a great range of cutting flowers to grow from seed, from Calendula to snapdragons, with plenty of different varieties to choose from. Their website is excellent, with useful information about each plant, including comprehensive cultivation notes and sowing instructions. Seedaholic.com.

- Special Plants
Special Plants is run by Derry Watkins, who has travelled widely looking for plants and who has introduced many new plants to cultivation that she has collected and grown from seed. Her online seed shop is one of the best places to find unusual plants to grow from seed, especially perennials. Specialplants.net.

Seed Sowing Kit
- Sarah Raven
This is a one-stop shop for all the paraphernalia you'll need for seed sowing and growing, from seed trays and pots to plant labels, organic fertilizer and lightweight dead-heading scissors. Also buy vases here to display your cut flowers. Sarahraven.com.

- Harrod Horticultural
For garden tools and other equipment you'll need to look after your flowers, Harrod Horticultural has a great range of good-quality products. Their website offers seven propagators including a self-watering propagation kit. Harrodhorticultural.com.

- Capital Garden Products
To display your flowers, Capital Gardens offers a wide range of tubs, window boxes and containers in lightweight fibreglass, with realistic-looking terracotta or faux-lead finishes. Capital-garden.com.

- McVeigh Parker
This agricultural company sells cattle
feeders and water troughs in heavy duty,
galvanized steel. Cheaper than other
bespoke trough planters, they are ideal
as containers. Just drill holes through the
base for drainage and fill with compost.
Mcveighparker.com.

Courses

- Derry Watkins of Special Plants runs
a Growing from Seed course each
autumn at her nursery in Somerset.
Specialplants.net.

- The RHS run Beginners Propagation
courses at RHS Wisley Garden.
Rhs.org.uk.

- West Dean Gardens offers a Sowing
and Growing your Garden course led
by Derry Watkins. Westdean.org.uk.

- Rachel Siegfried of Green and
Gorgeous cut flowers in Oxfordshire
runs Seed Propagation courses each
spring. Greenandgorgeousflowers.co.uk.

Index

Figures in *italics* refer to illustrations. See also Glossary (pp. 198–9)

Acknowledgements

We would like to thank our long-suffering husbands for putting up with our plant addictions. Thank you to Chiltern Seeds for sending us seeds to grow, and to growers Tamsin Borlase (bosleypatch.com), Tammy Hall (wildbunchflowers.co.uk), Rachel Siegfried (greenandgorgeousflowers.co.uk), Alice Tite (rhosorganic.co.uk) and everyone who kindly let us share their garden for photography. Huge thanks to photographer Eva Nemeth (evanemeth.com) for her lovely portrait in the Introduction. We would also like to thank Layla Robinson, whose annual garden inspired Sabina to grow from seed, and Laura Prioli, for her patience.